TAKE CARE
OF YOURSELF

IMPORTANT ADDRESSES & TELEPHONE NUMBERS

Emergency room _____

_____

Poison control center _____

_____

Ambulance _____

_____

Family doctor _____

_____

Pediatrician _____

_____

Specialist _____

_____

Dentist _____

_____

Dental emergency number _____

_____

Hospital _____

_____

Other _____

_____

HOW TO USE THIS BOOK

Welcome to *Take Care of Yourself*. We've tried to make this book very easy for you to use. We want you to be able to quickly find the information you want, from emergency advice to preventive measures that will help you stay healthy for a long time.

To help you get the most from this book, here's one useful way to read it:

Today

- Read the rest of this section and the next section, "Emergencies," so that you can develop a plan for dealing with a medical problem or emergency *before* one happens.
- Write the names and telephone numbers of your Emergency Room, Poison Control Center, and other resources on the opposite page.
- Read about what you need in your Home Pharmacy at the start of Chapter 2.
- Start a Family Medical Record for every member of your household (space is provided for this starting on page 350).
- Leaf through the rest of the book and read what interests you.

In the Next Month

- Read the Introduction and Part I. Consider the seven keys to health and what preventive steps you can take to keep yourself and your family healthy.
- Read Part III and consider your medical coverage. Review any questions about your health insurance with your coverage provider.
- Once again, leaf through the whole book and read what interests you.

If you follow the steps on the previous page, when a medical problem arises you'll quickly be able to find the advice about it in Part II, "Common Complaints." Then you can perform Home Treatment or contact your doctor, whichever the book advises.

With *Take Care of Yourself* you'll handle common medical problems effectively and confidently. You'll save money by not going to the doctor when you don't have to, and you'll save yourself grief by recognizing problems before they grow. Finally, by living a healthy life, you can live a happier life.

When you face a medical problem, consider these seven steps:

1. *Is emergency action necessary?*

Usually the answer is obvious. The most common emergency signs are listed in the box on page v. More advice on these problems is found in "Emergencies," right after this section. It's a good idea to read "Emergencies" *now* so that you're prepared. Fortunately, the great majority of complaints don't require emergency treatment.

2. *Look up your chief complaint or symptom.*

Part II contains more than 100 common medical problems. Determine your chief complaint or symptom — a cough, an earache, dizziness — and look up that problem. Don't jump to conclusions about the cause of the problem: chest pain, for instance, may indicate indigestion rather than a heart attack. (Look that problem up under Chest Pain, **S82**). Each problem is numbered so that it's easier to find. Each section also contains a decision chart to help you choose between home treatment and a call or visit to the doctor.

Use the list of chapters opposite to find the appropriate problem section. The chapters in Part II are organized by type of complaint and by area of the body: skin problems, neck pain, shoulder pain, arm pain, and so on. You can also look up a symptom in the contents or the index.

3. *If in doubt, turn to the section for your worst problem first.*

You may have more than one problem, such as abdominal pain, nausea, and diarrhea. In such cases, look up the most serious complaint first, then the next most serious, and so on. If you use more than one chart, play it safe: if one chart recommends home treatment and the other advises a call to the doctor, call the doctor.

4. *Read all of the general information in the section.*

The general information describes possible causes of each problem, methods for treating it at home, and what to expect at a doctor's office if

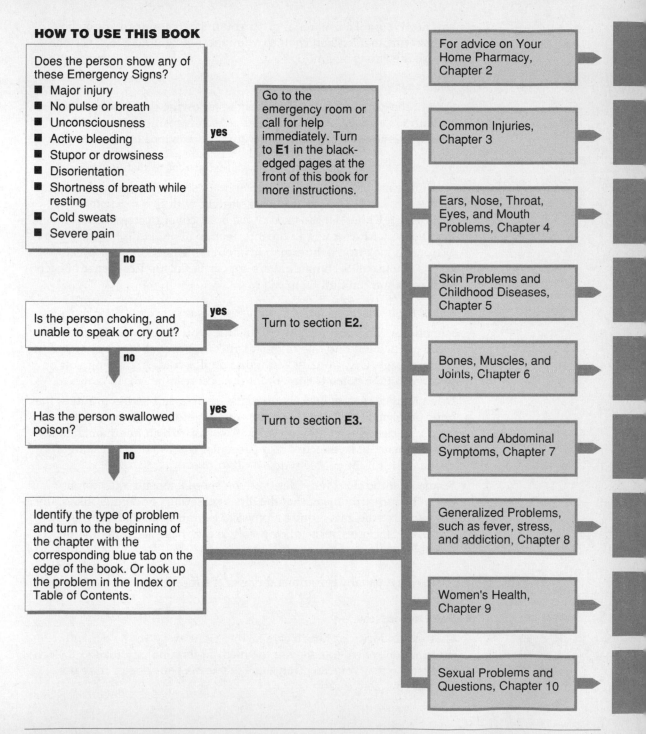

HOW TO USE THIS BOOK

Does the person show any of these Emergency Signs?
- Major injury
- No pulse or breath
- Unconsciousness
- Active bleeding
- Stupor or drowsiness
- Disorientation
- Shortness of breath while resting
- Cold sweats
- Severe pain

yes → Go to the emergency room or call for help immediately. Turn to **E1** in the black-edged pages at the front of this book for more instructions.

no ↓

Is the person choking, and unable to speak or cry out?

yes → Turn to section **E2.**

no ↓

Has the person swallowed poison?

yes → Turn to section **E3.**

no ↓

Identify the type of problem and turn to the beginning of the chapter with the corresponding blue tab on the edge of the book. Or look up the problem in the Index or Table of Contents.

For advice on Your Home Pharmacy, Chapter 2

Common Injuries, Chapter 3

Ears, Nose, Throat, Eyes, and Mouth Problems, Chapter 4

Skin Problems and Childhood Diseases, Chapter 5

Bones, Muscles, and Joints, Chapter 6

Chest and Abdominal Symptoms, Chapter 7

Generalized Problems, such as fever, stress, and addiction, Chapter 8

Women's Health, Chapter 9

Sexual Problems and Questions, Chapter 10

you need to go. This material gives you important information about interpreting the decision chart. If you ignore it, you may inadvertently choose the wrong action.

5. *Go through the decision chart.*

Start at the top. Answer every question, following the arrows indicated by your answers. Don't skip around: that may result in errors. Each question assumes that you've answered the previous question.

6. *If you see a number in boldface, flip to that section for related information.*

A number in boldface refers you to another section of the book. The sections in Part II all have numbers starting with **S,** for *symptoms.* Sections **E1–E3** here in the front of the book cover *emergencies.* Numbers starting with **M** refer you to the information about *medicines* in Chapter 2; look up the information about a medication or medical tool before you use it. Section numbers appear in the top left corner of each section so you can find them easily.

7. *Follow the treatment indicated by the decision chart.*

Sometimes the decision chart will instruct you to go to another section. More often you'll find one of the instruction boxes shown below and on the next page. Occasionally you'll find an illustration showing you how to carry out the home treatment for the best results.

Don't assume that an instruction to use home treatment guarantees that your problem is trivial and may be ignored. Home therapy must be used conscientiously if it is to work. Also, as with all treatments, home therapy may not be effective in a particular case, so don't hesitate to visit a doctor if the problem doesn't improve.

Similarly, if the chart indicates that you should consult a doctor, it doesn't necessarily mean that the illness is serious or dangerous. Many less serious problems require a physical examination to diagnose the cause, and facilities at the doctor's office can make accurate diagnosis possible.

The charts usually recommend one of the following actions:

■ **See Doctor Now**

Go to your doctor or health care facility right away. In the general information we try to give you the medical terminology related to each problem so that you can "translate" the terms your doctor may use during your conversation.

See Doctor Today

Call your doctor's office and say that you're coming in. Describe your problem over the phone as clearly as you can. Review the sections in Chapter 11 about communicating with your doctor so that you can get the most from your visit.

Make Appointment with Doctor

Schedule a visit to your doctor's office any time during the next few days. Before the appointment, review the sections in Chapter 11 about communicating with your doctor.

Call Doctor or Call Doctor Now

Often a phone conversation with your doctor or nurse will enable you to avoid an unnecessary visit, which is one way of using medical care more wisely. Remember that most doctors don't charge for telephone advice but regard it as part of their service to regular patients. Don't abuse this service in an attempt to avoid paying for necessary medical care.

If every call results in a recommendation for a visit, your doctor is probably sending you a message: come in and don't call. This is unfortunate, and you may want to look for a doctor willing to put the telephone to good use.

After your doctor's appointment, update your Family Medical Records, if necessary.

Use Home Treatment

Follow the instructions for home treatment closely, and keep it up. These steps are what most doctors recommend as a first approach to these problems.

There are times when home treatment is not effective even though you do it conscientiously. Think the problem through again, using the decision chart. The length of time you should wait before calling your doctor can be found in the general information in most sections. If you become seriously worried about your condition, call the doctor.

Emergencies

Emergencies require prompt action, not panic. What action you should take depends on the facilities available and the nature of the problem.

If there are massive injuries or if the victim is unconscious, you must get help immediately. Go to the emergency room if it is close. Have someone call ahead if you can.

If you can't reach the emergency room quickly, you can often obtain help by calling an emergency room or the rescue squad. Calling for help is especially important if you think that someone has swallowed poison. Poison control centers and emergency rooms can often tell you over the phone how to counteract the poison, thus beginning treatment as early as possible.

The most important thing is to *be prepared.* Work out a procedure for medical emergencies. Develop and test it before an actual emergency arises. Know the best way to reach the emergency room by car. If you plan emergency action ahead of time, you'll decrease the likelihood of panic and increase the probability of receiving the proper care quickly.

An **ambulance** isn't always the fastest way to reach a medical facility. It must travel to both your location and back and often isn't twice as fast as a private car. If the victim can readily move or be moved and a private car is available, use the car and have someone call ahead.

On the other hand, the ambulance brings with it a trained crew who know how to lift a victim to minimize chance of further injury. Intravenous fluids and oxygen are usually available; splints and bandages are provided; and in some instances, lifesaving resuscitation may be employed on the way to the hospital. Thus, care by ambulance attendants may most benefit a person who:

- Is gravely ill
- May have a back or head injury
- May have a serious heart attack
- Is severely short of breath

In our experience, ambulances are too often used as expensive taxis. An ambulance may be needed more urgently at another location, so use good judgment in deciding to call for one. Your community's EMT (emergency medical technician) program can be a great resource; use it wisely.

1 Emergency Signs

The decision charts for the common problems covered in Part II of this book assume that no emergency signs are present. *Emergency signs overrule the charts and dictate that you must seek medical help immediately.* Be familiar with the following emergency signs.

Major Injury

Common sense tells us that a person with a broken leg or large chest wound deserves immediate attention. Emergency facilities exist to take care of major injuries. They should be used promptly.

No Pulse or Breath

Again, someone whose heart or lungs aren't working needs help right away. Call for help. If you know CPR (cardiopulmonary resuscitation), start it after you call for help or direct someone else to call. If the person is choking, see section **E2,** Choking.

Unconsciousness

The person who is unconscious needs emergency care immediately.

Active Bleeding

Most cuts will stop bleeding if pressure is applied to the wound. This is the most important part of first aid for such wounds. Unless the bleeding is obviously minor, a wound that continues to bleed despite the application of pressure requires attention in order to prevent unnecessary loss of blood. The average adult can tolerate the loss of

several cups of blood with little ill effect, but children can tolerate only smaller amounts, relative to their body size.

Stupor or Drowsiness

A decreased level of mental activity, short of unconsciousness, is termed "stupor." A practical way of determining if the severity of stupor or drowsiness needs urgent treatment is to note the victim's ability to answer questions. If the victim is not sufficiently awake to answer questions concerning what has happened, then urgent action is necessary. Children are more difficult to judge, but the child who cannot be aroused needs immediate attention.

Disorientation

In medicine, disorientation is described and measured in terms of time, place, and person — that is, according to whether the person can answer these questions correctly:

- What is the date?
- Where are we?
- Who are you?

A person who doesn't know his or her identity is in more trouble than a person who doesn't know where he or she is, and that person is in more trouble than a person who can't give the correct date.

Disorientation may be part of a variety of illnesses and is especially common when the person has a high fever. The person who previously has been alert and then becomes disoriented and confused deserves immediate medical attention.

Shortness of Breath

We discuss shortness of breath more extensively in its own section **(S83).** As a general rule, immediate attention is needed if the person is short of breath even though resting. However, in young adults the most frequent cause of shortness of breath at rest is the hyperventilation syndrome, which is not a serious concern **(S101).** Nevertheless, if you can't confidently determine that shortness of breath is due to the hyperventilation syndrome, then the reasonable course of action is to seek immediate aid.

Cold Sweats

As an isolated symptom, sweating isn't likely to be serious. It's the normal response to elevated temperature. It's also the natural response to stress, either psychological or physical. Most people have experienced sweaty palms when "put on the spot" or stressed psychologically.

In contrast, a "cold sweat" in a person complaining of chest pain, abdominal pain, or light-headedness indicates a need for immediate attention. It's a common effect of severe pain or serious illness. Remember, however, that aspirin often causes sweating in lowering a fever. Sweating associated with the breaking of a fever is not the cold sweat referred to here.

Severe Pain

Surprisingly, severe pain by itself rarely determines if a problem is serious and urgent. Most often, pain is associated with other symptoms that indicate the urgency of the condition. The most obvious example is pain associated with major injury — like a broken leg — which itself clearly requires urgent care.

The severity of pain is subjective and depends on the individual; often the magnitude of the pain is altered by emotional and psychological factors. Nevertheless, severe pain demands urgent medical attention, if for no other reason than to relieve the pain.

We haven't tried to teach complex first aid procedures such as CPR (cardiopulmonary resuscitation) in this book. To use such procedures correctly, you need hands-on instruction and practice. Community organizations such as the American Red Cross and the American Heart Association offer training in these procedures. We urge you to take these classes.

Much of the art and science of medicine is directed at the relief of pain, and the use of emergency procedures to secure this relief is justified even if the cause of the pain eventually proves to be minor. However, the person who frequently complains of severe pain from minor causes is in much the same situation as the boy who cried "wolf"; calls for help will inevitably be taken less and less seriously by the doctor. This situation is a dangerous one, for the person may have difficulty obtaining help when it is most needed.

2 Choking

Your dinner companion can't breathe, can't talk, and is turning blue. He's gasping for air and puts his hand to his throat. These signs tell you he's choking. Do you know what to do?

Choking on a foreign object, usually food, is all too common. The most frequent setting for choking in adults is the evening meal, often in a restaurant or at a party. This situation increases the risk of choking in several ways: First, the victim is likely to have been drinking alcoholic beverages, and this may slow the reflexes that normally keep food from going down the wrong way. Second, the victim is likely to be distracted from the business of eating by conversation or entertainment. Finally, this is the time that solid meats such as steak are most commonly eaten, and these meats are usually the culprits in adult choking.

Children stick a much wider variety of objects into their mouths, are likely to do so at any time of the day or night, and are much less likely to complicate the situation with alcohol. Nevertheless, a child is still most likely to choke on food. The most likely foods are hot dogs, grapes, peanuts, and hard candy.

HOME TREATMENT

Choking is an emergency, but emergency medical services — doctors, EMTs, ambulances, emergency rooms, hospitals — play virtually no role in its treatment. In almost every case the victim's fate will be decided by the time such help can respond. Either someone knowledgeable steps forward and relieves the choking, or there's a very good chance the person won't survive.

You can be that knowledgeable someone. The most effective way to relieve choking is with the abdominal-thrust, or Heimlich, maneuver. Pushing on the lungs from below rapidly raises the air pressure inside the lungs and behind the foreign object that is causing the choking. This results in the forceful expulsion of the object from the throat back into the mouth. Done properly, an abdominal-thrust maneuver does not pose great risk of doing harm. Still, it's not the kind of thing you want to do to someone who won't benefit from it. The most important sign that a person should be treated with the abdominal-thrust maneuver is the inability to talk. If the person in difficulty can speak, forget about the abdominal-thrust maneuver.

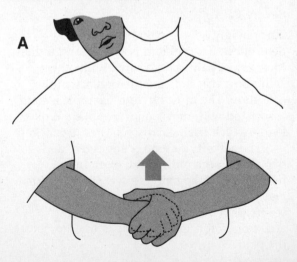

Abdominal-thrust (Heimlich) maneuver for adults. The figures show proper hand positions: *A (right):* standing position; *B (far right):* prone position.

CHOKING

Is the victim able to speak or cry out? —**yes**→ Consider problem other than choking.

no ↓

Is the victim a small child? —**yes**→ **USE EMERGENCY HOME TREATMENT ON PAGE XIV**

no ↓

Is the victim an infant? —**yes**→ **USE EMERGENCY HOME TREATMENT ON PAGE XV**

no ↓

USE EMERGENCY HOME TREATMENT ON THIS PAGE

B

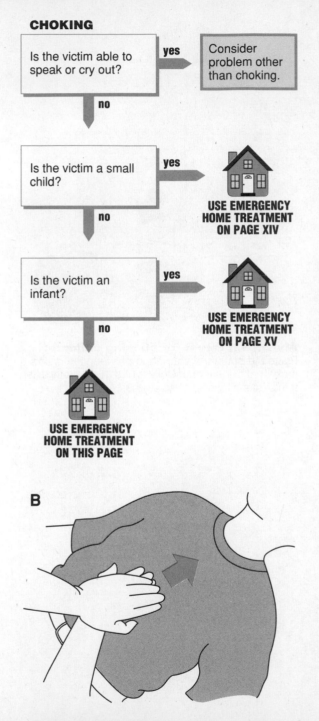

FOR ADULTS

1. Stand behind the choking victim and place your arms around him or her. Make a fist and place it against the victim's abdomen, thumb side in, between the navel and the breastbone.

2. Hold the fist with your other hand, and push upward and inward, four times quickly.

If the victim is pregnant or obese, place your arms around his or her chest and your hands over the middle of the breastbone. Give four quick chest thrusts.

If the victim is lying down, roll the victim over onto his or her back. Place your hands on the abdomen and push in the same direction on the body that you would if the victim were standing (inward and toward the upper body).

If the victim is much taller or heavier than you, make the victim lie on the floor and use the lying-down method described above.

3. If the victim doesn't start to breathe, open the mouth by moving the jaw and tongue, and look for the swallowed object. *If you can see the object,* sweep it out with your little finger. If you try to remove an object you can't see, you may only push it in more tightly.

4. If the victim doesn't begin to breathe after the object has been removed from the air passage, use mouth-to-mouth resuscitation.

5. Call for help, and repeat these steps until the object is dislodged and the victim is breathing normally.

FOR SMALL CHILDREN

1. Kneel next to the child, who should be lying on his or her back.

2. Position the heel of one hand on the child's abdomen between the navel and the breastbone. Deliver six to ten thrusts inward and toward the upper body.

3. If this doesn't work, open the mouth by moving the jaw and tongue and look for the swallowed object. *If you can see the object,* sweep it out of the throat using your little finger. If you try to remove an object you can't see, you may only push it in more tightly.

4. If the child doesn't begin to breathe after the object has been removed, use mouth-to-mouth resuscitation.

5. Call for assistance, and repeat these steps until the object is dislodged and the child is breathing normally or until help arrives.

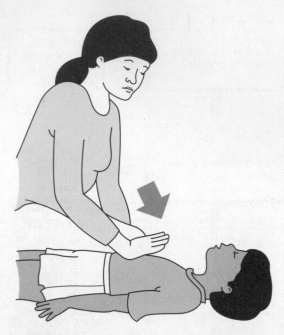

Abdominal thrust for choking children.
Place the bottom of your hand between the child's navel and breastbone. Deliver 6 to 10 quick thrusts. If this doesn't work, go to step 3.

In the past, we were uncertain about whether the abdominal-thrust (Heimlich) maneuver could be learned simply by reading about it. We're no longer in doubt. On January 17, 1988, Carolyn Tubbs used the abdominal-thrust maneuver to dislodge a piece of food from the throat of her husband, Eddie. Eddie was in real trouble, and we believe that Carolyn's quick action saved his life. Carolyn's only knowledge of this maneuver came from reading a self-care newsletter. We're quite certain about this episode because Carolyn was secretary to one of the authors at the time.

FOR INFANTS

1. Hold the infant along your forearm, face down, so that the head is lower than the feet.

2. Deliver four rapid blows to the back, between the shoulder blades, with the heel of your hand.

3. If this doesn't work, turn the baby over and, using two fingers, give four quick upward thrusts to the chest.

4. If you're still not successful, open the infant's mouth by moving the jaw and tongue and look for the swallowed object in the throat. *If you can see the object*, try to sweep it out gently with your little finger. If you try to remove an object you can't see, you may do more harm by pushing it in more tightly or triggering the child's gag reflex.

5. If the baby doesn't begin to breathe after the object has been removed, use mouth-to-nose-and-mouth resuscitation.

6. Call for assistance, and repeat these steps until the object is dislodged and the baby is breathing normally.

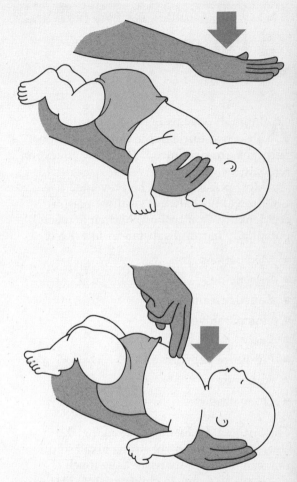

Abdominal thrust for choking infants. If 4 rapid blows to the infant's back don't work, deliver 4 quick thrusts to the infant's chest as shown above.

3 Poisoning

Although poisons may be inhaled or absorbed through the skin, for the most part they are swallowed. The term "ingestion" refers to swallowing.

Most poisoning can be prevented. Children almost always swallow poison accidentally. Don't allow children to reach potentially harmful substances like these:

- Medications
- Insecticides
- Caustic cleansers
- Organic solvents
- Fuels
- Furniture polishes
- Antifreezes
- Drain cleaners

The last item is the most damaging: drain cleaners like Drano are strong alkali solutions that can destroy any tissue they touch.

Keep all drugs in child-resistant bottles. Because there are no totally childproof bottles, keep drugs out of small children's reach. Aspirin overdoses have been responsible for more childhood deaths than any other medication.

Identifying the Problem

Treatment must be prompt to be effective, but identifying the poison is as important as speed. *Don't panic*. Try to identify the swallowed substance without taking up too much time. If you can't or if the victim is unconscious, go to the emergency room right away. If you can identify the poison, call the doctor or poison control center immediately and get advice on what to do. Always bring the container with you to the hospital. Life-support measures come first in the case of an unconscious victim, but doctors must identify the ingested substance before they can begin the proper therapy.

Many significant medication overdoses are due to suicide attempts. Any suicide attempt is an indication that the person needs help, even if he or she has physically recovered from the overdose itself and is in no immediate danger. Most successful suicides are preceded by unsuccessful attempts.

HOME TREATMENT

All cases of poisoning require professional help. Someone should call for help immediately. If the victim is conscious and alert and the ingredients swallowed are known, there are two types of treatment: those in which vomiting should be induced, and those in which it should not.

Do not induce vomiting if the victim has swallowed any of the following:

- **Acids:** battery acid, sulfuric acid, hydro-chloric acid, bleach, hair straightener, etc.
- **Alkalis:** Drano, drain cleaners, oven cleaners, etc.
- **Petroleum products:** gasoline, furniture polish, kerosene, lighter fluid, etc.

These substances can destroy the esophagus or damage the lungs as they are vomited. Neutralize them with milk while contacting the physician. If you don't have milk, use water or milk of magnesia.

Vomiting is a safe way to remove medications, plants, and suspicious materials

POISONING

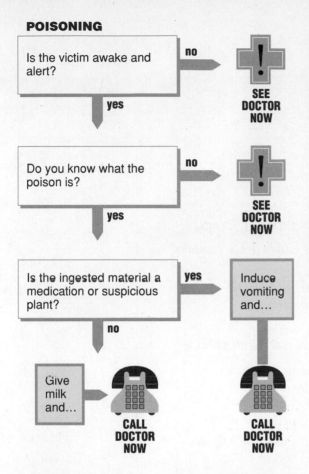

Is the victim awake and alert? — no → **SEE DOCTOR NOW**

yes ↓

Do you know what the poison is? — no → **SEE DOCTOR NOW**

yes ↓

Is the ingested material a medication or suspicious plant? — yes → Induce vomiting and... → **CALL DOCTOR NOW**

no ↓

Give milk and... → **CALL DOCTOR NOW**

Food poisoning is sometimes blamed for stomach or bowel problems that don't have any obvious explanation ("Must have been something I ate"). In reality, food poisoning due to bacteria (e.g., staphylococcus, streptococcus) is rare and causes symptoms that are seldom serious or long-lasting. Treat these symptoms as described in the appropriate sections: Diarrhea **(S86)** and Nausea and Vomiting **(S85)**. An exception is food poisoning due to botulism, but the main symptom of that disease is paralysis, starting with the muscles of the eyes, mouth, and throat, and then involving the entire body — that's obviously an emergency!

from the stomach. It's more effective and safer than using a stomach pump and doesn't require the doctor's help. Vomiting can sometimes be achieved immediately by touching the back of the throat with a finger. This is usually the fastest way, and time is important.

Another way to induce vomiting is to give two to four teaspoons (10–20 ml) of syrup (not extract) of ipecac **(M7)**, followed by as much liquid as the victim can drink. Vomiting usually follows within 20 minutes. Mustard mixed with warm water also works. If there's no vomiting within 25 minutes, repeat the dose. Collect what comes up so that the doctor can examine it.

Before, during, and after first aid for poisoning, contact a doctor.

If an accidental poisoning has occurred, make sure that it doesn't happen again. Put poisons where children cannot reach them. Flush old medications down the toilet.

WHAT TO EXPECT AT THE DOCTOR'S OFFICE

Significant poisoning is best managed at the emergency room. Treatment of the conscious victim depends on the particular poison and whether the person has vomited most of it back out. If indicated, the stomach will be emptied by vomiting or by the use of a stomach pump. Victims who are unconscious or have swallowed a strong acid or alkali will require admission to the hospital.

TAKE CARE OF YOURSELF

The Complete Illustrated Guide to Medical Self-Care

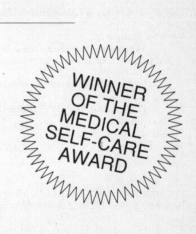

SIXTH EDITION

Donald M. Vickery, M.D.
James F. Fries, M.D.

ADDISON-WESLEY PUBLISHING COMPANY

Reading, Massachusetts ▪ Menlo Park, California ▪ New York
Don Mills, Ontario ▪ Harlow, England ▪ Amsterdam ▪ Bonn
Sydney ▪ Singapore ▪ Tokyo ▪ Madrid ▪ San Juan
Paris ▪ Seoul ▪ Milan ▪ Mexico City ▪ Taipei

Many of the designations used by manufacturers and sellers to distinguish their products are claimed as trademarks. Where those designations appear in this book and Addison-Wesley was aware of a trademark claim, the designations have been printed in initial capital letters (e.g., Excedrin).

Instructions on the abdominal-thrust maneuver for choking (pages xii–xv) have been adapted from the National Safety Council publication *Family Safety and Health*, Winter 1986–1987.

The drawing on fishhook removal from the foot (page 94) is adapted from George Hill, *Outpatient Surgery*. Philadelphia: Saunders, 1973.

The decision chart on alcoholism (page 297) has been adapted from J. A. Ewing, "Detecting Alcoholism: The CAGE Questionnaire," *Journal of the American Medical Association*, 252 (1984): 1905.

Information on substance abuse (pages 298–300) has been adapted from *Lifeplan: Your Own Master Plan for Maintaining Health and Preventing Illness*, by Donald M. Vickery (Reston, Va.: Vicktor, 1990).

Table on pages 318–319 adapted with permission from Pfeiffer, G. J. *Taking Care of Today and Tomorrow*. Reston, Va.: The Center for Corporate Health Promotion, 1989.

Table on page 328 adapted from Howard W. Ory, "Mortality Associated with Fertility and Fertility Control: 1983." *Family Planning Perspectives*, Vol. 15, No. 2, March/April 1983.

Library of Congress Cataloging-in-Publication Data

Vickery, Donald M.
    Take care of yourself : the complete illustrated guide to medical
self-care / Donald M. Vickery, James F. Fries. — 6th ed.
       p. cm.
    Includes bibliographical references and index.
    ISBN 0-201-48989-9
    1. Medicine, Popular. 2. Self-care, Health I. Fries, James F.
II. Title.
RC81.V51 1995
613—dc20
                                      95-49545
                                         CIP

Electronic page make-up: Mark Corsey, Nashua, N.H.

0-201-48989-9
0-201-95981-X

1 2 3 4 5 6 7 8 9-UG-0099989796

First Edition, 1976, Twenty-nine printings
Second Edition, 1981, Twenty-seven printings
Third Edition, 1986, Fourteen printings
Fourth Edition, 1989, Nineteen printings
Fifth Edition, 1993, Fifty-one printings
Sixth Edition, Second printing, February 1996

TO OUR READERS

*T*his book is strong medicine. It can be of great help to you. The medical advice is as sound as we can make it, but it will not always work. Like advice from your doctor, it won't always be right for you. This is our problem: If we don't give you direct advice, we can't help you. If we do, we'll sometimes be wrong. So here are some qualifications:

- If you're under the care of a doctor and receive advice contrary to this book, follow the doctor's advice; the individual characteristics of your problem can then be taken into account. This is especially important if you have been diagnosed with a chronic condition.

- If you have an allergy or a suspected allergy to a recommended medication, check with your doctor, at least by phone, before following the advice in this book.

- Read medicine label directions carefully; instructions vary from year to year, and you should follow the most recent.

- If your problem persists beyond a reasonable period, you should usually see a doctor.

CONTENTS

PART I   *The Habit of Health*   1

CONTENTS

CHAPTER 5 *Skin Problems and Childhood Diseases* 141

CONTENTS

CHAPTER 6   *Bones, Muscles, and Joints*   203

CONTENTS

PART III

Managing Your Professional Medical Care 333

PREFACE

*T*ake Care!" With this traditional parting phrase we express our feelings for our friends and show our priorities. When I see you again, be healthy. Keep your health. Not "Be rich!" or "Be famous!" but "Take care of yourself!"

This book is about how to take care of yourself. For us, the phrase has four meanings:

First, "take care of yourself" means maintaining the habits that lead to vigor and health. Your lifestyle is your most important guarantee of lifelong vigor, and you can postpone most serious chronic diseases by making the right choices about how to live. You can prevent bad health.

Second, "take care of yourself" means periodic monitoring for those few diseases that can sneak up on you without clear warning, such as high blood pressure, cancer of the breast or cervix, glaucoma, or dental decay. In such cases, taking care of yourself may mean going to a health professional for assistance.

Third, "take care of yourself" means responding decisively to new medical problems that arise. Most often your response should be self-care, and you can act as your own doctor. At other times, however, you need professional help. Responding decisively means that you pay particular attention to the decision about going, or not going, to see the doctor. This book helps you make that decision.

Many people think that all illness must be treated at the doctor's office, clinic, or hospital. In fact, over 80% of new problems are treated at home, and an even larger number could be. The public has had scant instruction in determining when outside help is needed and when it is not. In the United States, the average person sees a doctor slightly more than five times a year. Over 1.5 billion prescriptions are written each year, about eight for each man, woman, and child. Medical costs now average over $3,000 per person per year — over 14% of our gross national product. In total, $1 trillion each year. Among the billions of different medical services used each year, some are lifesaving, some result in great health improvement, and some give great comfort. But some are totally unnecessary, and some are even harmful.

In our national quest for a symptom-free existence, we make millions of unnecessary visits to doctors — as many as 70% of all visits are for new problems. For example, 11% of such visits are for uncomplicated colds. Many others are for minor cuts that do not require stitches, for tetanus shots despite current immunizations, for minor ankle sprains, and for the other problems discussed in this book. But while you don't need a doctor to treat most coughs, you do for some. For every ten or so cuts that don't require stitches, there is one that does. For every type of problem, there are some instances in which you should decide to see the doctor and some in which you should not.

Consider how important these decisions are. If you delay a visit to the doctor when you really need it, you may suffer unnecessary discomfort or leave an illness untreated. On the other hand, if you go to the doctor when you don't need to, you waste time, and you may lose money or dignity. More subtly, confidence in your own ability to judge your health and in the healing power of your own body begins to erode. You can even suffer physical harm if you receive a drug that you don't need or have a test that you don't require. Your doctor is in an uncomfortable position when you come in unnecessarily and may feel obligated to practice "defensive medicine" just in case you have a bad result and a good lawyer. This book, above all else, is intended to help you with the decision of when to see your doctor. It provides you with a "second opinion" within easy reach on your bookshelf. It contains information to help you make sound judgments about your own health.

The fourth meaning of the title of our book is this: Your health is your responsibility; it depends on your decisions. There is no other way to be healthy than to "take care of yourself." You have to decide how to live, whether to see a doctor, which doctor to see, how soon to go, whether to take the advice offered. No one else can make these decisions, and they profoundly direct the course of future events. To be healthy, you have to be in charge.

Take care of yourself!

Donald M. Vickery, M.D.
Evergreen, Colorado

James F. Fries, M.D.
Stanford, California

ACKNOWLEDGMENTS

We are grateful to many people for their help with this sixth edition, including the thousands of readers who have written with suggestions and encouragement and the hundreds of health workers who have used previous editions in their programs and practices. Special thanks to Lisa H. Schneck and Anita J. Waller for their diligence in revising and preparing this edition.

We would also like to thank Dr. William Bremer, Rick Carlson, Dr. William Carter, Dr. Grace Chickadonz, Dr. Peter Collis, Charlotte Crenson, Ann Dilworth, Dr. Edgar Engleman, William Fisher, Sarah Fries, Jo Ann Gibely, Harry Harrington, Dr. Halsted Holman, Dr. Robert Huntley, Dr. Donald Iverson, Dr. Julius Krevans, Dr. Kenneth Larsen, Dr. Kate Lorig, Professor Nathan Maccoby, Florence Mahoney, Michael Manley, Lawrence McPhee, Dr. Dennis McShane, Dr. Eugene Overton, Dr. Robert H. Pantell, Charles L. Parcell, Christian Paul, Clarence Pearson, William Peterson, George Pfeiffer, Gene Fauro Pratt, Dr. Robert Quinnell, Nancy Richardson, Dr. Robert Rosenberg, Dr. Ralph Rosenthal, Craig Russell, Dr. Douglas Solomon, Dr. Michael Soper, Warren Stone, Dr. Richard Tompkins, Dr. William Watson, Douglas Weiss, and Dr. Craig Wright for their advice and support.

INTRODUCTION

*Y*ou can do more for your health than your doctor can.

We introduced the first edition of *Take Care of Yourself* in 1976 with this phrase. The concept that health is more a personal responsibility than a professional one was controversial at that time, although it can be found in the earlier writings of René Dubois, Victor Fuchs, and John Knowles, among others. But the idea was still foreign to a society heavily dependent on experts of every kind and seemingly addicted to ever more complex gadgetry and medications.

What a difference twenty years can make! In 1981 the Surgeon General of the United States released a carefully worded report, *Health Promotion and Disease Prevention*, with this statement: "You, the individual, can do more for your own health and well being than any doctor, any hospital, any drugs, any exotic medical devices." The report goes on to detail a strategy for improved national health based on personal effort. The federal government now has a National Center for Chronic Disease Prevention and Health Promotion. The strategy of *Take Care of Yourself* is now a nationally accepted one. Your health depends on you. We are proud that this book has played a role in the changing national perception of health.

In 1991, the Department of Health and Human Services released an important document called *Healthy People 2000: National Health Promotion and Disease Prevention Objectives*. It laid out health goals for the nation for the year 2000; they have long been the goals of *Take Care of Yourself*. Some of the specific targets:

- Increase the number of people participating in moderate daily physical activity to at least 30% of people (currently 23%)
- Reduce overweight problems to no more than 20% of people (currently 25%)

- Reduce dietary fat intake to an average of less than 30% of calories (currently 36%)
- Reduce cigarette smoking to less than 15% of adults (currently 29%)
- Reduce alcohol intake by 20% (from 2.54 to 2.0 gallons, or 7.5 liters, per person per year)
- Increase fiber intake to five servings a day on average (currently two a day)

We are pleased to support these national goals fully, and you will find many specific suggestions in *Take Care of Yourself* for how to reduce your personal health risks in the direction of the national goals.

The first five editions of *Take Care of Yourself* included more than a hundred printings totaling well over nine million copies in North America alone. The book has been translated into ten languages. It has been the central feature of many health promotion programs sponsored by corporations, health insurance plans, and other institutions. Acceptance by professional review panels is testimony to the soundness of the medical advice provided here and is also a testament to far-sighted panels and program directors who saw the need for new approaches to health problems.

Evidence That This Book Works

But does *Take Care of Yourself* work? Can you improve your health with the aid of a book? Can you use the doctor less, use services more wisely, save money? Absolutely. *Take Care of Yourself* has been more carefully evaluated by critical scientists than any health book ever written, and the evaluations have been published in the major medical journals. The five largest studies involved an aggregate of many thousands of individuals and cost nearly $2 million in total to perform. The results of all the studies have been positive.

- A report in the *Journal of the American Medical Association* described a randomized study conducted in Woodland, California. As determined by lot, 460 families were given *Take Care of Yourself*, and 239 were not. The number of visits to doctors by those who were given *Take Care of Yourself* was reduced by 7.5% compared with those who were not given the book. Visits to doctors decreased 14% for upper respiratory tract infections (colds).

- A 1983 report in the *Journal of the American Medical Association* compared the use of *Take Care of Yourself* in a health maintenance organization with a random control group. Total medical visits were reduced 17%, and visits for minor illnesses were reduced 35%. This large study of 3,700 subjects over five years obtained its data directly from medical records, had a rigorous experimental design, and found statistically significant reductions in medical visits in both the Medicare and general populations.

- A major study reported in the journal *Medical Care* in 1985 detailed an experiment at 29 work sites that reduced visitation rates for households of 5,200 employees by 14% — 1.5 doctor visits per household per year — after distribution of *Take Care of Yourself.*

- In 1992, a report in the *American Journal of Health Promotion* analyzed health risk changes in over 250,000 people given *Take Care of Yourself* and Healthtrac materials and followed their health for up to 30 months. A decrease in health risks was consistent, at about 10% per year, and applied equally to young and old age groups and to those with less or more education.

- In 1993, the *American Journal of Medicine* reported a randomized two-year controlled trial of nearly 6,000 Bank of America retirees. The people who received *Take Care of Yourself* and the Senior Healthtrac program reduced health risks by 15% compared with control groups. Furthermore, they saved about $300 per person.

- In 1994, a randomized trial of 59,000 people reported in the *American Journal of Health Promotion* showed that the same materials improved health and saved over $8 million for the California Public Employees Retirement System.

We, as a nation, are in the midst of a health care cost crisis. Costs now average $3,000 per person per year — more than double those of many countries. Many people can no longer afford insurance. The *Take Care of Yourself* solution is simple:

- Stay healthy and reduce your need for medical care.
- Be a good purchaser and purchase only the services you truly need.

For every heart attack prevented, the system saves $50,000, and you may save your life. By preparing a Living Will you may save your family thousands of dollars, and you can increase the dignity of your care if you develop a terminal illness. Even that cold that you treat at home may save $100 or more of doctor bills, laboratory tests, X-rays, and medication.

Why should you work to reduce medical care costs when you have insurance? You paid for it; why not use it? We are reminded of the "tragedy of the commons." In a small mountainous village in Spain, each family had one goat, which represented their total wealth. The village goats grazed on the common land inside the circle of huts and provided milk and cheese. One man reasoned that if he had two goats he would be twice as wealthy, and the commons could surely support one more goat, so he raised two goats. Then another man did the same. And another. And another. Eventually the grass was all eaten up, the goats died, and the villagers starved.

The health care crisis can be controlled if we all work to decrease our need for and use of medical services. Now is a time to work for the common good: to preserve common resources. Moreover, your good health is its own reward. A vigorous lifestyle, a continuing sense of adventure and excitement, the exercise of personal will, and the acceptance of individual responsibility are essential to — and benefits of — the healthy life. Take care of yourself. You will help the broader society. And your loved ones will thank you for it.

PART I

The Habit of Health

CHAPTER 1

A Pound of Prevention: Your Actions, Your Future

You can do much more than any doctor to maintain your health and well-being. But you have to get into the habit of health. You must have a plan. At the age of 50, individuals with good health habits can be physically 30 years younger than those with poor health habits. In other words, at age 50 you can feel as if you're 65 years old or 35 years old. It's up to you. You'll feel better and accomplish more if you develop the habit of health. In this chapter we'll help you make the most important plan of your life, your plan for good health.

The major health problems in the United States are chronic, long-term illness in middle age and later, and trauma at young ages. These illnesses include heart disease, cancer, emphysema, and liver cirrhosis, and cause nearly 90% of all deaths. They also account for about 90% of all sickness in the United States. About two-thirds of cases of these illnesses can be prevented.

The illness and pain associated with disease, as well as the deaths, can be greatly reduced by a good plan for health. For example, only two years after your last cigarette you return to the normal risk level for heart attacks. After ten years you're back to nearly normal risk for lung cancer. In only a few weeks, exercise programs begin to contribute to your health and well-being. For most chronic diseases, not only can you slow the rate of progression, but you can also reverse part of the damage.

As a bonus, your plan for good health can prevent many nagging nonfatal health problems such as hernias, back pain, varicose veins, and osteoporosis. By developing the habit of health, you can reduce the amount of illness you'll have in your life. As an even bigger bonus, you'll feel much better and have more energy. Good health is its own reward.

An ounce of prevention is better than a pound of cure. Think of what a pound of prevention can do!

The Seven Keys to Health

Good news! There are only seven major ingredients in a plan for good health:

- Exercise
- Diet
- Not smoking
- Alcohol moderation
- Weight control
- Avoiding injury through common sense
- Professional prevention practices

In fact, most individuals don't even need to worry about all seven areas. You're probably already a nonsmoker. Quite possibly your body weight isn't too far from where it needs to be. Probably your alcohol intake is already moderate. Probably you already do some exercise, and probably you already have some good dietary practices. Most likely you already take some measures, such as using your automobile seat belts, to reduce your chances of serious injury. And you probably work with your doctor to have some of the periodic screening tests that you need.

EXERCISE

Exercise is the central ingredient of good health. It tones the muscles, strengthens the bones, and makes the heart and lungs work better. It increases your physical reserve and your vitality. Exercise eases depression, assists the function of the bowels, leads to sound sleep, and aids in every activity of daily life. Exercise helps prevent heart disease, high blood pressure, stroke, and many other diseases.

The Three Types of Exercise

Exercise comes in several different flavors. There are strengthening exercises, stretching exercises, and aerobic (or endurance) exercises. You need to know the merits and limits of each type.

Strengthening exercises are the traditional "body-building" exercises that build stronger muscles. Squeezing balls, lifting weights, and doing push-ups or pull-ups are examples. Strengthening exercises are only one part of a beneficial exercise program, however. These exercises can be very helpful in improving function in a particular body part after surgery (for example, knee surgery) where it's necessary to rebuild strength. They also help to strengthen your bones, since bones react to stress by becoming stronger; they can help strengthen bones even at advanced ages.

It should go without saying that you should never use anabolic steroids or any other drugs as part of a strengthening program. By so doing, you may damage your future health.

Stretching exercises are designed to help keep you loose. These are a bit more important; everyone should do some of them, but they don't have many direct effects on health. Be careful not to overdo these exercises. Toe-touching, for example, should be done gently, without bouncing. Stretch relatively slowly, to the point of discomfort and just a little bit beyond.

Stretching exercises can be of great benefit in these situations:

- If you have a joint that's stiff because of arthritis or injury
- If you've just had surgery on a joint
- If you have a disease condition that results in stiffness

There's nothing mysterious about the stretching process. Any body part that you can't completely straighten or completely bend needs to be frequently and repeatedly stretched; a good rule is twice daily. Over weeks or months, you can often regain motion of that body part.

For most people, however, stretching exercises are useful mainly as a warm-up for aerobic (endurance) exercise activity. Gently stretching before you begin aerobic exercise is important for three reasons:

- It warms up the muscles
- It makes the muscles looser
- It decreases the chances of injury

Stretching again after the aerobic exercise can help prevent stiffness.

Aerobic (endurance) exercise is the key to fitness and vitality. This is the most important kind of exercise. The word "aerobic" means that during the exercise period, the oxygen (air) that you breathe in balances the oxygen that you use up. During aerobic exercise, a number of good things happen. Your heart speeds up to pump larger amounts of blood. You breathe more frequently and more deeply to increase the oxygen transfer from the lungs to the blood. Your body develops increased heat and compensates by sweating to keep your temperature normal. You build endurance.

As a result of endurance exercise, the cells of the body develop the ability to extract a larger amount of oxygen from the blood. This improves the function of all of the cells of the body. As you become more fit, these effects increase. The heart becomes larger and stronger and can pump more blood with each stroke. The cells can take up oxygen more readily. As a result, your heart rate when you're resting doesn't need to be as rapid. This allows more time for the heart to repair itself between beats.

Your Aerobic Program

Aerobic exercise is important for all ages. It's never too soon to develop the habit of lifetime exercise. It's never too late to begin an aerobic exercise program and to experience the often dramatic benefits. There are, of course, a few difficulties in beginning a new exercise program. If you've been deconditioned by avoiding exercise for some time, start at a lower level of physical activity than a more active person would. You may have an underlying medical condition that limits your choice of exercises; if so, ask your doctor for advice about exactly how to proceed.

Some people worry that (1) exercise will increase their heart rates, (2) they have only so many heartbeats in a lifetime, so (3) they may be using them up. In fact, because of the decrease in their resting heart rates, fit individuals use 10 to 25% fewer heartbeats in the course of a day, even after allowing for the increase during exercise periods. Aerobic training also builds good muscle tone, improves reflexes, improves balance, burns fat, aids the bowels, and makes the bones stronger.

Other people worry about destroying their joints by too much exercise, or about sudden death while exercising. The truth is the opposite. Those who exercise have much less disability than those who don't, and the tissues around their joints become stronger. And while occasionally a person does have a heart attack during exercise, the overall chances of a heart attack are greatly decreased by aerobic exercise.

Heart Rate. Much has been made of reaching a particular heart rate during exercise, a rate that avoids too much stress on the heart and yet provides the desired training effect. Cardiologists (heart specialists) often suggest that a desirable exercise heart rate is 220 minus your age times 75%. For example, at age 40 your target exercise heart rate is 180 x .75 = 135 beats per minute. It can be difficult to count your pulse while you're exercising, but you can check it by counting the pulse in your wrist for 15 seconds immediately after you stop and then multiplying by 4.

As your training progresses, you may wish to count your resting pulse, perhaps in bed in the morning before you get up. The goal here (if you don't have an underlying heart problem and aren't taking a medication such as propranolol, which decreases the heart rate) is a resting heart rate of about 60 beats per minute. An individual who isn't fit will typically have a resting heart rate of 75 or so.

We generally find this whole heart rate business a bit of a bother and somewhat artificial. There really are no good medical data to justify particular target heart rates. You may wish to check your pulse rate a few times just to get a feel for what is happening, but it doesn't have to be something you watch extremely carefully. Aerobic exercise shouldn't be "all out"; if you can't talk to a companion while you're exercising, you're probably working too hard.

Aerobic Choices. Your choice of a particular aerobic activity depends on your own desires and your present level of fitness. You should be able to grade the activity; that is, you should be able to easily and gradually increase both the effort and the duration of the exercise.

Walking gently isn't a true aerobic exercise, but it provides important health benefits. If you haven't been exercising at all, start by walking. A gradual increase in walking activity, up to a level of 100 to 200 minutes per week, usually should precede attempting a more aerobic program. First get in the habit of putting in the exercise time, then increase the effort. Walking briskly can be aerobic, but you need to push the pace quite a bit to break a sweat and get your heart rate up. Walking uphill can quite quickly become aerobic.

Jogging, swimming, and brisk walking are appropriate for all ages. At home, stationary bicycles or cross-country ski machines are good. We have seen people confined to bed using a specially designed stationary bicycle. Some individuals like to use radio earphones while they exercise; others exercise indoors while watching the evening news. Almost any activity from gardening to tennis can be aerobic, but remember that aerobic exercise can't be "start and stop." Aerobic activity can't come in bursts; it must be sustained for at least 10 to 12 minutes during each exercise period. The most recent recommendations are for 20- to 30-minute exercise periods five to seven days a week.

Cautions. If you have a serious underlying illness, particularly one involving the heart or the joints, or if you're over age 70, ask your doctor for specific advice. Advice from your doctor should always take precedence over recommendations in this book. For most people, however, a doctor's advice isn't required in order to start exercising. We recommend mentioning your exercise program to your doctor while on a visit for some other reason. A good doctor will encourage your exercise program and perhaps assist you in choosing goals and activities.

Some doctors recommend that you have an electrocardiogram (EKG) or an exercise electrocardiogram before you start exercising, particularly if you're over 50 years of age. It is difficult to see what this accomplishes because (1) gentle, graded exercise is a treatment for heart problems anyway, and (2) the test produces up to 80% "false-positive" results, suggesting that you have problems when you don't. Many doctors (including us) don't think these tests are necessary, regardless of age, unless you (the patient) have specific, known problems. If a doctor recommends a coronary arteriogram (X-ray study of the arteries of the heart after injecting a dye into the arteries) before you begin an exercise program, you should seek a second opinion to see if this somewhat hazardous test is needed.

"Crash" exercise programs are always ill-advised. You have to start gently and go slowly. There's never a hurry, and there's a slight hazard in pushing yourself too far too fast. Age alone is not a deterrent to exercise. Many seniors who have achieved record levels of fitness, as indicated by world-class marathon times for their age, started exercising only in their 60s, 70s, or even 80s. Mount Fuji has been climbed by a man over 100 years of age.

Getting Started. Assess your present level of activity. This is where you start. Set goals for the level of fitness you want to achieve. Your final goal should be at least one year away, but you may want to develop in-between goals for one, three, and six months. Select the aerobic activity you want to pursue. Choose a time of day for your exercise. Develop exercise as a routine part of your day. We like to see exercise regularly performed for at least five out of seven days of the week; if you exercise all seven days, take it easy one or two days each week. Younger individuals can frequently condition with exercise periods three or four times a week. For seniors, more gentle activities performed daily are more beneficial and less likely to result in injury. You can make ordinary activities like walking or mowing the lawn aerobic by doing them at a faster and constant pace.

Start slowly and gently. Your total exercise activity shouldn't increase by more than about 10% each week. Each exercise period should be reasonably constant in effort. When you're walking, jogging, or whatever, you can use both distance and time to keep track of your progression. When starting out, it's a good idea to keep a brief diary of what you do each day to be sure you're on track. It's best to slowly increase your weekly exercise *time* to at least 90 or 100 minutes before you work to increase the *effort* level of the exercise. Get accustomed to the activity first and then begin to push it just a little bit. Again, progress slowly.

Be sure to loosen up with stretching exercises before and after exercise periods, and to wear clothing warm enough to keep your muscles from getting cold and cramping. The bottom line is patience and common sense.

Handling Setbacks. No exercise program ever progresses without any problems whatsoever. After all, you're asking your body to do something it hasn't done for a while. It will complain every now and again. Even after you have a well-established exercise program, there will be interruptions. You may be ill, take a vacation where it's difficult to exercise, or sustain an injury. There will be setbacks, but they shouldn't change your overall plan.

Common sense is the key to handling setbacks. Often you can substitute another activity for the one with which you're having trouble and thus maintain your fitness program. Sometimes you can't, and you just have to lay off for a while.

When you begin again, don't try to start immediately at your previous level of activity; deconditioning is a surprisingly rapid process. On the other hand, you don't have to start again at the beginning. The general rule is to take as long to get back to your previous level of activity as you were out. If you can't exercise for two weeks, gradually increase your activity over a two-week period to get back to your previous level.

Topping Out. After your exercise program is well established, you need to make sure that it becomes a habit you want to continue for a long time. Two hundred minutes of aerobic exercise a week (about half an hour a day) seems to give the best results. There is no medical evidence that more than 200 minutes a week is of additional value. Many people won't want to exercise this much, and that's perfectly fine. You can get most of the benefits with less activity. At 100 minutes a week, you get almost 90% of the gain that comes with 200 minutes. At 60 minutes a week, a total of one hour, you get about 75% of the benefit that you get with 200 minutes.

Exercise should be fun. Often it doesn't seem so at first, but after your exercise habits are well developed, you'll wonder how you ever got along without them. Once you're fit, you can take advantage of your body's increased reserve to vary your activity more than you did during the early months. You can change exercise activities or alternate hard exercise and easy exercise days. At that point, we hope you're a convert to exercise programs. You then can work to introduce others to the same benefits.

DIET AND NUTRITION

Diet is the second major factor for a healthy life. In general, you should move slowly in making changes from your present diet. Most people can't easily make sudden, radical changes in diet, so they may not maintain such changes. Instead, develop good dietary habits slowly over a long time span. The more changes you make, the greater the benefits. Table 1 provides guidelines for a healthy diet.

Fat Intake

Excessive total fat and saturated fat intake is the worst food habit in the typical American diet. Excessive fat intake is the major cause of atherosclerosis (hardening of the arteries' inner lining), which leads to heart attacks and strokes. The U.S. government's *Healthy People 2000* goals call for people to reduce their total fat intake to less than 30% of the total calories they consume and their saturated fat intake to less than 10%. The current U.S. average is 37% of calories as total fat and nearly 20% as saturated fat.

We think that you should try for 20% of calories as total fat and 7% as saturated fat since such stricter diets have been shown to actually *reverse* some early artery hardening. In some cases patches on the artery walls

TABLE 1	*Your Diet for Health*
Protein	Slightly decrease total protein. Reduce protein intake from red meat; increase protein from whole-grain foods, vegetables, poultry, and fish.
Fat and Cholesterol	Decrease total fat intake to less than 20% of total calories. Greatly decrease the saturated fats found in whole milk, most cheeses, and red meat. Switch to vegetable oils, canola oil, soybean oil, corn oil, peanut oil, or olive oil.
Carbohydrate	Increase total carbohydrates, emphasizing whole-grain foods, vegetables, cereals, fruit, pasta, and rice; these contain "complex" carbohydrates.
Alcohol	Moderate use or less; "moderate" is approximately two drinks daily.
Fiber	Increase fiber intake, with emphasis on fresh fruits and vegetables and whole-grain foods.
Salt	Decrease to about 4 grams per day (average intake in the United States is 12 grams per day). Avoid added salt in cooking or at the table and avoid heavily salted foods, such as most snack foods. Further decrease salt intake if medically recommended.
Caffeine	Limit to 300 milligrams (mg) or less per day, equivalent to three cups of coffee.
Calcium	Standard recommendations are for at least 1,000 mg per day for men after age 65 and 1,500 mg per day for women after menopause. For reference, nonfat milk has 250 mg per glass. Use powdered nonfat milk in foods such as soup. If necessary, consider calcium supplements.

nearly disappear. Such improvements have been seen both in monkeys given high-fat diets and then normal diets and exercise, and in X-ray dye studies of human hearts.

Cholesterol

An elevated serum cholesterol level is one sign warning you to reduce dietary fat. A good level is "200 or less" — that's 200 milligrams (mg) of cholesterol per deciliter (dl) of blood. Measurement of cholesterol is only a very rough guide to your dietary needs, however, and *everyone* will benefit from decreasing fat intake. The actual chemistry of fats in the body is very complicated. The waxy white cholesterol not only comes from your diet but is also manufactured in your liver. This cholesterol production in turn is related to the various other fats in your diet. Attached to the cholesterol itself are high-density lipoproteins (HDL), which actually help prevent atherosclerosis, and low-density lipoproteins (LDL), which make heart problems much more likely. The LDL (bad cholesterol) travels "outbound" from the liver and can deposit on the inside walls of blood vessels. The

HDL (good cholesterol) takes cholesterol "inbound" back to the liver for excretion and can help remove plaque from arterial walls. Many laboratories measure serum cholesterol quite inaccurately. Hence, we're not enthusiastic about using serum cholesterol levels as the sole measure of your dietary needs.

You can simplify this whole complicated business by simply cutting down on the largest sources of saturated fat in your diet. Fortunately, there are easy approaches to changing saturated fat intake.

- With **eggs,** you just have to cut down the number per week; two eggs a week or fewer is a good ration.

- Instead of butter, use soft or liquid **margarine.** Some evidence suggests that solid margarines are not much better for you than butter.

- Use **low-fat** or **nonfat milk** instead of whole milk. The calcium and other nutrients in milk are very good for you, but the saturated fat is bad.

- To reduce fat intake from **meats,** don't eat these foods often. A good rule for many people is to avoid having red meat two days in a row. This is easy, and it gets variety into your diet. Remember, it's really the white fat in the red meat that is the problem. Pork, bacon, hot dogs, and sausage are not colored "red" but usually contain a great deal of saturated animal fat. When you do have meat, trim the fat extensively before cooking, broil so that some fat burns or runs off, and cook the meat a little more well done. For meat lovers, a good (and economical) practice is to buy smaller cuts of meat; surround a smaller four- or five-ounce steak with larger portions of vegetables.

- **Don't fry foods;** this usually adds saturated fat. If you do fry, avoid saturated fats such as palm oil and coconut oil; although these are vegetable oils, they're also saturated fats and bad for your arteries. Monounsaturated fats — such as olive oil, peanut oil, and canola oil — may actually be good for you.

What about other ways to lower your serum cholesterol and other fats (lipids) in the bloodstream? As we discuss later, fiber (as in vegetables, celery, apples, beans, and whole-grain breads and cereals) actually acts to lower serum cholesterol by binding some cholesterol in the bowel before the cholesterol can be absorbed. Adequate calcium intake, needed for strong bones, also lowers blood pressure and probably the blood lipids. Your exercise program lowers your total cholesterol and also increases the good HDL in your blood. When you stop smoking, your HDL cholesterol goes up. Good health habits all seem to fit together.

Protein

What's the best protein for your diet? Probably that from whole-grain foods. Fish is excellent; you should plan at least two fish meals a week. Interestingly, the best fish for you are the high-fat fishes that live in cold water, such as salmon or mackerel. These contain a kind of fish oil that is good for your heart and actually lowers your serum cholesterol level.

Chicken and other poultry are good neutral foods. They contain less fat than red meat, though still some cholesterol; they have much less fat if you remove the skin.

The official national nutritional guidelines recommend that you substitute complex carbohydrates (such as whole-grain foods and cereals) for some of the fat and some of the protein in your diet. The complex carbohydrates are more slowly digested and provide a more even source of energy.

Salt Intake

Too much sodium (salt) in your system tends to retain fluid in your body, increasing your blood pressure and predisposing you to such problems as swollen legs. Your heart has to work harder with the increased amount of fluid volume. Thus, it's good to decrease your salt intake.

The average person in the United States takes in about 12 grams of sodium each day, one of the highest intakes in the world. Our convenience foods and fast foods are usually loaded with salt. Salt is in ketchup, in most sauces, and in hidden form in many foods. You need to read the labels to find it: look for "sodium," not "salt." The recommended amount of salt intake is 4 grams a day. You'll get plenty of salt in your food without adding more. People with problems of high blood pressure, heart failure, or some other difficulties may need to reduce salt much more radically, and should discuss desirable intake levels with their doctor.

Do you have a craving for junk foods? Don't despair — there are healthy snacks! One of our favorites: popcorn, air-cooked, sprayed with butter-flavored PAM instead of butter, and sprinkled with a little Parmesan cheese. Even better, try popcorn with olive oil instead of butter, unsalted peanuts in the shell, or French bread basted with olive oil and toasted with oregano or garlic. Try low-salt whole-grain pretzels. To add flavor to foods, use lemon juice, pepper, or herbs rather than salt. There are even hot dogs without any fat or cholesterol; check the labels.

Fiber

Adequate fiber intake is important to your future health. Fiber is the indigestible residue of food that passes through the entire bowel and is then eliminated in the stool. It's found in unrefined grains, cereals, vegetables (particularly celery), and most fruits.

The beneficial effects of fiber come from its actions as it passes through the bowel. Fiber attracts water and provides consistency to the stool so that it may pass easily. The increased regularity of bowel action that results turns out to be very important; it decreases the chances of diverticulitis, an inflammation of the colon wall. Fiber protects the bowel so that the development of precancerous polyps is greatly reduced, as is the risk of cancer of the colon. Fiber also acts to decrease problems with constipation, hemorrhoids, tears in the rectal wall, and other minor problems. Finally, fiber binds cholesterol and helps eliminate it from the body.

We must emphasize that the natural-fiber approach to maintaining regular bowel movements is much better than using laxatives and bowel stimulants, which have none of the advantages of fiber. You need to get the fiber habit and to avoid the stimulant and laxative habit.

Calcium

Everybody needs enough calcium. Sufficient calcium intake is particularly important for senior men and even more important for senior women. Our national trend toward better health habits has decreased our intake of calcium-containing milk and cheese. Hence, calcium intake for many people has dropped below what is desirable, and calcium supplements are often needed.

Women over age 50 should have at least 1,500 milligrams (mg) of calcium each day, and men over age 65 at least 1,000 mg. A glass of nonfat milk contains about 250 mg of calcium. Add in the odds and ends of calcium in various foods and a typical daily intake is usually around 500 mg. Therefore, many people need some sort of calcium supplement. The most popular forms are Tums and Oscal; each tablet contains 500 mg of calcium. One or two tablets a day will usually do it.

It's important for you to remember the "calcium paradox." Just taking enough calcium in your diet doesn't really help because the extra calcium is not, for the most part, absorbed by the body. You need both to take in enough calcium and to give your body a stimulus to absorb it. Weight-bearing exercise is a strong stimulus for your body to absorb more calcium and to develop stronger bones. Exercise is for everyone. For women after menopause, estrogen supplementation also can provide a strong stimulus for absorption of calcium, and this possible treatment should be discussed with your doctor.

Diet Supplements

What about fish oil capsules? These contain the good fish oils, such as those found in salmon and mackerel, which lower the serum cholesterol level. Five capsules are about equivalent to one serving of salmon, but they cost less than salmon. There's nothing really wrong with using them, but in general we're not much for taking pills. The capsules are big and hard to swallow. Besides, cats may start to follow you around.

The good effects of vitamin supplements, particularly vitamin E, have been supported by research. We discuss these in detail on page 60.

Aspirin Treatment

What about taking a tablet of baby aspirin (80 mg) every day to thin the blood? This regimen has benefits, but *don't do it instead of changing your diet.* Even very small doses of aspirin thin the blood and prevent clots in the arteries and veins, but these same doses can result in excessive bleeding. Studies of regular aspirin use have shown a decrease in the number of heart attacks, but this was partly compensated for by increases in other diseases, including hemorrhagic strokes. We believe that this regimen should be undertaken only after your doctor's advice, and generally not by those below age 40.

Drugs to Lower Cholesterol

The same recommendation holds for newer cholesterol-lowering drugs, such as lovastatin, as well as the older ones like niacin and cholestyramine. We recommend that you discuss such medications with your doctor if you continue to have high LDL cholesterol levels and if you're in one of the following groups:

- You've already had a heart attack
- You have a very high cholesterol level, over 260 mg/dl total cholesterol or over 180 mg/dl LDL cholesterol
- You have a family member who had an early heart attack (before age 40)

Nevertheless, try your diet and exercise program first, second, and third. Medication is the fourth step, if your doctor agrees.

NOT SMOKING

Cigarette smoking kills 307,000 people in the United States each year. Lung cancer and emphysema (chronic lung disease) are the best known and among the most miserable outcomes. However, smoking causes atherosclerosis to develop faster, and that problem affects smokers whether or not the other diseases mentioned occur. Atherosclerosis results in heart attacks and strokes, angina pectoris (heart pains), intermittent claudication (leg pains), and many other problems. Pipe and cigar smoking don't have the pulmonary (lung) consequences that cigarette smoking does, but can lead to cancer of the lips, tongue, and esophagus. Nicotine in any form has bad effects on the small blood vessels and thus increases your chance of heart attacks.

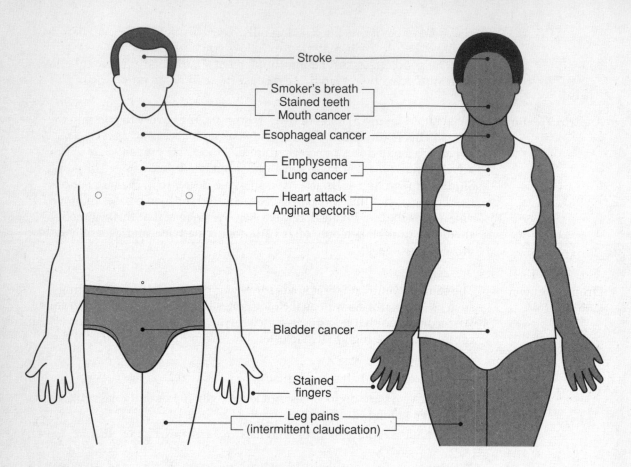

Stroke

Smoker's breath
Stained teeth
Mouth cancer

Esophageal cancer

Emphysema
Lung cancer

Heart attack
Angina pectoris

Bladder cancer

Stained
fingers

Leg pains
(intermittent claudication)

Smoking. The damage occurs at many sites throughout the body.

It's never too late to quit. Only two years after your last cigarette, your risk of heart attack returns to average. It has actually decreased substantially the very next week! After only two years, there's a decrease in lung cancer risk by perhaps one-third, and after ten years the risk is back to nearly normal. The development of emphysema is stopped for many people when they stop smoking, although this condition doesn't actually reverse. Most people who quit smoking will enjoy major health benefits the rest of their lives.

Moreover, you'll notice at once that your environment has become more friendly when you're not a smoker. A lot of the daily hassles that impair the quality of your life go away when you stop offending others by this habit.

Here are some tips for quitting:

■ Decide firmly that you really want to do it. You need to believe that you can. Set a date on which you will stop smoking. Announce this date to your friends. When the day comes, stop.

■ You can expect that the physical addiction to nicotine may make you nervous and irritable for about 48 hours. After that, there's no further physical addiction. There is, of course, the psychological craving that sometimes lasts a very long time. Often, however, this craving is quite short.

■ Reward yourself every week or so by buying something nice with what would have been cigarette money.

■ Combine your stop-smoking program with an increase in your exercise program. The two changes fit together naturally. Exercise will take your mind off the smoking change, and it will decrease the tendency to gain weight in the early weeks after you stop smoking; this weight gain is the only negative consequence of stopping smoking.

The immediate rewards of not smoking include better-tasting food, happier friends, less cough, better stamina, more money, fewer holes in your clothes, and membership in a larger world. If you have children, you become a better role model for them.

Many health educators are skeptical about cutting down slowly and stress that you need to stop completely. We don't think this is always true. For some people, rationing is a good way to get their smoking down to a much lower level, at which point it may be easier to stop entirely. For example, the simple decision not to smoke in public can help your health and decrease your daily hassles. To cut down, keep in the cigarette pack only those cigarettes that you'll allow yourself that day. Smoke the cigarettes only halfway down before extinguishing them.

Many good stop-smoking courses are offered through the American Cancer Society, the American Lung Association, and your local hospital. Most people actually don't need these, but if you do they can help you be successful. Try by yourself first. Then, if you still need help, there's a lot of it around.

Nicotine chewing gum or nicotine patches can help some people quit, and your doctor can give you a prescription and advice. Don't plan on this as a long-term solution because the nicotine in the gum or patch is just as bad for your arteries as is the nicotine in cigarettes.

Your decision to stop smoking is one example of your ability to make your own choices. If you're trapped by your addictions, even the minor ones, you can't make your own choices. Victory over smoking improves your mental health, in part because it is difficult. Winning this fight can open the door to success in other areas.

ALCOHOL MODERATION

Excessive alcohol intake is a serious problem for some people in every age group. Drinking too much leads to depression, danger, and disease. Among the potentially fatal complications are:

- Damage to the liver
- Delirium tremens (the DTs) from alcohol withdrawal
- Car, motorcycle, or other accidents in which alcohol plays a role

There are many other problems that aren't fatal but that decrease the quality of your life. A drinking problem makes a person dependent on the next drink, interferes with emotions and thinking, and burdens loved ones, diminishing everyone's quality of life.

Fortunately, alcoholism is a disease from which many people recover, although recovery is a lifelong process. There are about a million recovered alcoholics in the United States, and between half and three-quarters of the people who attempt rehabilitation succeed. Among some highly motivated groups, the success rate is much higher. For example, more than 90% of physicians and airline pilots who go into highly structured, monitored programs stay in recovery. Success depends on personal characteristics, early treatment, the quality of counselors or of a support program, access to the right medical services, and the strong support of family, friends, and coworkers.

We discuss the warning signs and treatment of alcoholism in **S104** (Alcoholism). Please refer to this section if you have any questions about your drinking. Usually this problem gets too little attention too late. Be alert for alcohol-related problems in family and friends, express your concerns to them, and cooperate in helping them establish a program for alcohol control or elimination. You can save their lives, and perhaps even save your own.

WEIGHT CONTROL

Excessive body weight compounds many health problems. It stresses the heart, the muscles, and the joints. It increases the likelihood of hernias, hemorrhoids, gallbladder disease, varicose veins, and many other problems. Excess weight makes breathing more difficult. It slows you down, makes you less effective in personal encounters, and lowers your self-image. You snore more if you're overweight. Fat people are hospitalized more frequently than people with normal weight; they have more heartburn, more surgical complications, more cases of breast cancer, more high blood pressure, more heart attacks, and more strokes.

Weight control is a difficult task. Think of "weight control" as "fat control," and it will fit in well with your other good health habits. For most of us, the problem and the solution are personal, not medical. (Excess weight is very seldom due to thyroid disease or other specific illness.) As with the other habits that change health, management of this problem begins with recognizing that it is a problem. Weight control requires your continued attention. There are genetic factors that act to make weight control very difficult for some. For those of us with a potential problem, we must have lifelong vigilance.

Increasingly, exercise is recognized as an important key to weight control. Part of every weight-control program should be an exercise program. Obesity isn't just the result of overeating; obese people, when studied carefully, are found to move around less and therefore to burn too few calories. There's nothing very mysterious about calories. Thirty-five hundred calories equals about one pound (450 g). If you take in 3,500 calories fewer than you burn, you lose a pound. If you take in 3,500 more than you burn, you gain a pound.

There are two important phases to weight control: the weight-reduction phase and the weight-maintenance phase. Surprisingly, the **weight-reduction phase** is the easiest. Here, the method you use to lose weight doesn't matter too much, although you should check with your doctor if you plan to lose a large amount of weight unusually quickly. You want to be sure that the diet you intend to follow is sound. Complex carbohydrates are important to most sound diets. During the weight-loss stage, many of your calories are provided by your own body fat and protein as they're being broken down and burned as fuel; thus, you need less fat and less protein in your diet during this period. Weight loss diets usually have a gimmick of some kind that encourages you and helps you remember the diet, and there are dozens of books available with "secret" tips.

Remember that weight loss is naturally slow; even a total fast will cause weight loss of less than one pound a day. More rapid changes in weight are generally due to loss of fluid. When you eat less, you usually eat less salt as well. The first few days of a diet often give you a false sense of accomplishment as you lose some of the fluid that the salt was retaining in your body. Then, when the rate of weight loss slows, you may think that the diet has failed. You have to be patient with this weight-loss phase.

Most people have some success in losing weight. If you set a target, tell people what you're trying to do, and stick with the effort for a while, you can probably lose weight. One pound a week is a reasonable goal. This requires elimination of the equivalent of one day's food each week.

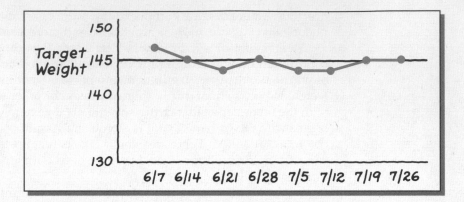

The **weight-maintenance phase** involves staying at the desirable weight you've achieved. This is more difficult, and it requires continual attention. Weigh yourself regularly and record the weight on a chart. Draw a red line at three pounds over your desired weight and maintain your weight below the line, using whatever method works best for you. Keep exercising. Accept no excuses for increasing weight; it's easier and healthier to make frequent small adjustments in what you eat than to try to counteract binges of overeating with crash diets. Keep yourself off the dietary roller coaster. Failure at weight maintenance accounts for most diet failures.

AVOIDING INJURY

Each year more than 400,000 Americans are killed or maimed as a result of preventable traumatic injury. More than half of all deaths before age 45 are due to injury! Yet somehow we all think that it can't happen to us. When a loved one, friend, or neighbor is killed or crippled, or when we read about tragedies in the newspaper, we tend not to associate them directly with our own lives. Because we get away with so many risky behaviors, we tend to feel immune from such "bad luck" ourselves. True, there are some unavoidable risks. But we can avoid 90% of our risk by our own actions.

Seat Belts

Automobile seat belts reduce death and injury by 75% — but only when people wear them! Wear seat belts all of the time, whether you're a driver or passenger. Strap the little kid into a secure infant car seat. Air bags are great, but you still need to buckle the belt. All the time. Thousands of people, mostly children and young adults, die or suffer severe head injuries because they neglected to wear a helmet while bicycling, motor-cycling, or skating. Wear one!

Seat belt and helmet use symbolize the other healthy actions you can take to avoid injury. This simple and easy-to-achieve habit greatly reduces health risks, and adopting the habit means that you've thought ahead, considered the probabilities and the risks, and taken action to preserve your future health. The same kind of thinking will help you reduce other risks. Studies show that people who always use their seat belts have also lowered their risks in other areas. They're less frequently smokers, for example, and they're less likely to drink and drive.

Impairment

The other extremely important preventable contribution to automotive injury is from alcohol, or less frequently, from impairment by other drugs. Often it seems the intoxicated driver survives intact, while passengers or innocents in the other car suffer. Your primary responsibility to yourself and those around you is not to drive when under the influence. You can wreck your life, not just your car. We believe, however, that responsibility extends to passengers as well. Don't ride with an impaired driver under any circumstances. Walk, call a cab, or go with someone else. Before the party appoint a "designated driver" whose responsibility is to stay sober. Hide the car keys from someone who has had too much to drink.

Water

Drownings are also usually preventable. Watch the kids whether they are in a pool, lake, or the sea. Wear life preservers on small boats. Don't go boating with an impaired captain, and don't be one yourself. Don't dive into hard objects or shallow depths. Watch out for the undertow. Use common sense.

Fire

Fires are usually preventable tragedies. They're started by overloaded electrical systems, faulty heaters, smoking in bed, hot ashes in garbage cans, careless use of fireworks, playing with matches, inadequate fireplace screening — all avoidable hazards. Fires have an even better chance to hurt people when there are no smoke alarms or no fire extinguishers. Having well-placed and functioning smoke alarms in your home is another proof that you're thinking ahead, considering probabilities and risks, and taking action to protect your future.

Falls

Most broken bones are caused by falls, and most falls are preventable. Clutter in the home, nothing to hold onto in the bathroom, poor lighting, wrong shoes, careless use of ladders, unsteady walking because of alcohol or other drugs — all are causes.

Firearms

Man shoots wife. Wife shoots husband. Kid shoots kid. Drunk shoots drunk. Accidents don't just happen. If you have guns in your house (and we personally hope that you don't), think ahead, consider the risks and probabilities, and take action to ensure that the wrong finger can't be on the trigger of a loaded gun at the wrong time. The safest way is to lock ammunition securely away from the firearm.

PROFESSIONAL PREVENTION

Most prevention is personal. But, to take care of yourself, you'll sometimes require professional help. Medicine in recent years has been oriented to "cure" rather than to "prevent," even though most of the greatest medical successes, such as eradication of smallpox and control of paralytic polio, have been achieved through preventive measures. We doctors have been crisis-oriented: our approach has been to wait for a consequence to appear and then to try to treat it.

Today doctors are becoming more interested in preventive medicine. The most important part of prevention, developing good health habits, has been discussed and is your personal responsibility. But the idea of preventive medicine also includes the following five strategies that involve health professionals, and it's important to understand both the strengths and the limitations of these strategies:

- The checkup or periodic health examination
- Screening for early problems
- Early treatment for problems
- Immunizations and other public health measures
- Health risk appraisal

Periodic
Checkups

The "annual checkup" is still recommended by some schools, camps, employers, and the army. However, doctors seldom go to each other for routine checkups. Checkups don't detect treatable diseases early with any regularity, and they may raise false confidence; that is, they may encourage the false belief that if you're regularly checked you don't need to concern yourself as much about developing good health habits.

Your primary interest is in finding conditions about which something can be done, and for this the checkup is unfortunately not very useful. If you use the techniques described above to reduce your health risks, and if you attend to new symptoms as discussed in Part II of this book, you'll gain few advantages from an annual "complete checkup."

Are "complete" checkups ever worthwhile? Yes. The first examination by a new doctor allows you to establish a relationship with him or her. Increasingly, the periodic checkup is being used not as much for the detection of disease as for the opportunity to counsel the patient about poor health habits, so that patients can do a better job of personal disease prevention. We applaud this change and look to doctors to further refine their skills at influencing their patients to take care of themselves.

Screening for Early Problems

Although complete checkups may offer limited benefits, periodic screening tests in several specific areas are important. Try to arrange these tests when you visit your doctor for another reason so as not to require a special trip.

- **High blood pressure** is a significant medical condition that gives little warning of its presence. During adult life, it's advisable to have your blood pressure checked at least every year or so. This measurement can easily be done by a nurse, physician's assistant, or nurse's aide, but a doctor's visit isn't required. If high blood pressure is found, a doctor should confirm it and you should carefully attend to the measures needed to keep it under control (see High Blood Pressure, S99).

- If you're a woman over age 20, you should have a **Pap smear** taken every year or so. Some authorities now recommend beginning annual Pap smear testing at the age of first sexual activity, decreasing its frequency to every three to five years after the first three tests are negative, and again increasing the frequency to every one or two years after age 40. This test detects cancer of the cervix, the portion of the womb (uterus) that protrudes into the vagina. In early stages this cancer is almost always curable. See Chapter 9, "Women's Health," for more information.

- Women over age 25 should practice **breast self-examination** monthly. Any suspicious changes should be checked out with a doctor; the great majority of breast cancers are first detected as suspicious lumps by the patient. Women with large breasts can't practice self-examination with as much reliability as other women and may wish to discuss other screening procedures with their doctor. In general, we don't like to recommend mammography as a yearly screening procedure for women below age 50, but others believe it should start at age 40. Women who have already had a breast tumor should follow their doctors' recommendations. Women with a strong history of breast cancer in their family should begin with mammography by age 40.

The importance of these few examinations is underscored by their availability as a public service, free of charge, at many city and county clinics. The National Blue Cross/Blue Shield Association recently commissioned 12 papers by leading experts to assess the clinical literature on

TABLE 2   *Recommended Adult Screening Procedures*

Procedure	*Recommendation*
Pap smear for cervical cancer (women)	Annually for 3 years starting at age 20, or when sexual activity begins, whichever is earlier. If these first 3 tests are negative, every 3 to 5 years from then on.
Fecal occult blood tests for colorectal cancer	Annually after age 50.
Sigmoidoscopy for colorectal cancer	Every 3 to 5 years after age 50. If a parent or sibling has had colon cancer, air-contrast barium enema and sigmoidoscopy every 3 to 5 years after age 40.
Breast cancer screening (women)	Monthly self-examination. Yearly physician examination after age 40. Annual mammography after age 50, or after age 40 if mother or a sister has had breast cancer.
Serum cholesterol and triglyceride screening	Cholesterol measured at intervals of 5 or more years up to age 70. Screening serum triglyceride is now controversial and currently *not recommended.*
High blood pressure screening	Recommended, incidental to other health-care services (no special visit is needed).
Diabetes screening	Glucose tolerance test recommended for pregnant women between the 24th and 28th week of gestation, or women with diabetes in their family who are planning to become pregnant. Otherwise *not recommended.*
Asymptomatic coronary artery disease screening	Screening with exercise stress testing *not recommended.*
Lung cancer screening	Screening *not recommended.*
Osteoporosis screening	Screening *not recommended.*

screening procedures. Its recommendations are summarized in Table 2 and closely parallel our views about screening.

The value of other screening tests is more dubious. Some doctors believe that routine glaucoma tests, tests for blood in the stool after age 30, and regular sigmoidoscopy after age 50 are worthwhile, and others don't.

Many news stories have suggested that screening with prostate specific antigen (PSA) determinations, with or without digital rectal examination, revolutionizes the outlook for prostate cancer and promises to save many men's lives. Unfortunately, there's no convincing evidence that this screening improves the outlook for prostate cancer.

Early Treatment

An effective health maintenance strategy includes seeking medical care promptly whenever an important new problem or finding appears. For example, you should seek medical attention without delay if you notice one of the following symptoms:

- A lump in your breast
- Unexplained weight loss
- A fever for more than a week
- Coughing up blood

These symptoms don't always represent true emergencies, but they do indicate a need for professional attention. Most times, nothing will be seriously wrong; on other occasions, however, an early cancer, tuberculosis, or other treatable disease will be found. You always need to carefully consider how to respond to some change you've noted in your body.

The guidelines in Part II of this book can help you select those instances in which you should seek medical care. In most cases, you can take care of yourself with home treatment. However, you must respond appropriately when professional care is needed.

To ensure timely treatment, you need to have a plan. Think things through ahead of time.

- Do you have a doctor?
- If you need emergency care, where will you go? To an emergency hospital? To the emergency room of a general hospital? To the on-call physician of a local medical group?
- If you're not sure what to do after consulting this book, whom can you call for further advice?
- Have you written down the phone numbers you need?

Only rarely will you need emergency services. But the time that you need them is not the time to begin wondering what to do. If you have a routine problem that requires medical care, where will you go? Is there a nearby doctor? Who has your medical records? Chapter 11, "Working With Your Doctor and Your Health Care System," will help you answer these questions. Plan ahead.

Immunizations

Immunizations have had far greater impact on health in the developed nations than all of the other health services put together. Only a few years ago smallpox, cholera, paralytic polio, diphtheria, whooping cough, and tetanus killed large numbers of people. These diseases have been effectively controlled by immunization in the United States and in most

TABLE 3

Recommended Immunization Schedule

Age	Immunization
Newborn	Hepatitis B (or later as directed by doctor)
2 months	DPT (diphtheria, pertussis, tetanus), OPV (oral polio virus), and HIB (hemophilus influenza type B)
4 months	DPT, OPV, and HIB
6 months	DPT, OPV (in certain areas only, not in the United States), and HIB
15 months	Measles, Mumps, Rubella
18 months	DPT and OPV
4–6 years	DTap (diphtheria, tetanus, acellular pertussis) and OPV
5–18 years	Measles, Mumps, Rubella
Every 10 years	T(d) (adult tetanus, diphtheria)

other developed nations. Smallpox has been eradicated from the entire world, and there's no longer any need for smallpox immunization. An incredible success story!

Unfortunately, many Americans have become lax about childhood immunizations. As a result, there has been a resurgence of measles, mumps, and rubella. You and your children can reap the benefits of immunizations while minimizing their risk by following the recommendations in Table 3.

Keep a record of your immunizations in the back of this book. Don't allow yourself to be reinoculated just because you've lost records of previous immunizations. If you haven't had a tetanus shot for ten years or so, ask for a booster shot while visiting the doctor for another reason. You can save future trips to the doctor by being protected for the next ten years.

In general, don't seek out the optional immunizations. Flu shots, for example, are only partially effective and often cause a degree of fever and aching; they're recommended only for the elderly and for those with severe major diseases. We recommend that the optional immunizations (including pneumonia and flu) be taken only on the recommendation of your doctor. They have a definite role for some people, but not for all.

Health Risk Appraisal

Your future health is largely determined by what you do now. Your lifestyle and your habits have a dominant influence on how healthy you are, how healthy you'll be, how much time you'll spend in hospitals, and how rapidly you'll "physiologically" age.

Recently techniques have been developed for mathematically estimating your future health risks, and these techniques are variously termed "health risk appraisal," "health hazard appraisal," or "health assessment." You complete a questionnaire or otherwise provide information about your lifestyle and health habits. Your responses are mathematically combined to estimate your likelihood of developing major medical problems such as heart disease and cancer. Other estimates such as your "physiologic" age also may be calculated. These techniques form an increasingly important part of comprehensive health education programs such as Healthtrac,

Senior Healthtrac, and Informed Choice. They also have a potentially large role in helping you shape your own personal health program.

You should know several things about health risk appraisals:

- The results are only estimates. Even though they're based on the best medical studies, data are incomplete and may not apply equally to all populations. In general, the estimates may be accurate to within 10 or 20%. Think of health risk scores as similar to IQ or achievement test scores; they're approximately correct but not exact.

- The predictions are only averages. Some people will do better than the tests predict and others worse.

- Any single assessment represents you at one point in time, but your actual risks depend on the changes you make and your average lifetime health habits as well. Regular repeated assessments can reveal your current status and the benefits you've achieved through lifestyle changes.

- A good health risk appraisal should be based only on those relatively few risk factors that are scientifically well established and associated with major health problems. These include cigarette smoking, exercise, automobile seat belt use, helmet use, alcohol intake, obesity, dietary fiber, salt, fat intake, blood pressure, cholesterol levels, and stress level.

- The health risk assessment itself provides no health benefits unless it results in changes in your health-related behaviors, and the risk assessment might even frighten you unnecessarily. Therefore, these assessments are best used as part of a program that not only identifies risk but also educates you, motivates you for change, provides suggestions and recommendations, and reinforces positive changes.

We're enthusiastic about the growing role of health promotion programs that focus attention on prevention of disease and about the use of good health assessment tools. Well-designed programs are already having a large effect, decreasing human illness. As a bonus, they also reduce medical care costs.

The Power of Prevention: How It Works

Now you can put together a master plan for illness prevention. The plan is simple. First, you need to prevent the fatal illnesses mentioned at the beginning of this chapter. Second, you need to prevent the nonfatal illnesses.

Table 4 summarizes the ways that you can substantially reduce risks for 23 serious and very common conditions. You may be surprised to learn

TABLE 4

Your Master Plan for Preserving Your Health

	Exercise	Diet and Nutrition	Not Smoking	Alcohol Moderation	Weight Control	Avoiding Injury
POTENTIALLY FATAL DISEASE						
Heart Attack and Stroke	X	X	X		X	
Lung Cancer			X			
Breast Cancer		X			X	
Colon Cancer	X	X				
Mouth Cancer			X			
Liver Cancer			X	X		
Esophageal Cancer			X	X		
Cervical Cancer						
Emphysema			X			
Cirrhosis		X		X		
Diabetes	X	X			X	
Trauma				X		X
NONFATAL DISEASE						
Osteoarthritis	X				X	
Hernias	X		X		X	
Hemorrhoids	X				X	
Varicose Veins	X		X		X	
Thrombophlebitis	X		X		X	
Gallbladder Disease		X			X	
Stomach Ulcers		X	X	X		
Dental Problems		X	X			
Osteoporosis	X	X				
Falls and Fractures	X					X

TABLE 4   *Your Master Plan for Preserving Your Health*

	Treat High Blood Pressure	Screening Tests	Estimated Risk Reduction	Notes
POTENTIALLY FATAL DISEASE				
Heart Attack and Stroke	X		70%	Diet: low in saturated fat and salt, high in fiber; vitamin E and aspirin as advised
Lung Cancer			90%	Smoking causes nearly all cases
Breast Cancer		X	50%	Screening: self-examination, annual doctor's exam, mammography
Colon Cancer		X	50%	Diet: low in satured fat, high in fiber. Screening: colonoscopy.
Mouth Cancer			90%	Smoking (pipes and cigars) causes nearly all cases
Liver Cancer			50%	Alcohol causes many cases
Esophageal Cancer			50%	Smoking causes many cases
Cervical Cancer		X	90%	Screening: Pap smears
Emphysema			90%	Smoking causes nearly all cases
Cirrhosis			90%	Alcohol, together with poor nutrition, causes nearly all cases
Diabetes			50%	Much diabetes occurring late in life can be prevented
Trauma			75%	Failure to wear seat belts and drunk driving are the largest factors
NONFATAL DISEASE				
Osteoarthritis			50%	You can prevent the disability, not necessarily the arthritis
Hernias			50%	Poor muscle tone, a big belly, and coughing are a bad combination
Hemorrhoids			50%	Sitting around while overweight causes much of the problem; hygiene is also important
Varicose Veins			50%	Inactivity lets the fluid drop to the lowest point; using leg muscles helps blood flow in legs
Thrombophlebitis			50%	The factors for this condition can also cause blood clots in the legs
Gallbladder Disease			40%	Dietary fat and obesity are the causes in many cases
Stomach Ulcers			70%	Also be aware that aspirin and other drugs can cause stomach problems
Dental Problems		X	80%	Diet: low in sugar. Screening: dental checkups. Brush and floss.
Osteoporosis			50%	Diet: high in calcium. Exercise: weight-bearing. Estrogen and other drugs may help.
Falls and Fractures			50%	Keep your body and bones strong; make your environment friendly

how many different health problems can be prevented. If you do everything right to reduce your risk for individual conditions, you can reduce your risk for all diseases combined by about 70%. That's the power of prevention!

THE HABIT OF HEALTH

An old joke maintains that everything pleasurable is either illegal, immoral, or fattening. This is exactly the wrong idea. Health is pleasurable; ill health is miserable. Good health habits have their own immediate reward. If changing your behavior for health is making you fell less well, you're doing something wrong. Exercise makes you feel better. Good diets make you feel better. Avoiding nicotine makes you feel better. Having a good body weight makes your life activities easier and more pleasurable.

Much of what's written about healthy behaviors makes the whole process seem mysterious and complicated. The supermarket tabloids are always reporting some new threat to your health. There is indeed a long list of possible threats to health, but trying to keep track of them all overlooks two important facts. First, these threats often aren't adequately proven. Second, even if they do prove to be true, they aren't that important. For instance, barbecued foods may pose cancer-causing risks, and we suggest moderating the amount of barbecued foods you eat — but only if you eat such meals more than 30 times a year. Many people find a benefit in controlling caffeine intake, particularly in the evening, but this is a minor problem compared with drinking alcohol.

Here we've tried to emphasize only the important and the proven. As we said before, only seven areas require your attention.

- **Exercise:** work up to a regular aerobic (endurance) exercise program
- **Diet:** especially cut down fat
- **Not smoking**
- **Alcohol moderation:** no more than two drinks a day
- **Weight control:** maintain a healthy weight instead of losing and gaining
- **Avoiding injury:** exercise your common sense
- **Professional prevention practices:** work alongside your doctor

CHAPTER 2

Your Home Pharmacy

*T*o effectively treat the minor illnesses that appear from time to time in your family, you need to have certain medications on hand and know where to obtain others. Your stock should include only the most inexpensive and frequently needed medications. Medications deteriorate with time, so you should replace them at least every three years.

Table 5 gives a comprehensive list of products for a home medical shelf. Only those in the top section are essential: bandages, antiseptic cleanser, a thermometer, acetaminophen (or another pain and fever reliever), an antacid, baking soda, and syrup of ipecac (in households with children under 12). Note that only six items in this list are essential for adults, and only two (acetaminophen and antacid) are drugs people take internally. You don't need most of the items currently in your medicine cabinet.

Nearly all of the home treatment recommended in this book may be carried out with the items in Table 5. We refer to them again and again in the guidelines for common medical problems in Part II, indicating when and why to use each medication. (Look for references to section numbers beginning with **M.**)

In this chapter, we discuss drug dosage and side effects to add some perspective to the instructions the manufacturers include with their products. Because dosages change and because we often discover new things even about common drugs, you should carefully read the instructions that come with each medication. Always remember:

- Used in effective dosages, all drugs have the potential for side effects. Many common drugs have some side effects, such as drowsiness, that are impossible to avoid at effective dosages.

- Misuse of over-the-counter drugs can have serious consequences. Do *not* assume that a product is safe because it doesn't require a prescription.

- The drugs in this chapter act only to control symptoms. They don't do anything to change the basic problem. If you can get along without them, it's usually best to do so.

- Because there are no totally childproof bottles, keep all drugs out of small children's reach. Aspirin overdoses have been responsible for more childhood deaths than any other medication.

Hundreds of over-the-counter medicines are available at your supermarket or drugstore. For most medicines, several nearly identical products exist as competing brands. This has posed a problem for us in organizing this chapter. If we discuss drugs by chemical name, the terms are long and confusing; if we use brand names, we may appear to favor a particular product when there are equally satisfactory alternatives. We decided to give you some clues to reading the list of ingredients on the package so that you can figure out what the drug is likely to do. We don't list all available drugs, but we do mention some representative alternatives. The brand names listed in this chapter are vigorously marketed and should be available almost everywhere. They aren't necessarily superior to alternatives containing similar formulas that aren't listed.

TABLE 5   *Home Pharmacy*

Section	Medication or Tool	Use
ESSENTIAL		
M1	**Bandages and Adhesive Tape**	To close and protect minor wounds
M2	**Antiseptic Cleanser** (3% hydrogen peroxide, iodine)	To cleanse minor wounds
M3	**Thermometer**	To measure body temperature
M4	**Pain and Fever Medications** (acetaminophen, aspirin, ibuprofen, or naproxen)	To relieve pain, to lower fever
M5	**Antacid** (nonabsorbable)	To relieve upset stomach
M6	**Baking Soda**	To treat skin irritation and soak wounds
RECOMMENDED FOR FAMILIES WITH SMALL CHILDREN		
M7	**Syrup of Ipecac**	To induce vomiting in some cases of poisoning
See **M4**	**Liquid Acetaminophen**	To relieve pain and fever in small children
See **M4**	**Aspirin Rectal Suppositories**	To relieve fever in small children who can't keep down other medicine
OPTIONAL		
M8	**Antihistamines and Decongestants**	To treat allergy symptoms
M9	**Nose Drops and Sprays**	To treat runny nose
M10	**Cold Tablets**	To treat cold symptoms
M11	**Cough Syrups**	To treat coughing
M12	**Bulk Laxatives**	To treat constipation
M13	**Diarrhea Remedies**	To treat diarrhea
M14	**Sodium Fluoride**	To prevent dental problems
M15	**"Artificial Tears" Eye Drops**	To treat irritated eyes
M16	**Zinc Oxide**	To treat hemorrhoids
M17	**Antifungal Preparations**	To treat skin fungus
M18	**Hydrocortisone Cream**	To treat rashes
M19	**Sunscreen Agents**	To prevent sunburn
M20	**Wart Removers**	To remove some warts
M21	**Elastic Bandages**	To treat sprains

1 Bandages and Adhesive Tape

Purpose

To close and protect minor wounds. Bandages really don't "make it better." Sometimes it's better to leave a minor wound open to the air than to cover it. Still, a home medical shelf wouldn't be complete without a tin of assorted adhesive bandages. To fashion larger bandages, you also need adhesive tape and gauze. Bandages are useful for covering tender blisters, keeping dirt out of wounds, and keeping the edges of a cut together. They have some value in keeping the wound out of sight and thus are of cosmetic importance.

Dosage

For smaller cuts and sores, use a bandage from the tin. Leaving the bandage on for a day or so is usually long enough; change the bandage daily if you wish to keep the wound covered longer. For cuts, apply the bandage perpendicular to the cut, and draw the skin toward the cut from both sides to relax skin tension before applying the bandage. The bandage should then act to keep the edges together during healing. For larger injuries, make a bandage from a roll of sterile gauze or from sterile 2"x2" (5x5 cm) or 4"x4" (10x10 cm) gauze pads, and firmly tape it in place with adhesive tape. Change the bandage daily. If you see white fat protruding from the cut, see your doctor.

Side Effects

If the wound isn't clean when you cover it with a bandage, you may hide a developing infection from early discovery. Clean the wound with antiseptics and keep it clean. Change the bandage if it becomes wet. Some people are allergic to adhesive tape and should use nonallergenic paper tape. If adhesive tape is left on for a week or so, it will irritate almost anyone's skin, so give the skin a rest.

Some people leave a bandage on too long because they're afraid of the pain as they remove it — particularly if their hairs are stuck to the tape. For painless removal, apply nail polish remover to the back of the adhesive tape and let it soak for five minutes. This will dissolve the adhesive and release both the skin and hair.

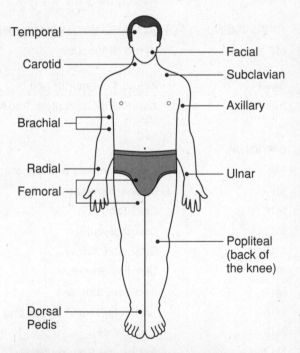

Temporal
Carotid
Brachial
Radial
Femoral
Dorsal Pedis

Facial
Subclavian
Axillary
Ulnar
Popliteal (back of the knee)

Pressure points. If a bandage doesn't stop a person's wound from bleeding, slow the flow of blood to that part of the body by squeezing on a pressure point. Choose the nearest pressure point between the wound and the person's heart. The most commonly used pressure points are **inside the upper arm** and **inside the thigh.**

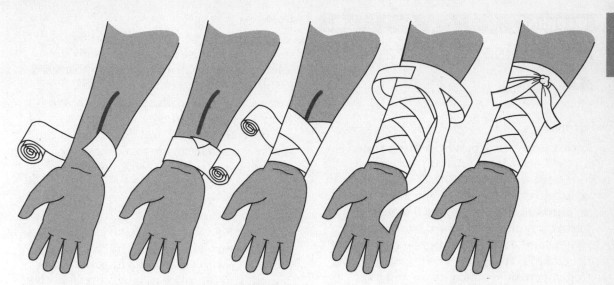

Wraparound bandage. This type of bandage makes a neat, long-lasting wrap for a large wound. It is easier to tape the end of the bandage, but if you have no tape you can tie the bandage as shown.

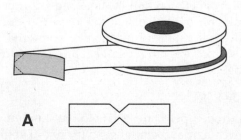

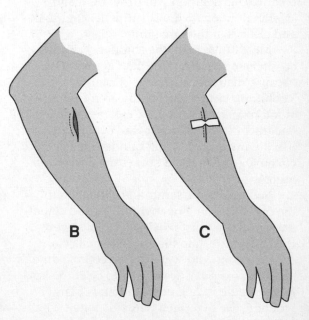

Butterfly bandage. This type of bandage allows a short, shallow wound to heal quickly.
(A) Fold a length of adhesive tape in two and snip off the folded corners.
(B) Make sure the wound is clean, and that one edge is not lying over the other.
(C) Tape the wound together so that its edges meet and the narrow part of the bandage lies over the cut.
Use this only in the first six hours after injury; otherwise bacteria may grow in the wound.

2 Antiseptic Cleansers

Purpose

To cleanse minor wounds. A dirty wound often becomes infected. If dirt or foreign bodies are trapped beneath the skin, they can fester and delay healing. Only a few germs are introduced at the time of a wound, but they may multiply to a very large number over several days. An antiseptic removes the dirt and kills the germs. A solution of 3% hydrogen peroxide, which foams and cleans as you work it into the wound, is a good cleansing agent, and iodine is a reasonably good agent with which to kill germs. A strong baking soda solution will draw fluid and swelling out of a wound and will act to soak and clean it at the same time.

Most of the time, the solutions' cleansing action is more important than germ killing because many preparations (Listerine, Zephiran, Bactine, etc.) really aren't very good at killing germs. Antibiotic creams (such as Bacitracin and Neosporin) are expensive, usually unnecessary, and of questionable effectiveness. First-aid sprays are a waste of money.

You must give scrupulous attention to the initial cleaning of a wound and scrub out any embedded dirt particles. Do this even though it hurts and bleeds. For small, clean cuts, use soap and water followed by iodine and then soap and water again. Betadine is a non-stinging iodine preparation. For larger wounds, use hydrogen peroxide with vigorous scrubbing.

Dosage

Most hydrogen peroxide is sold at the 3% strength. Don't use a hydrogen peroxide solution stronger than 3%, such as that used for bleaching hair. Pour the solution on the wound and scrub with a rough cloth. Wash it off and repeat. Continue until you can see no dirt beneath the level of the skin. If you can't get the wound clean, go to a doctor.

Iodine is painted or wiped onto the wound and the surrounding area. Wash it off within a few minutes, leaving a trace of the iodine color on the skin.

To soak a wound in a baking soda solution, use one tablespoon (15 ml) in one cup (250 ml) of warm water. If a finger or toe is injured, you can place it in the cup. For other wounds, soak a wash cloth with the solution and place over the wound as a compress. Generally, a wound should be soaked for five to ten minutes at a time, twice a day. If the skin is puckered and "water-logged" after the soak, it has been soaked too long. You can place cellophane or plastic wrap over the cloth compress to retain heat and moisture longer.

Side Effects

Hydrogen peroxide is safe to the skin but can bleach hair and clothing, so try not to spill it.

Iodine can burn the skin if left on full strength, so be careful. Iodine is also poisonous if swallowed; keep it away from children. Some people are allergic to iodine; discontinue use if you get a rash.

Baking soda is completely safe as long as it's used on the skin, not swallowed.

3 Thermometer

Purpose

To measure body temperatures. Fever is an important clue in diagnosing illness, and a very high body temperature may lead to problems. The best places to measure body temperature are the rectum and the mouth. Rectal temperatures are about 0.5°F (0.25°C) higher than oral (mouth) temperatures and usually reflect the body's condition more accurately. Oral temperature can be affected by hot or cold foods, routine breathing, and smoking.

Mercury thermometers are designed in different ways to make taking oral and rectal temperatures easier. Generally, oral thermometers have a longer bulb at the business end, providing a greater surface area for a faster reading. Rectal thermometers have a shorter, rounder bulb to facilitate entry into the rectum. Both Fahrenheit and Celsius thermometers are acceptable.

Rectal thermometers are best for young children because it's hard for them to hold an oral thermometer under the tongue.

Lubricants, such as Vaseline, can make inserting rectal thermometers easier. Place the child on his or her stomach and hold one hand on the buttocks to prevent movement. Insert the thermometer an inch or so (2–3 cm) inside the rectum. The mercury will begin to rise within seconds. Remove the thermometer when the mercury is no longer rising, after a minute or two.

You can take oral temperature with a rectal thermometer after sterilizing it for five to ten minutes in a 10:1 water:bleach solution. This will require a longer period in the mouth than an oral thermometer to achieve the same degree of accuracy. Oral thermometers can also be used to take rectal temperatures, but we don't recommend using them in children because of their shape.

Electronic thermometers, including those that take temperatures from the ear, have the advantage of quicker readings, which is useful for younger children. They're more expensive than mercury thermometers, however. Contact thermometers—strips of plastic held against the forehead—aren't as accurate.

Side Effects

The mercury in thermometers is poisonous, so people should never bite down while having an oral temperature taken.

Oral thermometer.
Note the long, thin bulb. In this example the mercury needs to be shaken down towards the bulb before use.

Rectal thermometer.
The rounded bulb makes it easier to put into the rectum. This drawing shows a thermometer ready to use, its mercury shaken down.

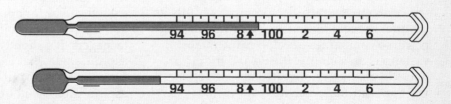

4 Pain and Fever Medications

Purpose

To relieve pain and to lower fever. There are four major over-the-counter drugs that do these tasks: acetaminophen, aspirin, ibuprofen, and naproxen. Acetaminophen is the safest; the other three can cause severe or even fatal bleeding of the stomach, although only rarely if just a few tablets are taken. On the other hand, acetaminophen doesn't reduce inflammation; aspirin, ibuprofen, and naproxen do, if taken in substantial dosage. Ibuprofen and naproxen are better than the other two for relief of menstrual cramps.

In addition, ketoprofen (Orudis) has just been approved for over-the-counter sale. Its uses and side effects are similar to naproxen. In high doses it appears to be more toxic than the four main drugs, so use it sparingly. Do not exceed the recommended dose.

Most of the time, a pain reliever maker conceals the key drug in the pain relief medication somewhere in the fine print under "active ingredients," and refers obliquely to the amount of analgesic, or pain reliever, present in each tablet. It's often surprisingly hard to find out what is in the drug from the box. There are really only four drugs, and many manufacturers. Each company wants its product to seem unique in a crowded market-place, so companies develop many minor variations on a similar theme and try to develop distinctive advertising.

For example: Anacin is aspirin and caffeine (caffeine improves pain relief but may make you jittery); Anacin 3 is acetaminophen;

Excedrin is half aspirin and half acetaminophen. Some pain relievers include other ingredients. For example, an antacid may be added (as in Bufferin or Ascriptin) in an attempt to cut down on stomach distress. Other than these variations, there's little medical reason to prefer one product over another in most cases. If you like a particular formulation, use it. If you want to save money, read the labels carefully and look for the best buys.

On some pain reliever bottles you may see the initials U.S.P., which stand for "United States Pharmacopoeia." Although not an absolute guarantee that the drug is the best, it does mean that the drug has met certain standards in composition and physical characteristics. The same is true of the designation N.F., which stands for "National Formulary."

Finally, remember that acetaminophen, ibuprofen, and naproxen are available by doctor's prescription at up to twice the strength of the nonprescription formulas. If you have the stronger type of one drug in your medicine cabinet, don't confuse it with the weaker over-the-counter formula.

ACETAMINOPHEN

Acetaminophen is available in several brand-name preparations (Tylenol, Datril, Liquiprin, Tempra, etc.). In the British Commonwealth, it's known as paracetamol. Acetaminophen is a good choice for adults because of its safety, and it's our first choice for children and teenagers. It's slightly less predictable than aspirin, somewhat less powerful, and doesn't have the anti-inflammatory action that makes aspirin valuable in treatment of arthritis and some other diseases. On the other hand, it doesn't cause ringing in the ears or upset stomach, common side effects with aspirin. Nor can it cause Reye's syndrome, a rare but serious potential side effect of aspirin when taken by children with chicken pox or the flu.

Dosage

Acetaminophen is used in doses identical to those of aspirin. For adults, two 325 mg tablets every three to four hours is standard. In children, 65 mg per year of age every four hours is satisfactory. There's never a reason to exceed these doses because there's no additional benefit in taking higher amounts. Like aspirin, acetaminophen comes combined with other ingredients in products that offer little advantage over acetaminophen.

Side Effects

People seldom experience side effects from acetaminophen. If you suspect a side effect, call your doctor. A variety of rare toxic effects have been reported, but none are definitely related to the use of this drug. A truly major overdose can cause liver failure, particularly in children, and this can be fatal. Keep the bottle where children can't get at it. If you abuse alcohol, severe liver toxicity can occur at as little as 4,000 to 6,000 mg a day.

LIQUID ACETAMINOPHEN FOR SMALL CHILDREN

Most pediatricians prefer liquid acetaminophen or sodium salicylate to aspirin for the small child, because these liquid preparations are easier to administer and are better tolerated by the stomach. If the child can't keep these medications down because of vomiting, call your doctor for advice; aspirin rectal suppositories, which require a prescription in most places, may work better.

Dosage

Liquid acetaminophen comes in varying concentrations, so read the label on your bottle for the correct dosage. In general, use a dropper to give 65 mg of acetaminophen for every year of the child's age every four hours. From noon to midnight, awaken the child if necessary. After midnight the fever will usually break by itself and become less of a problem, so if you miss a dose it's less important. But check the child's temperature at least once during the night to make sure. Remember, acetaminophen lasts only about four hours in the body, and you must keep repeating the dose or you'll lose the effect.

ASPIRIN

Expensive aspirin preparations may use coated tablets for easier swallowing or they may dissolve faster, but this usually doesn't make them more effective than cheaper brands.

If an aspirin bottle contains a vinegary odor when opened, the pills have begun to deteriorate and should be discarded. Aspirin usually has a shelf life of about three years, although shorter periods are sometimes quoted.

Dosage

In adults, the standard dose for pain relief is two tablets taken every three to four hours as required. The maximum effect occurs in about two hours. Each standard tablet is 5 grains, or 325 mg. If you use a nonstandard concoction, you'll have to do the arithmetic to calculate equivalent doses. The terms "extra strength," "arthritis pain formula," and the like merely indicate a greater amount of aspirin per tablet. This is medically trivial. You can take more tablets of the cheaper aspirin and still save money. When you read that a product "contains more of the ingredient that doctors recommend most," you may be sure that the product contains a little bit more aspirin per tablet; perhaps 400 to 500 mg instead of 325.

Here are some hints for good aspirin usage. Aspirin treats symptoms; it doesn't cure problems. Thus, for symptoms such as headache or muscle pain or menstrual cramps, don't take it unless you hurt. On the other hand, for control of fever, you'll be more comfortable if you repeat the dose every four hours during the day because this prevents fever from moving up and down. The afternoon and evening are the worst for fever, so try not to miss a dose during these hours. If you need aspirin for relief from some symptom over a prolonged period, check the symptom with your doctor. Relief from pain or fever is not improved if you increase the dose, and you're more likely to irritate your stomach, so take only the standard dose (650 mg every four hours) even if you still have some discomfort.

To control inflammation, as in serious arthritis, the dose of aspirin must be high, often 16 to 20 tablets daily, and must continue over a prolonged period. A doctor should monitor such treatment; it's relatively safe, but problems sometimes occur.

To be safe, avoid using aspirin for children or teenagers with a fever because of the possibility they may later develop Reye's syndrome, a potentially fatal disease of the liver and brain. We recommend acetaminophen instead. If aspirin is all that's available for a child under age ten, give no more than 65 mg for every year of the child's age. Thus, a six-year-old child should receive no more than 380 mg (65 x 6 = 380) every four hours. Each "baby aspirin" tablet contains 81 mg of aspirin.

Aspirin is also used to prevent complications of high blood pressure in pregnant women and to prevent heart attacks. The dose for this use is very low: 81 mg (one baby aspirin) every other day. Ask your doctor before trying it.

Side Effects

In addition to Reye's syndrome in children, aspirin can cause an upset stomach or ringing in the ears in adults and children. If your ears ring, reduce the dose.

Serious gastrointestinal hemorrhage or a perforated (ruptured) stomach can occur; aspirin more than doubles your risk of a bleeding ulcer. If your stomach is upset, try taking aspirin a half-hour after meals, when the food in the stomach will act as a buffer. Coated aspirin (such as Ecotrin) can help protect the stomach. However, some people don't digest coated aspirin and so receive no benefit. Buffers are sometimes added to aspirin to protect the stomach and may help a little. If you take a lot of aspirin and want a buffered preparation, we recommend one made with a nonabsorbable antacid. In the short term buffers make little difference, and there's controversy as to whether they work at all.

Asthma, nasal polyps, deafness, serious bleeding from the digestive tract, ulcers, and other major problems have been associated with aspirin.

ASPIRIN RECTAL SUPPOSITORIES FOR SMALL CHILDREN

Aspirin rectal suppositories are available only by prescription in most places. If you have a small child, ask your doctor about aspirin rectal suppositories on a routine visit. Use them only when vomiting prevents the child from keeping medication down. Suppositories allow medicine to be absorbed through the mucous membranes of the rectum. Because of their side effects, and because of the risk of Reye's syndrome, aspirin rectal suppositories should be a last resort.

Dosage

You can give small children slightly more aspirin with suppositories than with tablets — 81 mg for each year of the child's age every four to six hours. After age ten, use the adult dose. Read the suppository label. Most contain 325 mg of aspirin; to create a safe dosage for young children you may need to cut them lengthwise with a warm knife. Then remove the label (many parents neglect to). As you insert the suppository into the rectum, firm but gentle pressure will cause the muscles around it to relax. Be patient. In small children the buttocks may need to be held together gently to keep the suppository in.

Side Effects

In addition to the potential side effects of aspirin taken by mouth, aspirin suppositories can irritate the rectum and cause local bleeding. Therefore, you should use them only if taking aspirin by mouth is impossible. Even then, call your doctor for advice if more than two or three doses seem to be required.

IBUPROFEN

Ibuprofen (Advil, Motrin, Nuprin, etc.) has long been used as a prescription drug for arthritis and is approved for over-the-counter use for pain and fever. Ibuprofen is about as toxic to the stomach as aspirin, and more so than acetaminophen. It doesn't cause ringing of the ears like aspirin or severe liver disease like acetaminophen (in rare cases). It appears to be almost impossible to commit suicide by overdose with ibuprofen. But concern has

been raised about kidney problems (mild and reversible), and ibuprofen is sometimes more expensive than the alternatives. It's the best over-the-counter preparation for menstrual cramps.

Dosage

Ibuprofen comes in 200 mg tablets, and the maximum recommended dose is 1,200 mg (six tablets) per day. This is about one-half the recommended dose for the prescription equivalent, but this dose is effective for minor problems and shouldn't be exceeded without a doctor's advice.

Side Effects

Gastrointestinal upset is the most frequent problem and is reason to stop or to call the doctor. Serious gastrointestinal hemorrhage or a perforated stomach can result. The rare patient with aspirin allergy may also react to ibuprofen. Read the label carefully.

NAPROXEN

Naproxen (Naprosyn and Anaprox by prescription; Aleve over-the-counter) has recently become available without prescription. Its main advantage is a longer "half-life" than other pain relievers, so you need to take it only twice a day. It is effective against pain, fever, and inflammation.

Dosage

Naproxen comes in 200 mg tablets. Read the label carefully. Because naproxen is slightly more toxic to the stomach than ibuprofen, don't take more than three tablets in 24 hours or more than two if you're over 65 years old.

Side Effects

Stop taking the drug and call your doctor if you experience gastrointestinal upset.

5 Antacids

Purpose

To relieve upset stomach. We recommend nonabsorbable antacids because they bring fewer bad consequences down the road.

NONABSORBABLE ANTACIDS

Maalox, Gelusil, Mylanta, Di-Gel, and Amphojel are examples of nonabsorbable antacids. They're an important part of the home pharmacy. They help neutralize stomach acid and thus decrease heartburn, ulcer pain, gas pains, and stomach upset. Because they aren't absorbed by the body, they usually don't upset the acid-base balance of the body and are quite safe.

Almost all these antacids are available in both liquid and tablet form. For most purposes, the liquid form is superior. It coats more of the surface area of the gullet and stomach than the tablets do. Indeed, if not well chewed, tablets may be almost worthless. Still, during work or play, a bottle can be cumbersome, and a few tablets in a shirt pocket or handbag may help with midday doses.

ABSORBABLE ANTACIDS

Baking soda, Alka-Seltzer, Rolaids, and Tums contain absorbable antacids. The main ingredient in these products is sodium bicarbonate (Alka-Seltzer, baking soda), dihydroxyaluminum sodium carbonate (Rolaids), or calcium carbonate (Tums). These medicines are more powerful acid neutralizers than nonabsorbable antacids, and they come in convenient tablet form. However, they're absorbed through the walls of the stomach, and this may cause problems. For this reason, we recommend the nonabsorbable antacids or a combination of nonabsorbable and absorbable. However, calcium carbonate is also an excellent source of supplemental calcium.

Reading the Labels

Nonabsorbable antacids contain magnesium or aluminum or both. As a general rule, magnesium causes diarrhea and aluminum causes constipation. Different brands are slightly different mixtures of the salts of these two metals, designed to avoid both diarrhea and constipation. A few brands also contain calcium, which can be mildly constipating.

Different products differ in taste. While there are some differences in potency, most people will ultimately select the particular antacid that has a taste they can tolerate and that doesn't upset their bowels. Keep trying different brands until you're satisfied.

Dosage

The standard adult dose is two tablespoons (30 ml) or two well-chewed tablets. Use one-half the adult dose for children of ages six to twelve, and one-fourth the adult dose for children of ages three to six. The frequency of the dose depends on the severity of the problem. For stomach upset or heartburn, one or two doses will often suffice. For gastritis, several doses a day for several days may be needed. For ulcers, six weeks or more may be needed, with the medication taken as frequently as every hour or so; this type of program should be supervised by a doctor.

If you wish to use baking soda as an antacid, use one teaspoonful (5 ml) in a glass of water every four hours as needed—but only occasionally. Baking soda is absorbable.

Side Effects

In general, the only problem is the effect on the bowel movements. Maalox tends to loosen the stools slightly, Mylanta and Gelusil are about average, and Amphojel and Aludrox (with more aluminum) tend to be more constipating. Aluminum intake has been linked to Alzheimer's disease, but this is far from certain. Adjust the dose and change brands as needed. Check with your doctor before using these compounds if you have kidney disease, heart disease, or high blood pressure. Some brands contain significant quantities of salt and should be avoided by people on a low-salt diet. Di-Gel has the lowest salt content of the popular brands.

Be careful if you take baking soda by mouth. First, there's a lot of sodium in it. If you have heart trouble or high blood pressure or are on a low-salt diet, you can get into trouble. Second, if you take baking soda for many months on a regular basis, there's some evidence that it may result in calcium deposits in the kidneys and thus cause kidney damage.

STOMACH ACID BLOCKERS

Tagamet (cimetidine) and Pepcid AC are prescription drugs widely used for stomach ulcers and have recently been approved for over-the-counter use in lower doses to treat heartburn. Rather than neutralize stomach acid like antacids, they act to block the body's production of the acid. Most people won't need Tagamet and Pepcid AC, but you can consider them if antacids aren't effective. If you take other medications, check with your doctor before taking Tagamet; it can increase the potency of a number of other medications, including some taken for blood thinning (warfarin), asthma (theophylline), and seizures. Pepcid AC may be slightly better in this regard. Don't exceed the recommended dose.

6 Baking Soda

Purpose

Baking soda (sodium bicarbonate, $NaHCO_3$) is a very useful household chemical. It has three principal medical uses:

- As a weak solution, it acts to soothe the skin and reduce itching; thus, it's helpful in conditions ranging from sunburn to poison oak to chicken pox. This is the usage we discuss on this page.

- As a strong solution, it will draw fluid and swelling out of a wound and will act to soak and clean the wound at the same time. (See **M2,** Antiseptic Cleansers.)

- If taken by mouth, it serves as an antacid and may help alleviate heartburn or stomach upset. Because the sodium in baking soda is absorbed by the body, however, we recommend using a nonabsorbable antacid instead. (See **M5,** Antacids.)

Dosage

To soothe the skin, use from two tablespoons to a half cup (30–120 ml) in a bath of warm water. Blot skin gently after the bath and allow solution to dry on the skin. Repeat this procedure as often as necessary.

Side Effects

There are none as long as the baking soda is applied only to the skin.

SKIN CREAMS AND MOISTURIZING LOTIONS

There's little to be said about the various artificial materials — for example, Lubriderm, Vaseline, Alpha-Keri — that people apply to their skin in an attempt to temporarily improve its appearance or retard its aging. The various claims of such products are not scientifically based, and long-term benefits have not been demonstrated.

Sometimes dry skin can actually cause symptoms, thus becoming a medical problem. Remember that bathing or exposure to detergents may contribute to the drying of skin. Decreasing the frequency of baths or showers, wearing gloves when working with cleansing agents, and other similar measures are more important than using any lotion or cream.

Moisturizing creams and lotions may make your skin feel better to you; this is the "soothing" action. Use such creams as the product labels state. They have essentially no side effects, except that some people are allergic to the lanolin in some of these products.

7 Syrup of Ipecac

Purpose

To induce vomiting if someone has been poisoned by a plant or a drug. Vomiting will empty the stomach of any poison that has not already been absorbed. Syrup of ipecac is especially useful if you have small children.

Don't use ipecac or anything else to induce vomiting if the poison swallowed is a petroleum-based compound or a strong acid or alkali. Call the Poison Control Center immediately. See **E3**, Poisoning, at the front of this book for more advice on poisoning.

It's far better to keep toxic chemicals out of a child's reach than to have to use ipecac. When you buy ipecac, use the purchase as a reminder to check the house for toxic materials that a child might reach; move them to a safer place. If your child does swallow something, the sooner the stomach is emptied, the milder the problem will be, with the exceptions listed above. There's no time to buy ipecac after your child has swallowed poison; therefore, you should have it on hand just in case you ever need it.

Dosage

One tablespoon (15 ml) of ipecac may suffice for a small child; two to four teaspoons (10–20 ml) are necessary for older children and adults. Follow the dose with as much warm water as can be given, until vomiting occurs. Repeat the dose in 15 minutes if you haven't had any results.

Side Effects

This is an uncomfortable medication, but it's not hazardous unless vomiting causes material to be thrown down the windpipe into the lungs. This can cause pneumonia, so do *not* induce vomiting in a victim who is unconscious or nearly unconscious. Do *not* cause vomiting of volatile materials, such as petroleum compounds or drain cleaner, that can be inhaled into the lungs and cause damage.

MEDICINE M8

8 Antihistamines and Decongestants

Purpose

To treat allergy symptoms. Allerest, Chlor-Trimeton, Sinarest, Actifed, Benadryl, Sudafed, and Dimetapp are among the over-the-counter drugs designed for treatment of minor allergic symptoms. They're similar to the cold compounds described in **M10,** but they less frequently contain pain and fever agents like aspirin, acetaminophen, naproxen, or ibuprofen. Usually these drug compounds contain an antihistamine and a decongestant agent, and sometimes acetaminophen. These ingredients can be identified from the label.

If you tolerate one of these drugs well and get relief, you may continue to take it for several weeks (for example, through a hay fever season) without seeing a doctor. However, the same sort of drug taken as nose drops or nasal spray should be used more sparingly and only for short periods, as detailed below in **M9,** Nose Drops and Sprays.

Reading the Labels

The decongestant is usually pseudoephedrine or phenylpropanolamine. If the compound name is not familiar, the suffix "-ephrine" or "-edrine" usually identifies a decongestant. The antihistamine is often chlorpheniramine, diphenhydramine, or brompheniramine. If not, the antihistamine is sometimes identifiable on the label by the suffix "-amine."

Dosage

Take according to product directions. Reduce the dose if you note side effects, or try another compound.

Side Effects

These are usually minor and disappear after the drug is stopped or decreased in dose. Agitation and insomnia usually indicate too much of the decongestant. Drowsiness usually indicates too much antihistamine. If you can avoid the substances to which you are allergic, it's far superior to taking drugs. Drugs, to a certain degree, inevitably impair your functioning.

9 Nose Drops and Sprays

Purpose

To treat a runny nose. A runny nose is often the worst symptom of a cold or allergy. Because this complaint is so common, remedies are big business, and there are many advertised as decreasing your nasal drip: Afrin, Neo-Synephrine, Vicks, Sinarest, and other drops or sprays.

The active ingredient in these compounds is a decongestant drug, often ephedrine or phenylephrine. These preparations are "topical," meaning that you apply them directly to the inflamed tissue. You can then feel the membranes shrinking down and "drawing," and you will note a decrease in the amount of secretion. However, there are some problems associated with using these compounds.

The major drawback is that the relief is temporary. Usually the symptoms return in a couple of hours, so you repeat the dose. This is fine for a while. But these drugs work by causing the muscle in the walls of the blood vessels to shrink, decreasing blood flow, and after many applications these small muscles become fatigued and fail to respond. Finally, they're so fatigued that they relax entirely, and the situation becomes worse than it was in the beginning. This is medically termed "rebound vasodilation" and can occur if you use these drugs steadily for three days or more. Many patients interpret these increased symptoms as a need for more medication, but taking more only makes the problem worse. Therefore, *use nose drops or sprays for only three days at a time.* After several days' rest, you may use them again for three more days.

Dosage

These drugs are almost always used in the wrong way. If you don't bathe the swollen membranes on the side surface of the inner nose, you won't get the desired effect. If you can taste the drug, you've applied it to the wrong area. Apply small amounts to one nostril while lying down on that side for a few minutes so that the medicine will bathe the membranes. Then apply the agent to the other nostril while lying on that side (see diagram below). Treat four times a day if needed, but don't continue for more than three days without interrupting the therapy.

Side Effects

Rebound vasodilation from prolonged use is the most common problem. If you apply these agents incorrectly and swallow a large amount of the drug, you may experience a rapid heart rate and an uneasy, agitated feeling. The drying effect of the drug can result in nosebleeds.

Try to avoid the substances to which you're allergic rather than treating the consequences of exposure. Often, simple measures like changing a furnace filter, using a vaporizer, or using an air conditioner to filter the air can improve allergic symptoms.

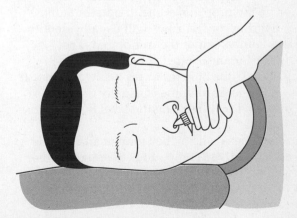

10 Cold Tablets

Purpose

To relieve some symptoms of colds and flu. Coricidin, Actifed, Triaminic, Contac, Dimetapp, and dozens of other products are widely advertised as being effective against the common cold. Surprisingly, many give satisfactory symptomatic relief. We don't think that these compounds add much to standard treatment with acetaminophen or aspirin and fluids, but some people believe otherwise. We don't discourage their use for short periods.

These compounds usually have three basic ingredients. The most important is a fever and pain reducer: acetaminophen, aspirin, or ibuprofen. In addition, there is a decongestant drug to shrink the swollen membranes and the small blood vessels, and an antihistamine to block any allergy and to dry mucus.

Reading the Labels

The decongestant is often pseudoephedrine or phenylpropanolamine. If not, the suffix "-ephrine" or "-edrine" will usually identify this component of the compound. The antihistamine is often chlorpheniramine (Chlor-Trimeton, etc.) or diphenhydramine. If not, the antihistamine is usually (but not always) identifiable on the label by the suffix "-amine."

Occasionally a "belladonna alkaloid" is added to these compounds to enhance other actions and reduce stomach spasms. In the small doses used, there's little effect from such a drug. It is listed as "scopolamine," "belladonna," or something similar. Other ingredients that may be listed contribute little. Don't use products with caffeine if you have heart trouble or difficulty sleeping.

These products take the much promoted "combination-of-ingredients" approach. As a rule, single drugs are preferable to combinations of drugs; they allow you to be more selective in treatment of symptoms, and consequently you take fewer drugs. The ingredients in combination products are available separately, and these individual products should be considered as alternatives. For example, the major ingredient in combination products is usually aspirin or acetaminophen. Pseudoephedrine is an excellent decongestant and is available without prescription in 30 mg and 60 mg tablets. Chlorpheniramine, a strong antihistamine, is available without prescription in the standard 4 mg size. When possible, consider applying medicine directly to the affected area, as with nose drops or sprays for a runny nose.

Finally, note that the commonly prescribed cold medicines (Sudafed, Actifed, Dimetapp) are really just more concentrated and expensive formulations of the same type of drugs that are available over the counter (often even under the same names). Is it worth a trip to the doctor just for that?

Dosage

Try the recommended dosage. If you feel no effect, you may increase the dosage by one-half. Don't exceed twice the recommended dosage. Remember that you're trying to find a compromise between desired effects and side effects. Increasing the dosage gives some chance of increased beneficial effects, but it guarantees a greater probability of side effects.

Side Effects

Drugs that put one person to sleep will keep another awake. The most frequent side effects of cold tablets are either drowsiness or agitation. The drowsiness is usually caused by the antihistamine component, and the insomnia or agitation results from the decongestant component. You can try another compound that has less or none of the offending chemical, or you can reduce the dose. There are no frequent serious side effects; the most dangerous is drowsiness if you intend to drive or operate machinery. In rare cases, the "belladonna" component will cause a dry mouth, blurred vision, or inability to urinate. You may experience aspirin's usual side effects — upset stomach, ringing in the ears, or, rarely, bleeding from the stomach.

11 Cough Syrups

We'll discuss Guaifenesin (Robitussin, Benylin expectorant, Vicks, etc.) and dextromethorphan (Vicks Formula 44, Robitussin-DM, etc.) specifically; follow the label instructions for other agents.

Purpose

Cough medication is a confusing area, with many products from which to choose. To simplify, consider two major categories:

- **Expectorants** are usually preferable because they liquefy the secretions the body produces while fighting illness and allow the body's defenses to get rid of the bad material by coughing it up more easily.

- **Cough suppressants** should be avoided if the cough is bringing up any material or if there's a lot of mucus. In the late stages of a cough, when it's dry and hacking, compounds containing a cough suppressant may be useful.

We prefer cough compounds that don't contain an antihistamine, which dries mucus and can harm as much as help.

Reading the Labels

Guaifenesin (Robitussin, Benylin expectorant, Vicks, etc.), potassium iodide, and several other frequently used chemicals cause an expectorant action.

Cough-suppressant action comes principally from narcotics, such as codeine. Over-the-counter cough suppressants cannot contain codeine. They often contain dextromethorphan hydrobromide, which is not a narcotic but is a close chemical relative.

Many commercial mixtures contain a little of everything and may have some of the ingredients of the cold compounds as well.

GUAIFENESIN

Guaifenesin draws more liquid into the mucus that triggers a cough. Thus, the cough medicine liquefies these mucus secretions so that they may be coughed free. The resulting cough is easier and less irritating. For a dry, hacking cough remaining after a cold, the lubrication alone often soothes the inflamed area. Guaifenesin doesn't suppress the cough reflex but encourages the natural defense mechanisms of the body. There's controversy over its effectiveness, but it appears to be safe. It isn't as powerful as the codeine-containing preparations, but for routine use we prefer it to prescription drugs. Pepper and garlic, not usually thought of as medicines, have a similar effect.

Reading the Labels

Guaifenesin is also available in combination with decongestants and cough suppressants; the decongestants may carry a "-PE" suffix for "phenylephrine" and the cough suppressants a "-DM" for "dextromethorphan."

Dosage

Follow directions on the label. Call your doctor if you have a sick and coughing child less than one year old.

Side Effects

No significant problems have been reported. If you use preparations containing other drugs, you may feel side effects from the other components of the combination.

DEXTROMETHORPHAN

Robitussin-DM, Triaminic-DM, Vicks Formula 44, and others contain dextromethorphan, a drug that "calms the cough center." The drug makes the areas of the brain that control coughs less sensitive to the stimuli that trigger coughs. No matter how much you use, it will seldom decrease a cough by more than 50%. Thus, you usually can't totally suppress a cough; this is actually good for you because the cough is a protective reflex. Dextromethorphan is best used with dry, hacking coughs that are preventing sleep or work.

Dosage

See directions on the label. Adults may require up to twice the recommended dosage to obtain any effect, but don't exceed this amount. A higher dose may produce problems, not further benefit.

Side Effects

Drowsiness is the only side effect that has been frequently reported.

12 Bulk Laxatives

Purpose

To treat constipation. We prefer a natural diet, with natural vegetable fiber residue, to the use of any laxative. But if you must use a laxative, the most attractive alternative is psyllium as a bulk laxative to hold water in the bowel and soften the stool.

Metamucil, EfferSyllium, and similar preparations contain substances refined from the psyllium seed. They can help both diarrhea and constipation. Psyllium draws water into the stool, forms a gel or thick solution, and thus provides bulk. It isn't absorbed by the digestive tract but only passes through; thus, it's a natural product and essentially has no side effects. However, it doesn't always work. A similar effect probably can be obtained by eating enough celery.

Dosage

One teaspoonful (5 ml), stirred in a glass of water, taken twice daily is a typical dose. A second glass of water or juice should also be taken. Psyllium is also available in more expensive, individual-dose packets, for when you don't have a measuring spoon. The effervescent versions mix a bit more rapidly and taste better to some people.

Side Effects

If you take a bulk laxative without sufficient water, the gel that is formed could conceivably lodge in your esophagus (the tube that leads from the mouth to the stomach). Sufficient liquid will prevent this problem.

13 Diarrhea Remedies

Purpose

To treat diarrhea. For occasional loose stools, no medication is required. A clear liquid diet (for example, water or ginger ale) is the first remedy for any diarrhea; it rests the bowel and replaces lost fluid. When diarrhea persists, products with kaolin, pectin, or bismuth are often helpful. If these don't control the diarrhea, stronger agents containing substances such as paregoric may be prescribed. Long-term or severe diarrhea may require the help of a doctor and antibiotic treatments.

To prevent "Traveler's Diarrhea," it's best to use antibiotics, such as tetracycline, doxycycline, or others. Consult your doctor before the trip for a prescription. Sometimes you can just do this by phone.

ATTAPULGITE

Diasorb, Rheaban, and similar medicines contain a mineral called attapulgite. This ingredient has a gelling effect that helps form a solid stool.

Dosage

Follow the directions on the label. For children below age three, call your doctor to ask for the correct dosage. In general, more severe diarrhea is treated more vigorously, whereas minor problems require less medicine.

Side Effects

None have been reported.

BISMUTH SUBSALICYLATE (PEPTO-BISMOL)

Dosage

Follow label directions. For children below age three, call the doctor for dosage.

Side Effects

Bismuth may cause a temporary, harmless darkening of the tongue and/or stool.

14 Sodium Fluoride

Purpose

To protect teeth from decay. Take care of your teeth; they help you chew. There's good evidence that preventive measures can save teeth. Brush your teeth with a toothpaste that contains fluoride as recommended by your dentist. Many doctors feel that daily flossing is the most important way to prevent adult tooth decay. Adult tooth loss is usually due to plaque buildup, gum disease, and bone loss. Water jets (such as Water Pik) remove food products from between the teeth, but they're less effective than proper flossing.

SODIUM FLUORIDE SUPPLEMENTS

If your water supply is fluoridated, your fluoride intake is adequate and you don't need to supplement your diet. The ground water in many areas is naturally fluoridated. Find out if your water is fluoridated; your local health department usually has the answer. If it isn't fluoridated, it's important for you to supplement your children's diet with fluoride. Arguments remain about whether fluoride is needed after the teeth have been formed, but all authorities agree that fluoride is needed through age ten. Adults probably don't require dietary fluoride, although painting teeth with sodium fluoride paste by the dentist is still felt to be helpful, as is use of a fluoride toothpaste.

Dosage

Fortunately it's relatively easy to supplement with fluoride when the water supply isn't treated. Buy a large bottle of soluble fluoride tablets. Most tablets are 2.2 mg and contain 2 mg of fluoride; the rest is a soluble sugar. A child under the age of three needs approximately 0.5 mg (one-fourth tablet) per day, and a child between the ages of three and ten needs 1 mg, or one-half tablet. The tablets can be chewed or swallowed. They may also be taken in milk; they don't alter its taste. In states where fluoride is available only by prescription, request a prescription from your doctor or dentist on a routine visit.

Side Effects

Too much fluoride will mottle the teeth (make gray spots) and won't give them additional strength, so don't exceed the recommended dosage. At the recommended dosage, there are no known side effects; fluoride is a natural mineral present in many natural water supplies.

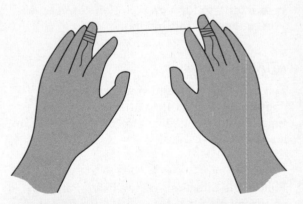

Dental floss. Wrap floss around your two middle fingers. Use your index fingers to guide the floss into the spaces between your teeth. This way you don't need to wrap the floss tightly. Rub the floss up and down against the teeth's surfaces.

15 "Artificial Tears" Eye Drops

Purpose

To treat irritated eyes. The tear mechanism normally soothes, cleans, and lubricates the eye. Occasionally, the environment can overwhelm this mechanism, or not enough tears may flow. In these cases the eye becomes "tired," feels dry or gritty, and may itch. A number of compounds that may aid this problem are available.

There are two general classes of eye preparations. One class contains compounds intended to soothe the eye (Murine, Prefrin, etc.). Added to these compounds may be decongestants that shrink blood vessels and thus "get the red out" (Visine, Murine Plus, Visine LR). Their capacity to soothe is debatable. The use of decongestants to get rid of a bloodshot appearance is totally cosmetic. It's even possible that such preparations interfere with the normal healing process, so we don't recommend them.

The other class of preparations makes no claims of special soothing effects and contains no decongestants. Their purpose is to lubricate the eye, to be "artificial tears." These are chemical solutions similar to those of the body, so that no irritation occurs. Ophthalmologists prefer such preparations for minor eye irritation. Murine Lubricating Eyedrops is one example.

Dosage

Use as frequently as needed in the quantity required. You can't use too much, although usually a few drops give just as much relief as a bottleful. If you have a constant problem of dry eyes, check it out with your doctor because it may indicate an underlying problem. Usually the symptom of dry eyes lasts only a few hours and is readily relieved. Too much sun, wind, or dust usually causes the minor irritation.

Side Effects

No serious side effects have been reported. Visine and other drugs containing decongestants tend to sting a bit.

None of these drugs treats eye infections or injuries or removes foreign bodies from the eye. In Part II, "Common Complaints," we give instructions for more severe eye complaints (S29–S33).

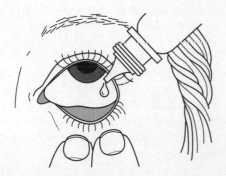

Inserting eye drops. Gently pull down the lower lid. Drip the solution into the sac formed by the lid, not on the eyeball itself. Blink a few times.

16 Zinc Oxide

Purpose

To treat hemorrhoids. Zinc oxide powders and creams soothe the irritated area while the body heals the inflamed vein. They also help toughen the skin over the hemorrhoids so that it's less easily irritated. Many people get relief with Preparation H, Anusol, or others, but these offer little advantage.

Reading the Labels

We don't advocate the use of creams that contain ingredients identified by the suffix "-caine" because repeated use of these local anesthetics can cause further irritation.

Dosage

Apply as needed, following label directions. Don't trap bacteria beneath the creams; apply them after a bath when you have carefully cleaned and dried the area. Remember to clean the area thoroughly with soap and water each day.

Side Effects

Essentially none.

17 Antifungal Preparations

Purpose

To treat fungus infecting the skin. Fungal infections of the skin aren't serious, so treatment isn't urgent. In general the fungus needs moist, undisturbed areas to grow and will often disappear with regular cleansing, drying, and application of powder to keep the area dry. Clean the area twice daily.

If you need a medication, there are effective nontoxic agents available. For athlete's foot, try one of the zinc undecylenate creams or powders, such as Desenex. In difficult cases, tolnaftate (Tinactin, etc.) and clotrimazole (Lotrimin, etc.) are useful for almost all skin fungus problems, but they are more expensive.

Dosage

For athlete's foot, use as directed on the label. For other skin problems, selenium sulfide is effective. It's available by prescription in a 2.5% solution but also over-the-counter in a 1% solution as Selsun Blue shampoo. Use the shampoo as a cream and let it dry on the skin; repeat several times a day to compensate for the solution's weaker strength.

Side Effects

There are very few. Selenium sulfide can burn the skin if used to excess, so decrease application if you notice any irritation. Selenium may discolor hair and will stain clothes. Be very careful when applying any of these products around the eyes. Don't take them by mouth.

18 Hydrocortisone Cream

Purpose

To temporarily relieve skin itching and rashes such as poison ivy and poison oak. Brand names of over-the-counter hydrocortisone cream include CaldeCORT, Cortizone-10, and Benadryl Itch Relief Cream. These are strong, local anti-inflammatory preparations; in general, they're as effective as anything that your doctor can prescribe. Used for a short period, these creams are safe and almost totally nontoxic. They'll clear up many minor rashes, but they "suppress" a condition rather than "cure" it.

Dosage

Rub a very small amount into the rash. If you can see any cream remaining on the skin, you've used too much. Repeat as frequently as needed, which often is every two to four hours.

Side Effects

Over the long term, these creams can cause skin atrophy (thinning of the skin), so limit their use to a two-week period. Beyond this time, check with your doctor. Theoretically, these creams can make an infection worse, so be careful about using them if it is possible the "rash" might be infected. Don't use these creams around the eyes, and don't take them by mouth.

19 Sunscreen Agents

Purpose

To prevent sunburn. Dermatologists continually remind us that sun is bad for the skin. Exposure to the sun accelerates skin aging and increases the chance of skin cancer. Advertisements, on the other hand, keep extolling the virtues of a suntan. As a nation, we spend much of our youth trying to achieve a pleasing skin tone, disregarding the later consequences.

Sunscreen agents can prevent burning but allow you to be in the sun. If your skin is unusually sensitive to the sun's effects, it's best to block the rays; this is achieved with a strong sunscreen agent, like Presun, or any PABA-containing agent with a high sunscreen number. The rating numbers on the label are a good guide to the blocking power of the different agents. The higher the number, the better the blocking power. Suntan lotions that aren't sunscreen agents block relatively little solar radiation.

The length of time an agent stays on the skin is important. Even the strongest cream or lotion won't help after it has washed off, so look for the non-water-soluble products if you plan to be in and out of the water.

Dosage

Apply evenly to exposed areas of skin as directed on the label.

Side Effects

Very rare skin irritation and allergy have been reported.

MEDICINE M20

20 Wart Removers

Purpose

To remove some warts. Warts are a curious little problem. The capricious way in which they form and disappear has led to countless myths and home therapies. They can be surgically removed, burned off, or frozen off, but they'll also go away by themselves or after treatment by hypnosis. Warts are caused by a virus and are a reaction to a minor local viral infection. If you get one, you're likely to get more. When one disappears, the others often follow. The exception is plantar warts, on the sole of the foot, which won't go away by themselves and sometimes not even with home treatment; the doctor may be needed.

Over-the-counter chemicals, such as Compound W and Wart-Off, are moderately effective for treatment of warts. They contain a mild skin irritant. By repeated application they slowly burn off the top layers of the wart and eventually the virus is destroyed.

Dosage

Apply repeatedly, as directed on the product label. Persistence is necessary.

Side Effects

These products are effective because they are caustic to the skin. Be careful to apply them only to the wart, and be very careful around your eyes or mouth.

21 Elastic Bandages

Purpose

To treat sprains and similar injuries. Any family periodically needs elastic (Ace, etc.) bandages. You'll probably need both a narrow and a broad width. If problems recur, the one-piece devices designed specifically for knee and ankle are sometimes more convenient. All these bandages primarily provide gentle support, but they also act to reduce swelling. The support given is minimal, and it's possible to reinjure the body part despite the bandage. Thus, an elastic bandage isn't a substitute for a splint, a cast, or a proper adhesive-type dressing. Perhaps the most important function of these bandages is to remind yourself that you have a problem so that you're less likely to reinjure yourself.

Dosage

When wrapping with the bandage, start at the far end of the area to be bandaged and work toward the trunk of the body, making each loop a little looser than the one before. Thus, a knee bandage should be tighter below the knee than above, and an ankle bandage should be tighter on the foot than on the lower leg. Many people think that because a bandage is elastic it must be stretched. That's wrong. The stretchability is to allow the person to move. Simply wrap the bandage as you would a roll of gauze.

Continue using the bandage as support well past the time of active discomfort to allow complete healing and to help prevent reinjury; this usually takes about six weeks. During the latter part of this period, you can stop using the bandage except during activities that will likely stress the injured part. Remember that reinjury is still possible while these bandages are being used.

Side Effects

The simple elastic bandage can cause trouble when it is applied too tightly. Problems arise when circulation in the limb beyond the bandage is impaired. The bandage should be firm but not tight. The limb shouldn't swell, hurt, or be cooler beyond the bandage. The skin shouldn't have any blue or purple color.

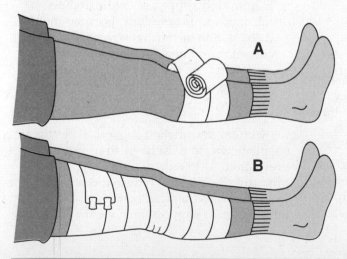

Wrapping an elastic bandage.
(A) Start wrapping the bandage on the far end of the joint (in this case, the knee). Don't stretch the bandage as you wrap. (B) Wrap past the joint, firmly at first then more loosely the farther up you go. Use the clips that come with most elastic bandages to fasten the loose end.

Vitamin Preparations

The use of vitamin supplements has always been controversial. In the past there was theoretical reason to believe that supplements might have benefits; there were also good reasons to believe that these benefits might only be theoretical. Classic diseases of vitamin deficiency (scurvy, beriberi, pellagra, etc.) are rare and occur only in people whose diets are inadequate in virtually every respect, or who have diseases or take medications that interfere with natural vitamins. Most past research on vitamin intake studied diet only and didn't directly address the issue of supplements to the diet. This research suggested that a well-balanced diet should provide adequate amounts of vitamins and minerals.

On the other hand, it's now known that there are specific situations in which vitamin supplements are appropriate. There are good studies indicating that supplements may be useful in individuals with "average" diets outside the special circumstances mentioned above. Here's a summary of current information on vitamin supplements.

- **Vitamin A:** One study has suggested that modest vitamin A supplementation may lower the risk of breast cancer, but that this benefit might occur only in women who had low amounts of vitamin A in their diet.

- **Vitamin C:** A Canadian study indicated that people over age 55 who took vitamin C supplements (at least 300 mg daily for five years) have a 70% lower risk for eye cataracts.

- **Vitamin D:** Most pediatricians recommend vitamin D supplements for infants who are breast feeding.

- **Vitamin E:** Several studies now suggest that vitamin E supplements (400 mg or more per day) may reduce the risk of heart disease by as much as one-half by preventing the oxidation of LDL cholesterol. The Canadian study that looked at vitamin C supplements and cataracts also investigated vitamin E supplementation (400 mg daily) and found a 50% lower risk of cataracts.

- **Folic acid:** Several studies have demonstrated that the use of a folic acid supplement (1 mg per day) before and during early pregnancy greatly reduces the risk of severe defects of the nervous system in the baby.

- **Multivitamins and minerals:** One study suggested that the use of a multivitamin and mineral preparation by healthy adults over 65 reduced the number of illness days by more than half. This supplement contained vitamin A, beta-carotene, thiamine, riboflavin, niacin, vitamin B_6, folic acid, vitamin B_{12}, vitamin C, vitamin D, vitamin E, iron, zinc, copper, selenium, iodine, calcium, and magnesium. The amount of each vitamin or mineral was similar to the current recommended daily allowances except for beta-carotene and vitamin E, which were above the usual recommended allowances.

Current information suggests that vitamin supplements are most likely to be useful in prevention. Although vitamin C appears promising as a way to reduce the side effects of some cancer therapies, there's still little information to support the hope that vitamins will cure disease ranging from colds to cancer, or that they're capable of providing benefits such as more energy or an improved sex life.

The use of vitamin supplements for purposes other than those indicated above is entirely optional. They're unlikely to cause problems when taken in reasonable dosages, but consider the cautions listed below. If you do buy vitamins, the cheaper "house" brands usually are of similar quality to those that are heavily advertised.

Dosage

Multivitamin preparations usually contain the current recommended daily allowance of each vitamin. Other dosages are indicated above.

Side Effects

Vitamin A, vitamin D, and vitamin B_6 (pyridoxine) can cause severe problems when taken in excessively large doses. Large doses of vitamin C have been reported to be associated with kidney problems in rare instances. Other vitamins have not been as well studied, but serious side effects appear to be rare.

PART II

Common Complaints

CHAPTER 3

Common Injuries

1 Cuts

Most cuts (lacerations) affect only the skin and the fatty tissue beneath it and heal without permanent damage. However, injury to internal structures such as muscles, tendons, blood vessels, ligaments, or nerves can bring permanent damage. Your doctor can decrease this chance. These are the signs that normally call for a cut to be examined by a doctor:

- Bleeding that you can't control with pressure — this is an emergency **(E1)**
- Numbness or weakness in the limb beyond the wound
- Inability to move fingers or toes

Signs of infection — such as pus oozing from the wound, fever, or extensive redness and swelling — won't appear for at least 24 hours. Bacteria need time to grow and multiply. If these signs do appear, you must consult a doctor.

Stitches

The only purpose of stitching (suturing) a wound is to pull the edges together to hasten healing and minimize scarring. Stitches injure tissue to some extent, so they aren't recommended if the wound can be held closed without them. Stitching should be done within eight hours of the injury. Otherwise, the edges of the wound are less likely to heal together and germs are more likely to be trapped under the skin. Stitching is often required in young children who are apt to pull off bandages, or in areas that are subject to a great deal of motion, such as the fingers or joints.

Difficult Cuts

Unless the cut is very small or shallow, call your doctor about cuts in these areas:

- On the chest, abdomen, or back
- On the face — facial wounds can be disfiguring
- On the palm — hand wounds can be difficult to treat if they become infected

HOME TREATMENT

Cleanse the wound. Soap and water will do, but be vigorous. You may also use 3% hydrogen peroxide or a commercial antiseptic such as Merthiolate. Make sure no dirt, glass, or other foreign material remains in the wound.

The edges of a clean, minor cut can usually be held together by "butterfly" bandages or, preferably, by "steristrips" — strips of sterile paper tape **(M1)**. Apply either of these bandages so that the edges of the wound join without "rolling under."

See the doctor if the edges of the wound can't be kept together, if signs of infection appear (pus, fever, extensive redness and swelling), or if the cut isn't healing well within two weeks.

WHAT TO EXPECT AT THE DOCTOR'S OFFICE

The wound will be thoroughly cleansed and explored to be sure that no foreign particles are left and that blood vessels, nerves, and tendons are undamaged. Since the doctor may use an anesthetic to numb the area, report any possible allergy to local anesthetics

CUTS

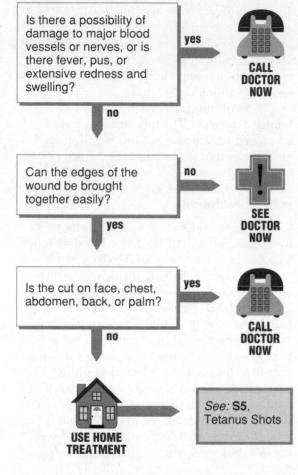

Is there a possibility of damage to major blood vessels or nerves, or is there fever, pus, or extensive redness and swelling?

yes → **CALL DOCTOR NOW**

no ↓

Can the edges of the wound be brought together easily?

no → **SEE DOCTOR NOW**

yes ↓

Is the cut on face, chest, abdomen, back, or palm?

yes → **CALL DOCTOR NOW**

no ↓

USE HOME TREATMENT

See: **S5,** Tetanus Shots

(Xylocaine, for example). The doctor will give a tetanus shot **(S5)** and antibiotics if needed.

Lacerations that may require a surgical specialist include those with injury to tendons or major vessels, especially in the hand, and those on the face.

Your doctor will tell you when stitches are to be removed. You can often perform this simple procedure at home with a clean pair of small, sharp scissors or a fingernail clipper.

1. Clean the skin and the stitches. Sometimes a scab must be removed by soaking.

2. Gently lift the stitch away from the skin by grasping a loose end of the knot with tweezers.

3. Cut the stitch as close to the skin as possible, so that a minimum amount of the stitch that was outside the skin will be pulled through. This reduces the chance of infection.

4. Lift the tweezers to pull the stitch out.

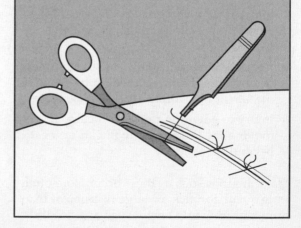

2 Puncture Wounds

Puncture wounds are those caused by nails, pins, tacks, and other sharp objects. Usually, the most important question is whether a tetanus shot is needed. See Tetanus Shots **(S5)** whenever a puncture wound occurs.

Signs to Call the Doctor

Most minor puncture wounds are located on the body's extremities: arms, hands, legs, and particularly feet. If the puncture wound is located elsewhere, a hidden internal injury may have occurred. Call the doctor for advice.

Many doctors feel that puncture wounds of the hand, if not minor, should be treated with antibiotics. Once started, infections deep in the hand are difficult to treat and may lead to loss of function. Call the doctor for hand wounds other than very minor ones.

Injury to a tendon, nerve, or major blood vessel is rare but can be serious.

- Injury to an **artery** may be indicated by blood pumping vigorously from the wound.

- Injury to a **nerve** usually causes numbness or tingling in the wounded limb beyond the site of the wound.

- Injury to a **tendon** causes difficulty in moving the limb (usually fingers or toes) beyond the wound.

Major injuries such as these occur more often from a nail, ice pick, or large instrument than from a narrow implement such as a needle.

Infection

To avoid infection, be absolutely sure that nothing has been left in the wound. Sometimes, for example, part of a needle will break off and remain in the foot. If there's any question of a foreign body remaining, a doctor should examine the wound.

Signs of infection usually take at least 24 hours to develop. The formation of pus, a fever, and severe redness and swelling are indications that you should see a doctor.

HOME TREATMENT

Clean the wound with soap and water or 3% hydrogen peroxide **(M2)**. Let it bleed as much as possible to carry out foreign material because you can't scrub the inside of a puncture wound. Don't apply pressure to stop the bleeding unless you see a large amount of blood loss or a "pumping" type of bleeding.

Soak the wound in warm water or a baking soda solution several times a day for four to five days **(M2)**. The object of the soaking is to keep the skin puncture open as long as possible so that any germs or foreign debris can drain from the open wound. If the wound closes, an infection may form beneath the skin but not become apparent for several days.

See the doctor if there are signs of infection or if the wound hasn't healed within two weeks.

WHAT TO EXPECT AT THE DOCTOR'S OFFICE

The doctor will be most concerned about the same questions that appear in the decision chart. If a metallic foreign body is suspected, X-rays may be taken; glass and wood don't show up on X-rays and may be difficult to

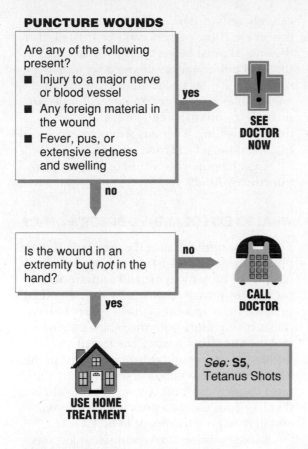

PUNCTURE WOUNDS

Are any of the following present?
- Injury to a major nerve or blood vessel
- Any foreign material in the wound
- Fever, pus, or extensive redness and swelling

yes → **SEE DOCTOR NOW**

no

Is the wound in an extremity but *not* in the hand?

no → **CALL DOCTOR**

yes

USE HOME TREATMENT

See: **S5**, Tetanus Shots

locate. Be prepared to tell the doctor of possible allergies to local anesthetics (Xylocaine, for example). The wound will be surgically explored if necessary. Most doctors will recommend home treatment. Antibiotics are only rarely suggested.

3 Animal Bites

The biggest concern after an animal bite is rabies, a very serious viral infection. The main carriers of rabies are skunks, foxes, bats, raccoons, and opossums. Rabies is also carried — though rarely — by cattle, dogs, and cats, and it's extremely rare in squirrels, chipmunks, rats, and mice. Although 3,000 to 4,000 animals with rabies are found in the United States each year, only one or two people contract the disease. Rabid animals act strangely, attack without provocation, and may drool or "foam at the mouth."

Any bite by an animal other than a pet dog or cat requires consultation with the doctor as to whether or not an antirabies vaccine is required. If the bite is by a dog or a cat, the animal is being reliably observed for sickness by its owner, and its immunizations are up to date, then you don't need to consult the doctor.

If the bite has left a wound that might require stitching or other treatment, consult Cuts (S1) or Puncture Wounds (S2). Although tetanus from an animal bite is rare, you should also check Tetanus Shots (S5).

This book has separate sections for Insect Bites or Stings (S13), Snake Bites (S14), Ticks (S53), and Chiggers (S54).

HOME TREATMENT

An animal whose immunizations are up to date is, of course, unlikely to have rabies. However, arrange for the animal to be observed for the next 15 days to make sure that it doesn't develop rabies. Most often, you can rely on the owners of the animal to observe it. If the owners can't be trusted, then the animal must be kept for observation by the local public agency charged with that responsibility. Many localities require that animal bites be reported to the health department. If the animal should develop rabies during this time, a serious situation exists and treatment must be started immediately.

Treat bites as you would other cuts or puncture wounds.

WHAT TO EXPECT AT THE DOCTOR'S OFFICE

The doctor must balance the generally remote possibility of exposure to rabies against the hazards of rabies vaccine and antirabies serum. An unprovoked attack by a wild animal or a bite from an animal that appears to have rabies may require both the rabies vaccine and the antirabies serum. The extent and location of the wounds also play a part in this decision; severe wounds of the head are the most dangerous. A bite caused by an animal that has since escaped presents a dilemma, and may require treatment to be safe.

Rabies vaccine is given in five injections, one as soon as possible and four over the next 28 days. The vaccine may cause local skin reactions as well as fever, headache, and nausea. Severe reactions to the vaccine are rare. The antirabies serum, unfortunately, has a high risk of serious reactions. The serum is given both directly into the wound and by injection into muscle.

Many physicians give a tetanus shot if the patient isn't "up to date," even though it's rare for tetanus bacteria to be introduced by an animal bite. Antibiotics are usually not needed.

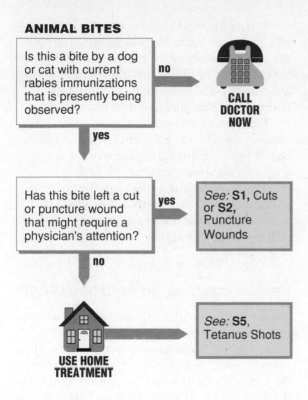

ANIMAL BITES

Is this a bite by a dog or cat with current rabies immunizations that is presently being observed?

no → CALL DOCTOR NOW

yes ↓

Has this bite left a cut or puncture wound that might require a physician's attention?

yes → *See:* **S1**, Cuts or **S2**, Puncture Wounds

no ↓

USE HOME TREATMENT → *See:* **S5**, Tetanus Shots

4 Scrapes and Abrasions

Scrapes and abrasions are shallow wounds. Several layers of the skin may be torn or even totally scraped off, but the wound doesn't go far beneath the skin. Abrasions are usually caused by falls onto the hands, elbows, or knees; but skateboard and bicycle riders can get abrasions on just about any part of the body. Because abrasions expose millions of nerve endings, all of which send pain impulses to the brain, they're usually much more painful than cuts.

HOME TREATMENT

Remove all dirt and foreign matter. Washing the wound with soap and warm water is the most important step in treatment. You can also use 3% hydrogen peroxide to cleanse the wound **(M2).** Most scrapes will scab rather quickly; this is nature's way of "dressing" the wound. Using Mercurochrome, iodine, and other antiseptics does little good and is sometimes painful.

Adhesive bandages may be used as necessary for a wound that continues to ooze blood; they must be removed if they get wet **(M1).** Antibacterial ointments (Neosporin, Bacitracin, etc.) are optional; their main advantage is in keeping bandages from sticking to the wound.

Loose skin flaps, if they aren't dirty, may be left to help form a natural dressing. If the skin flap is dirty, cut it off carefully with nail scissors. (If it hurts, stop! You're cutting the wrong tissue.)

Watch the wound for signs of infection — pus, fever, or severe redness or swelling — but don't be worried by redness around the edges; this is an indication of normal healing. Infection won't be obvious in the first 24 hours; fever may indicate a serious infection.

Pain can be treated for the first few minutes with an ice pack enclosed in a plastic bag or towel applied over the wound as needed. The worst pain subsides fairly quickly, and acetaminophen or other pain medication can then be used if needed **(M4).**

See the doctor if signs of infection appear or if the scrape or abrasion isn't healed within two weeks.

WHAT TO EXPECT AT THE DOCTOR'S OFFICE

The doctor will make sure that the wound is free of dirt and foreign matter. Soap and water and 3% hydrogen peroxide **(M2)** will often be used. Sometimes a local anesthetic (Xylocaine, for example) is required to reduce the pain of the cleansing process. Tell the doctor of possible allergies to such anesthetics.

An antibacterial ointment such as Neosporin or Bacitracin is sometimes applied after cleansing the wound. Betadine is a painless iodine preparation that is also occasionally used **(M2).** Tetanus shots aren't required for simple scrapes, but if the patient is overdue, it is a good chance to get caught up **(S5).**

SCRAPES

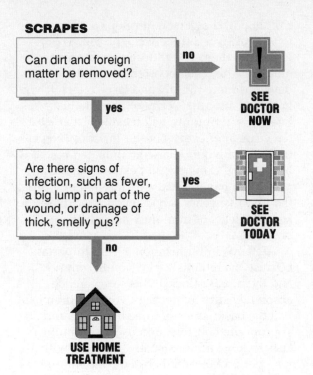

Can dirt and foreign matter be removed?

no → **SEE DOCTOR NOW**

yes

Are there signs of infection, such as fever, a big lump in part of the wound, or drainage of thick, smelly pus?

yes → **SEE DOCTOR TODAY**

no

USE HOME TREATMENT

5 Tetanus Shots

People may come to the doctor's office or emergency room to get a tetanus shot even though it isn't needed. This section's decision chart illustrates the essentials of the current U.S. Public Health Service recommendations. It can save you and your family several visits to the doctor. See the advice on immunizations (page 23) and Cuts (S1).

The question of whether or not a wound is "clean" and "minor" may be troublesome. Wounds caused by sharp, clean objects such as knives or razor blades have less chance of becoming infected than those in which dirt or foreign bodies have penetrated and lodged beneath the skin. Abrasions and minor burns won't result in tetanus. The tetanus germ can't grow in the presence of air, so the skin must be cut or punctured for the germ to reach an airless location.

IMMUNIZATION

If you've never received a basic series of three tetanus shots, you should see your doctor. Sometimes a different kind of tetanus shot is required if you haven't been adequately immunized. This shot is called "tetanus immune globulin" and is used when immunization isn't complete and there is a significant risk of tetanus. It is more expensive, more painful, and more likely to cause an allergic reaction than the tetanus booster. So keep a record of your family's immunizations in the back of this book and know the dates.

During the first tetanus shots (usually a series of three injections given in early childhood), the person develops a resistance to tetanus over a three-week period. This immunity then slowly declines over many months. After each booster, immunity develops more rapidly and lasts longer. If you have had an initial series of five tetanus injections, immunity will usually last at least ten years after every booster injection. Nevertheless, if a wound has contaminated material beneath the skin and isn't exposed to the air, and if you haven't had a tetanus shot within the past five years, a booster shot is advised to keep the level of immunity as high as possible.

Tetanus immunization is very important because the tetanus germ is quite common and the disease (lockjaw) is so severe. Be absolutely sure that each of your children has had the basic series of three injections and appropriate boosters. Because the immunity lasts so long, adults usually get away with a long period between boosters, but immunization of children should be "by the book."

TETANUS SHOTS

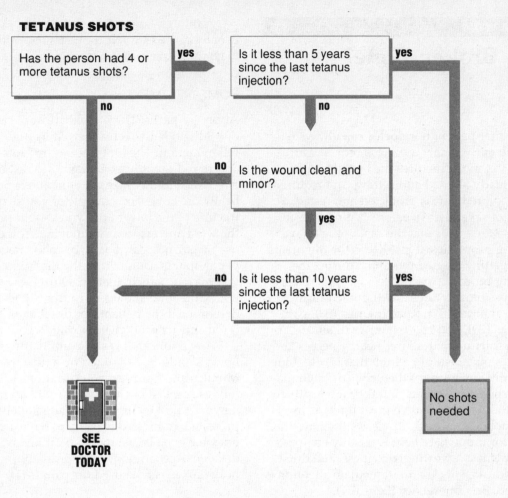

Has the person had 4 or more tetanus shots? **yes** → Is it less than 5 years since the last tetanus injection? **yes** → No shots needed

no ↓ (from first box) → SEE DOCTOR TODAY

Is it less than 5 years since the last tetanus injection? **no** ↓

no ← Is the wound clean and minor? **yes** ↓

no ← Is it less than 10 years since the last tetanus injection? **yes** → No shots needed

SEE DOCTOR TODAY

No shots needed

6 Broken Bone?

Neither patient nor doctor can always tell by eye whether a bone is broken. Fortunately, in most fractures the bone fragments are already aligned and setting isn't required. If the injured part is protected and rested, a delay of several days before casting does no harm. Remember that the cast doesn't have healing properties; it just keeps the fragments from getting joggled too much during the healing process.

Possible fractures are discussed further in Ankle Injuries **(S7)**, Knee Injuries **(S8)**, Arm Injuries **(S9),** and Head Injuries **(S10).**

A fracture that injures nearby nerves and arteries may result in a limb that is cold, blue, or numb. Fractures of the pelvis or thigh may be particularly serious, but they are relatively rare and usually involve great force, as in automobile accidents. In these situations, the need for immediate help is usually obvious.

Paleness, sweating, dizziness, and thirst can indicate shock, and immediate attention is needed. See Emergency Signs **(E1).**

Although broken ribs are generally diagnosed with X-rays, no particular treatment, other than taping and resting the affected ribs, is indicated. If you experience shortness of breath associated with a chest injury, there may have been an injury to the lung and a visit to the doctor is recommended; see Shortness of Breath **(S83).**

A crooked limb is an obvious reason to check for fracture. Pain that prevents any use of the injured limb suggests the need for an X-ray. Soft-tissue injuries, such as painful sprains, usually allow some use of the limb.

Although large bruises under the skin are usually caused by soft-tissue injuries alone, major bruising means a fracture is more likely.

HOME TREATMENT

Apply ice packs. The immediate application of cold will help decrease swelling and inflammation. The limb should be protected and rested for at least 48 hours. To rest a bone effectively, immobilize the joint above and below the bone. For example, if you suspect a fracture of the lower arm, you should prevent the wrist and elbow from moving. You can use magazines, cardboard, or rolled newspaper as splints. Don't wrap the limb tightly or you may cut off circulation. During this 48 hours, the limb should be cautiously tested to determine if the patient can use it at all and if it remains painful when moved.

Any injury that is still painful after 48 hours should be examined by a doctor. Minutes and hours aren't crucial unless the limb is crooked or there is injury to arteries or nerves. A broken limb that is adequately protected and rested is likely to have a good outcome even if casting or splinting is delayed. Acetaminophen, aspirin, ibuprofen, or naproxen can be used for pain **(M4).**

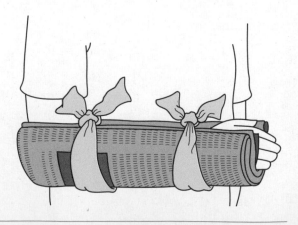

BROKEN BONE

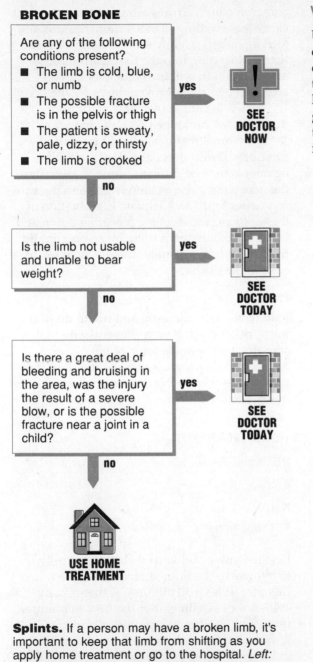

Are any of the following conditions present?
- The limb is cold, blue, or numb
- The possible fracture is in the pelvis or thigh
- The patient is sweaty, pale, dizzy, or thirsty
- The limb is crooked

yes →

SEE DOCTOR NOW

↓ **no**

Is the limb not usable and unable to bear weight?

yes →

SEE DOCTOR TODAY

↓ **no**

Is there a great deal of bleeding and bruising in the area, was the injury the result of a severe blow, or is the possible fracture near a joint in a child?

yes →

SEE DOCTOR TODAY

↓ **no**

USE HOME TREATMENT

Splints. If a person may have a broken limb, it's important to keep that limb from shifting as you apply home treatment or go to the hospital. *Left:* forearm splint made of rolled newspapers and cloths. *Right:* splint for one leg anchored by the other leg and by a board wrapped with a towel.

WHAT TO EXPECT AT THE DOCTOR'S OFFICE

Usually an X-ray will be required. In many offices and emergency rooms, a nurse or doctor's assistant will order the X-ray before the patient is even seen by a doctor. A crooked limb must be set, which sometimes requires general anesthesia. Pinning the fragments together surgically so that they will heal well is required for certain fractures.

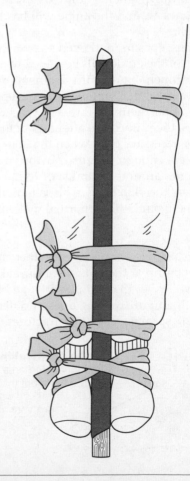

7 Ankle Injuries

Ligaments are tissues that connect the bones of a joint to provide stability during the joint's action. When the ankle is twisted severely, either the ligament or the bone must give way. If the ligaments give way, they may be stretched (strained), partially torn (sprained), or completely torn (torn ligaments). If the ligaments don't give way, one of the bones around the ankle will break (fracture).

Strains, sprains, and even some minor fractures of the ankle will heal well with home treatment. Some torn ligaments do well without a great deal of medical care; operations to repair them are rare. For practical purposes, the immediate attention of the doctor is necessary only when the injury has been severe enough to cause obvious fracture to the bones around the ankle or to cause a completely torn ligament. This is indicated by a deformed joint with abnormal motion.

Swelling

The typical ankle sprain swells either around the bony bump at the outside of the ankle or about two inches (5 cm) in front of and below it. The amount of swelling doesn't differentiate among sprains, tears, and fractures. The common chip fractures around the ankle often cause less swelling than a sprain. Sprains and torn ligaments usually swell quickly because there is bleeding into the tissue around the ankle. The skin will turn blue-black in the area as the blood is broken down by the body.

A swollen ankle that isn't deformed doesn't need prolonged rest, casting, or X-rays. Home treatment should be started promptly. Detection of any damage to the ligaments may be difficult immediately after the injury if much swelling is present. Because it is easier to do an adequate examination of the foot after the swelling has gone down and because no damage is done by resting a mild fracture or torn ligament, there is no need to rush to the doctor.

Pain

Pain tells you what to do and not to do. If it hurts, don't do it. If pain prevents any standing on the ankle after 24 hours, see a doctor. If little progress is being made so that pain makes weight-bearing difficult at 72 hours, see the doctor.

HOME TREATMENT

RIP is the key word:

- Rest
- Ice
- Protection

Rest the ankle and keep it elevated. Apply ice in a towel to the injured area and leave it there for at least 30 minutes. If there is any evidence of swelling after the first 30 minutes, then apply ice for 30 minutes on and 15 minutes off through the next few hours. If the ankle stops being painful while elevated, you may cautiously try to put weight on that leg. If the ankle is still painful when bearing

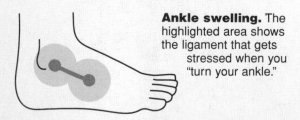

Ankle swelling. The highlighted area shows the ligament that gets stressed when you "turn your ankle."

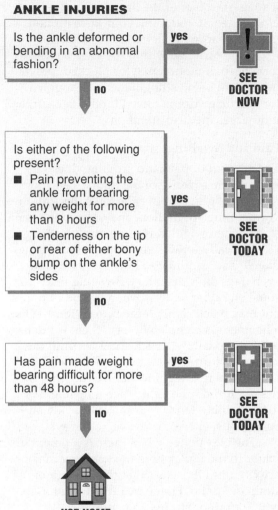

ANKLE INJURIES

Is the ankle deformed or bending in an abnormal fashion?

yes → SEE DOCTOR NOW

no ↓

Is either of the following present?
- Pain preventing the ankle from bearing any weight for more than 8 hours
- Tenderness on the tip or rear of either bony bump on the ankle's sides

yes → SEE DOCTOR TODAY

no ↓

Has pain made weight bearing difficult for more than 48 hours?

yes → SEE DOCTOR TODAY

no ↓

USE HOME TREATMENT

weight, you should avoid putting weight on that leg for the first 24 hours. Heat may be applied, but only after 24 hours.

An elastic bandage can help but won't prevent reinjury if you resume full activity **(M21).** Don't stretch the bandage so that it's very tight and interferes with blood circulation. You generally shouldn't try taping on children; if it's done incorrectly, it may cut off circulation to the foot.

The ankle should feel relatively normal in about ten days. Be warned, however, that full healing won't take place for four to six weeks. If strenuous activity, such as organized athletics, is to be pursued during this time, the ankle should be taped by someone experienced in this technique.

WHAT TO EXPECT AT THE DOCTOR'S OFFICE

The doctor will examine the motions of the ankle to see if they are abnormal and may have an X-ray taken. If there is no fracture or only a minor chip fracture, it is likely that a continuation of home treatment will be recommended. For other fractures, a cast will be necessary or, rarely, an operation to put the bones back together. An operation may be required to repair a completely torn ligament.

8 Knee Injuries

The ligaments of the knee may be stretched (strained), partially torn (sprained), or completely torn (torn ligaments). Unlike ankle ligament injuries, torn ligaments in the knee need to be repaired surgically as soon as possible after the injury occurs. If surgery is delayed, the operation is more difficult and less likely to be successful. For this reason, the approach to knee injuries is more cautious than for ankle injuries. If there is any possibility of a torn ligament, go to the doctor.

Fractures in the area of the knee are less common than around the ankle; they always need to be cared for by a doctor.

Knee injuries usually occur during sports, when the knee is more likely to experience twisting and side contact. (Deep knee bends stretch ligaments and may contribute to injuries; they should be avoided.) Serious knee injuries occur when the leg is planted on the ground and a blow is received to the knee from the side. If the foot can't give way, the knee will. There is no way to totally avoid this possibility in athletics. The use of shorter spikes and cleats helps, but knee braces and supports give little protection.

Abnormal Motion

When ligaments are completely torn, the lower leg can be wiggled from side to side when the leg is straight. Compare the injured knee to the opposite knee to get some idea of what amount of side-to-side motion is normal. If the knee slides front to back (called "the drawer sign"), this is even more serious, since it suggests a tear of the ligament in the front of the knee. If you think your knee motion may be abnormally loose, see a doctor.

If the cartilage within the knee has been torn, normal motion may be blocked, preventing it from being straightened. Although a torn cartilage doesn't need immediate surgery, it deserves medical attention.

Pain and Swelling

The amount of pain and swelling doesn't indicate the severity of the injury. The ability to bear weight, to move the knee through the normal range of motion, and to keep the knee stable when wiggled is more important.

Typically, strains and sprains hurt immediately and continue to hurt for hours and even days after the injury. Swelling tends to come on rather slowly over a period of hours but may reach rather large proportions. When a ligament is completely torn, there is intense pain immediately, which subsides until the knee may hurt little or not at all for a while. Usually there is significant bleeding into the tissues around the joint when a ligament is torn; swelling tends to come on quickly and be obvious, even impressive, to the eye.

The best policy when there is a potential injury to the ligament is to avoid any major activity until it is clear that this is a minor strain or sprain. Home treatment is intended only for minor strains and sprains.

HOME TREATMENT

RIP is the key word: rest, ice, and protection. Rest the knee and elevate it. Apply an ice pack, enclosed in a plastic bag or towel, for at least 30 minutes to minimize swelling. If there is more than slight swelling or pain despite the fact that the knee was immediately rested and ice was applied, see the doctor. If this

KNEE INJURIES

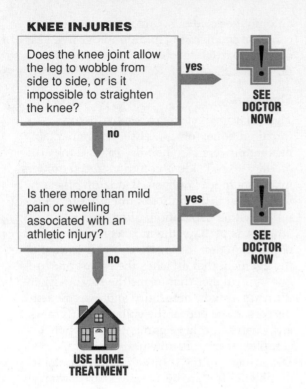

Does the knee joint allow the leg to wobble from side to side, or is it impossible to straighten the knee?

yes → SEE DOCTOR NOW

no

Is there more than mild pain or swelling associated with an athletic injury?

yes → SEE DOCTOR NOW

no

USE HOME TREATMENT

WHAT TO EXPECT AT THE DOCTOR'S OFFICE

The knee will be examined for abnormal motion. A massively swollen knee may have blood removed from the joint with a needle. Torn ligaments need surgical repair. X-rays may be taken but usually aren't helpful. For injuries that appear minor, home treatment will be advised. Pain medications are sometimes, but not often, required **(M4).**

isn't the case, apply the ice treatment on the knee for 30 minutes and then off for 15 minutes for the next several hours. Limited weight-bearing may be attempted during this time with a close watch for increased swelling and pain.

Heat can be applied after 24 hours. By then, the knee should look and feel relatively normal; after 72 hours this should clearly be the case. Remember, however, that a strain or sprain isn't completely healed for four to six weeks and requires protection during this healing period. Elastic bandages won't prevent reinjury but will ease symptoms a bit and remind the injured person to be careful with the knee **(M21).**

9 Arm Injuries

The ligaments of the wrist, shoulder, and elbow joints may be stretched (strained) or partially torn (sprained), but complete tears are rare. Fractures may occur at the wrist, are less frequent around the elbow, and are uncommon around the shoulder. Injuries often occur during a fall, when the weight of the body is caught on the outstretched arm.

Wrists

The wrist is the most frequently injured joint in the arm. Strains and sprains are common, and the small bones in the wrist may be fractured. Fractures of these small bones may be difficult to see on an X-ray. The most frequent fracture of the wrist involves the ends of the long bones of the forearm and is easily recognized because it causes an unnatural bend near the wrist. Physicians refer to this as the "silver fork deformity."

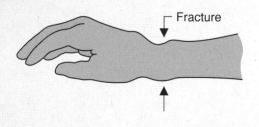

⌐ Fracture

Elbows

"Tennis elbow" is the most frequent elbow injury; if you think this is the problem, consult Elbow Pain **(S70).** Other injuries are much less frequent and usually result from falls, automobile accidents, or contact sports. A common problem in children under five years of age is partial dislocations due to adults pulling on the arm.

Shoulders

The collarbone (clavicle) is a frequently fractured bone; fortunately, it has remarkable healing powers. An inability to raise the arm on the affected side is common; the shoulders may also appear uneven. Bandaging the arm to the chest is the only treatment required.

Shoulder separation, often seen in athletes, is perhaps the most common injury of the shoulder. It is a stretching or tearing of the ligament that attaches the collarbone to one of the bones that forms the shoulder joint. It causes a slight deformity and extreme tenderness at the end of the collarbone. Sprains and strains of other ligaments occur, but complete tearing is unusual, as are fractures. Dislocations of the shoulder are rare outside of athletics but are best treated early when they do occur.

In summary, severe fractures and dislocations are best treated early. These usually cause deformity and severe pain and limit movement. Other fractures won't be harmed by delayed treatment if the injured limb is rested and protected. Complete tears of ligaments are rare; strains and sprains will heal with home treatment.

HOME TREATMENT

RIP is the key word: rest, ice, and protection. Rest the arm and apply ice wrapped in a towel for at least 30 minutes. If the pain is gone and there is no swelling at the end of this time, you can stop the ice treatment. A sling for shoulder and elbow injuries and a partial splint for wrist injuries will give protection and rest to the injury while

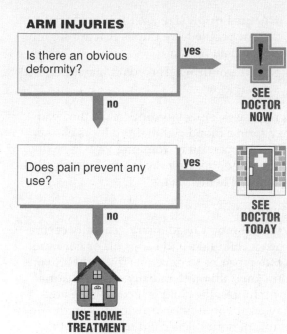

ARM INJURIES

Is there an obvious deformity?

yes → SEE DOCTOR NOW

no ↓

Does pain prevent any use?

yes → SEE DOCTOR TODAY

no ↓

USE HOME TREATMENT

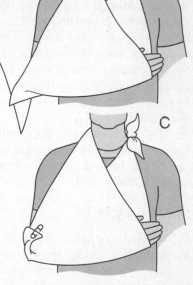

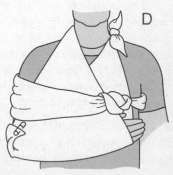

Tying an arm sling.

(A) Use a triangular piece of cloth (or a folded square sheet). A small folded towel adds support.

(B) Tie as shown.

(C) A safety pin will hold it securely.

(D) To add even greater security, tie another strip of cloth around the chest and arm as shown.

allowing the patient to move around. Continue ice treatment for 30 minutes on and 15 minutes off through the first eight hours if swelling appears.

Heat can be applied after 24 hours. The injured joint should be usable with little pain within 24 hours and should be almost normal by 72 hours. If not, see the doctor. Complete healing takes from four to six weeks, and activities with a likelihood of reinjury should be avoided during this time.

WHAT TO EXPECT AT THE DOCTOR'S OFFICE

An examination and sometimes X-rays will be performed. A cast or sling can be applied. Pain medication is sometimes given, but acetaminophen or other nonprescription medication (**M4**) is usually adequate. Certain fractures, especially those around the elbow, may require surgery.

10 Head Injuries

Head injuries are potentially serious, but few lead to problems. A concussion or a head injury that has led to a loss of consciousness requires emergency care.

If the skull isn't obviously damaged, bleeding inside the skull is the major concern. The accumulation of blood inside the skull may eventually put pressure on the brain and cause damage. Fortunately, the valuable contents of the skull are carefully cushioned. Careful observation is the most valuable tool for diagnosing serious head injury. Usually this can be done as well at home as in the hospital; there is some risk either way, so it is your choice.

The questions in the decision chart will help you distinguish between a brain injury, which can be serious, and a head injury, which usually isn't.

HOME TREATMENT

Ice applied to a bruised area may minimize swelling, but "goose eggs" often develop anyway. The size of the bump doesn't indicate the severity of the injury.

The initial observation period is crucial. Symptoms of bleeding inside the head usually occur within the first 24 to 72 hours. Check the patient every 2 hours during the first 24 hours, every 4 hours during the second 24, and every 8 hours during the third. Look for the following symptoms:

- **Loss of alertness:** Increasing lethargy, unresponsiveness, and *abnormally* deep sleep can precede coma.

- **Unequal pupil size** *after* **injury:** About 25% of people have pupils that are slightly unequal all the time.

- **Severe vomiting:** The vomit may be ejected several feet.

In rare cases, slow bleeding inside the head may form a blood clot that produces chronic headache, persistent vomiting, or personality changes months after the injury. This is called a subdural hematoma.

Minor Injury

A typical minor head injury generally occurs when a child falls and bangs his or her head. A bump begins to develop. The child remains conscious, although initially stunned. For a few minutes, the child is inconsolable and may even vomit once or twice during the first couple of hours. The child may nap but is easily aroused. Neither pupil is enlarged, and the vomiting ceases after a short time. Within eight hours, the child is back to normal except for the tender "goose egg." If bleeding occurs after such a head injury, see Cuts **(S1).**

Severe Injury

In a more severe head injury, symptoms usually take longer to develop. Two or more of the danger signs are often present at the same time. The individual remains lethargic and isn't easily aroused. A pupil may enlarge. Vomiting is usually forceful, repeated, and progressively worse. If in doubt, call your doctor.

Because most accidents occur in the evening hours, the injured person will generally be asleep several hours after the accident. You can look in on the person periodically to check pulse, pupils, and arousability if you are concerned. With minor head bumps and no signs of brain injury, nighttime checking is usually not necessary.

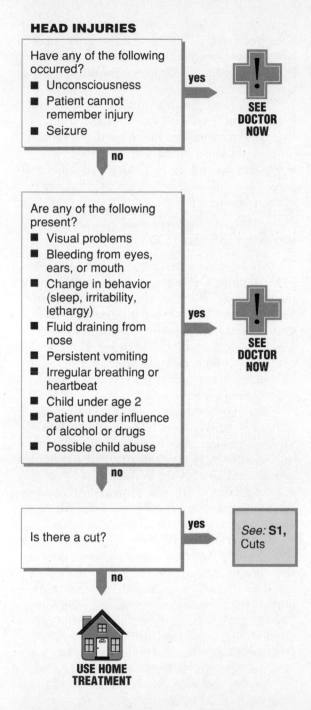

HEAD INJURIES

Have any of the following occurred?
- Unconsciousness
- Patient cannot remember injury
- Seizure

yes → **SEE DOCTOR NOW**

no ↓

Are any of the following present?
- Visual problems
- Bleeding from eyes, ears, or mouth
- Change in behavior (sleep, irritability, lethargy)
- Fluid draining from nose
- Persistent vomiting
- Irregular breathing or heartbeat
- Child under age 2
- Patient under influence of alcohol or drugs
- Possible child abuse

yes → **SEE DOCTOR NOW**

no ↓

Is there a cut?

yes → *See:* **S1,** Cuts

no ↓

USE HOME TREATMENT

WHAT TO EXPECT AT THE DOCTOR'S OFFICE

It is hard to diagnose bleeding within the skull with great accuracy. Skull X-rays are seldom helpful except in detecting whether a fragment of bone from the skull has been pushed into the brain, but this situation is rare. A CT scan or MRI can be helpful but is expensive and may miss early accumulations of blood. With severe injuries, neck X-rays may be required.

The doctor will ask for a description of the accident, assess the patient's appearance, and check blood pressure and pulse rate. In addition, the head, eyes, ears, nose, throat, neck, and nervous system will be examined. The doctor will also check for other possible sites of injury. When internal bleeding is possible but not certain, the patient may be hospitalized for observation. During this observation period the pulse, pupils, and blood pressure will be checked periodically. In short, the doctor will observe and wait, much as would be done at home. The doctor will avoid giving the patient medicines that may hide symptoms.

11 Burns

How can you tell how bad a burn is? Burns are classified according to depth.

First-degree Burns

First-degree burns are superficial and cause the skin to turn red. A sunburn is usually a first-degree burn; for more information on sunburn, see Sunburn (S51).

First-degree burns may cause a lot of pain but aren't a major medical problem. Even when they are extensive, they seldom result in lasting problems and seldom need a doctor's attention.

Second-degree Burns

Second-degree burns are deeper and result in splitting of the skin layers or blistering. Scalding with hot water and a very severe sunburn with blisters are common instances of second-degree burns.

Second-degree burns are also painful and, if extensive, may cause significant fluid loss. Scarring, however, is usually minimal, and infection usually isn't a problem.

Second-degree burns can be treated at home if they aren't extensive. Any second-degree burn that involves an area larger than the patient's hand should be seen by a doctor. In addition, a second-degree burn that involves the face or hands should be seen by a doctor. It might result in cosmetic problems or loss of function.

Third-degree Burns

Third-degree burns destroy all layers of the skin and extend into the deeper tissues. Such areas are painless because nerve endings have been destroyed. (Painless third-degree burns may be surrounded by painful second-degree burns, however.) Charring of the burned tissue is usually obvious.

Third-degree burns result in scarring and present problems with infection and fluid loss. The more extensive the burn, the more difficult these problems. All third-degree burns should be seen by a doctor because of these problems and because skin grafts are often needed.

HOME TREATMENT

Apply cold water or ice immediately. This reduces the amount of skin damage caused by the burn and also eases pain. The cold should be applied for at least five minutes and continued until pain is relieved or for one hour, whichever comes first. Be careful not to apply cold so long that the burned area turns numb — that could cause frostbite! Reapply treatment if pain returns.

You may use acetaminophen, aspirin, ibuprofen, or naproxen to reduce pain (M4).

Blisters shouldn't be broken. If they burst by themselves, as they often do, the overlying skin should be allowed to remain as a wet dressing. Let the skin underneath toughen up, keep the area clean, and protect yourself against the cause of the blisters next time.

Local anesthetic creams or sprays may relieve pain, but some doctors believe they slow healing. Also, some patients develop an irritation or allergy to these drugs. Don't use butter, cream, or ointments (such as Vaseline). They may slow healing and increase the possibility of infection. Antibiotic creams (Neosporin, Bacitracin, etc.) probably neither help nor hurt minor burns.

Any burn that stays painful for more than 48 hours should be seen by a doctor.

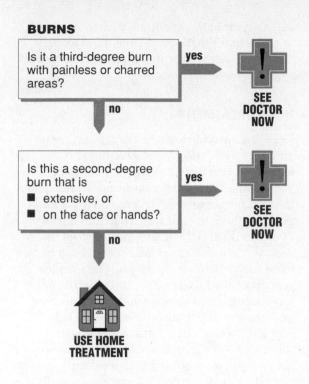

BURNS

Is it a third-degree burn with painless or charred areas? — **yes** → **SEE DOCTOR NOW**

no ↓

Is this a second-degree burn that is
- extensive, or
- on the face or hands?

yes → **SEE DOCTOR NOW**

no ↓

USE HOME TREATMENT

WHAT TO EXPECT AT THE DOCTOR'S OFFICE

The doctor will establish the extent and degree of the burn and will determine if the patient needs antibiotics, hospitalization, and skin grafting. A doctor may recommend a dressing (bandage) with an antibacterial ointment. This dressing must be changed, and the burn checked for infection frequently. Extensive burns may require hospitalization, and third-degree burns may eventually require skin grafts.

12 Infected Wounds and Blood Poisoning

To a doctor, blood poisoning means bacterial infection in the bloodstream and is termed "septicemia." This is a serious condition. Fever is an indication of this rare complication of an infected wound. The patient usually feels terrible, not simply because of the pain from the wound.

An infected wound usually festers beneath the surface of the skin, resulting in pain and swelling. Bacterial infection requires at least a day, and usually two or three days, to develop. Therefore, a late increase in pain or swelling is a legitimate cause for concern. If the festering wound bursts open, pus will drain out. This is good, and the wound will usually heal well. Still, this demonstrates that an infection was present, and a doctor should evaluate the situation unless it is clearly minor.

Normal Wound Healing

An explanation of normal wound healing will be helpful.

1. The body pours out serum into a wound area. Serum is yellowish and clear, and later turns into a scab. Serum is frequently mistaken for pus. Pus is thick, cheesy, smelly, and never seen in the first day or so.

2. The edges of a wound will be pink or red, and the wound area may be warm. Such inflammation is normal.

3. The lymphatic system helps remove dead cells from the wound. Thus, pain along lymph channels or in the lymph nodes can occur without infection.

HOME TREATMENT

Keep the wound clean. Leave it open to the air unless it is unsightly, oozes blood or serum, or gets dirty easily. If so, bandage it, but change the bandage daily. Soak and clean the wound gently with warm water for short periods, three or four times daily, to remove debris and keep the scab soft. Children like to pick at scabs and often fall on a scab. In these instances, a bandage is useful. The simplest wound of the face requires three to five days for healing. The healing period for the chest and arms is five to nine days, for the legs it is seven to twelve days. Larger wounds, or those that have gaped open and must heal across a space, require correspondingly longer periods to heal. Children heal more rapidly than adults. If a wound fails to heal within the expected time, call the doctor.

WHAT TO EXPECT AT THE DOCTOR'S OFFICE

An examination of the wound and regional lymph nodes will be done, and the patient's temperature will be taken. Sometimes cultures of the blood or the wound are performed, and antibiotics may be prescribed. If there is a suspicion of bacterial infection, cultures may be taken before the antibiotics are given. If a wound is festering, it may be drained either with a needle or a scalpel. This is not very painful and actually relieves discomfort. For severe wound infections, the patient may need to stay in the hospital.

INFECTED WOUNDS

Is there fever above 99.9°F (37.7°C), and does the person feel generally ill?

yes → 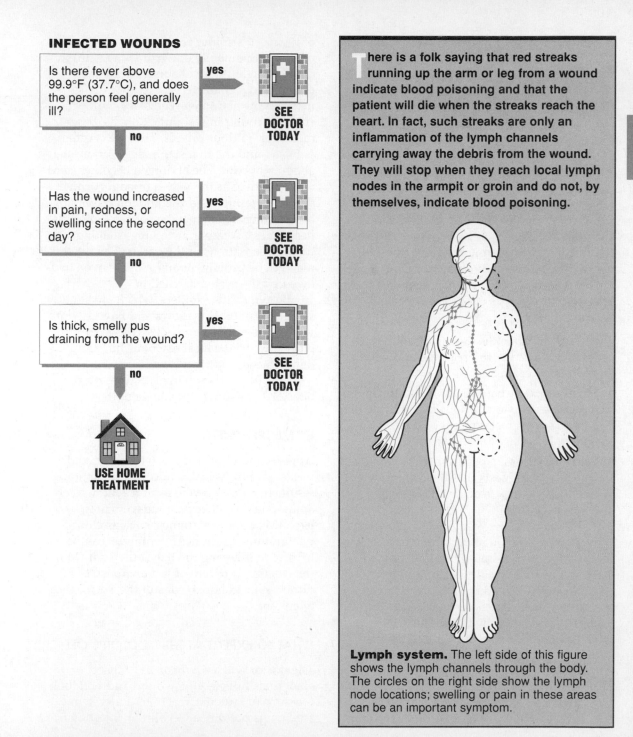 **SEE DOCTOR TODAY**

no ↓

Has the wound increased in pain, redness, or swelling since the second day?

yes → **SEE DOCTOR TODAY**

no ↓

Is thick, smelly pus draining from the wound?

yes → **SEE DOCTOR TODAY**

no ↓

USE HOME TREATMENT

There is a folk saying that red streaks running up the arm or leg from a wound indicate blood poisoning and that the patient will die when the streaks reach the heart. In fact, such streaks are only an inflammation of the lymph channels carrying away the debris from the wound. They will stop when they reach local lymph nodes in the armpit or groin and do not, by themselves, indicate blood poisoning.

Lymph system. The left side of this figure shows the lymph channels through the body. The circles on the right side show the lymph node locations; swelling or pain in these areas can be an important symptom.

13 Insect Bites or Stings

Most insect bites are trivial, but some bites or stings may cause reactions. Local reactions consist of pain, swelling, and redness at the site of the bite or sting. They are uncomfortable but don't pose a serious hazard.

In contrast, systemic reactions (those that involve the whole body) may occasionally be serious and may require emergency treatment. There are three types of systemic reaction. All are rare.

- An **asthma attack** is the most common, causing difficulty in breathing and perhaps audible wheezing.

- **Hives** or extensive skin rashes following insect bites are less serious but indicate that a more severe reaction might occur if the patient is bitten or stung again.

- **Fainting** or loss of consciousness rarely occurs and suggests that the collapse is due to an allergic reaction. This is an emergency **(E1).**

If the person has had any of these reactions in the past, he or she should be taken immediately to a medical facility if stung or bitten.

If the local reaction to a bite or sting is severe or a deep sore is developing, a doctor should be consulted by telephone. Children often have more severe local reactions than adults.

Spider Bites

Bites from poisonous spiders are rare. The female black widow spider accounts for many of them. This spider is glossy black with a body approximately one-half inch (1 cm) in diameter, a leg span of about two inches (5 cm), and a characteristic red hourglass mark on the abdomen. The black widow spider is found in woodpiles, sheds, basements, or outdoor privies. The bite is often painless, and the first sign may be cramping abdominal pain. The abdomen becomes hard and boardlike as the waves of pain become severe. Breathing is difficult and accompanied by grunting. There may be nausea, vomiting, headaches, sweating, twitching, shaking, and tingling sensations of the hands. The bite itself may not be prominent and may be overshadowed by the systemic reaction.

Brown recluse spiders, which are slightly smaller than black widows and have a white violin pattern on their backs, cause painful bites and serious local reactions but aren't as dangerous as black widows.

This book has separate sections on the bites of Ticks **(S53)** and Chiggers **(S54).**

HOME TREATMENT

Apply something cold, such as ice or cold packs, promptly. Delay in cold applications results in a more severe local reaction. Acetaminophen or other pain relievers may be used **(M4).** Antihistamines, such as chlorpheniramine or diphenhydramine, can be helpful in relieving the itch somewhat **(M8).** If the reaction is severe or if pain doesn't diminish in 48 hours, consult the doctor by telephone.

WHAT TO EXPECT AT THE DOCTOR'S OFFICE

The doctor will ask what sort of insect or spider has inflicted the wound and will look for signs of systemic reaction. If a systemic reaction is present, adrenalin by injection is

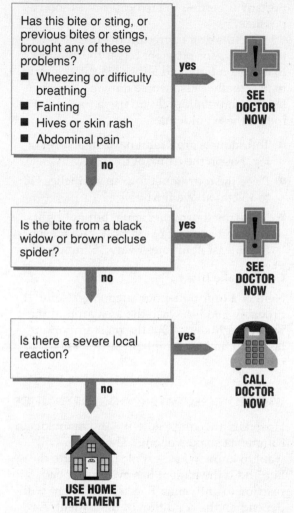

INSECT BITES

Has this bite or sting, or previous bites or stings, brought any of these problems?
- Wheezing or difficulty breathing
- Fainting
- Hives or skin rash
- Abdominal pain

yes → **SEE DOCTOR NOW**

no ↓

Is the bite from a black widow or brown recluse spider?

yes → **SEE DOCTOR NOW**

no ↓

Is there a severe local reaction?

yes → **CALL DOCTOR NOW**

no ↓

USE HOME TREATMENT

other cases pain relievers or antihistamines may make the patient more comfortable. Adrenalin injections are occasionally used for very severe local reactions.

If a systemic reaction has occurred, the doctor may give shots to try to desensitize the patient's body to the insect's poison. People with serious allergies to insect bites can buy emergency kits (such as EpiPen) to cut off systemic reactions.

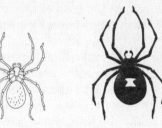

Poisonous spiders. *Left:* Brown recluse, shown from above. *Right:* Black widow, shown from below. Both spiders appear at approximate actual size.

usually necessary. Rarely, measures to support breathing or blood pressure will be needed; these measures require an emergency room or hospital.

If the problem is a local reaction, the doctor will examine the wound for signs of dead tissue or infection. Occasionally the wound will need to be drained surgically. In

14 Snake Bites

North America's poisonous snakes come in two groups: coral snakes and pit vipers, which include rattlesnakes, copperheads, and cottonmouths. At least one species of poisonous snake is found in each of the contiguous United States except Maine, Delaware, and Michigan.

Of the 45,000 snake bites reported each year in the U.S., only 20% are made by poisonous snakes. Those snakes don't inject venom with every bite. All told, fewer than 20 people actually die from snake bite each year. The major damage caused by poisonous snake bites is loss of function in an arm or leg.

HOME TREATMENT

Experts agree that the most important steps for snake bites are:

1. Correct identification of the snake
2. A quick trip to the hospital

Pit viper bites

Most experts believe that trying to suck the venom out of the wound makes sense if you can do it within three minutes after the bite. Use a suction cup, if possible, but in emergencies you can use your mouth, quickly spitting out the venom and blood. Experts don't agree on the benefit of making cuts over the bite in an attempt to remove venom. Don't apply cold to the bite. Don't lie flat; keep the bite lower than the heart. It is helpful for the patient not to use the arm or leg with the bite

and to rest, but these actions aren't as important as getting to medical care as soon as possible.

Doctors don't agree on the use of tourniquets for pit viper bites. Tourniquets that are too tight and left in place too long may actually cause worse damage and even lead to amputation. If you use a tourniquet, follow these guidelines:

- Tourniquets are useful only on an arm or leg, not on the trunk of the body.
- Place the tourniquet four to six inches (10 to 15 cm) above the bite.
- Make the tourniquet snug, but not tight enough to cut off blood flow, and loosen it for at least 2 minutes every 15 minutes.

Coral snake bites

Neither a tourniquet nor suction is useful. It's probably good to wash the area around the wound right away. But the most important task is to find medical help as quickly as possible.

WHAT TO EXPECT AT THE DOCTOR'S OFFICE

Hospitals are equipped with antivenin kits to counteract snake venoms. The doctor will want to know what sort of snake made the bite and if the patient has ever had a bad reaction to antivenin. Further treatment will depend on the condition of the patient. As stated above, most snake bites, even from poisonous snakes, are not fatal.

SNAKE BITES

Did the bite come from a coral snake? — yes → **SEE DOCTOR NOW**

no ↓

Did the bite come from a pit viper? — yes → If the bite occurred less than 3 minutes before, suck out the poison, and… → **SEE DOCTOR NOW**

no ↓

Have you identified the type of snake? — yes → *See:* **S2,** Puncture Wounds

no ↓

SEE DOCTOR NOW

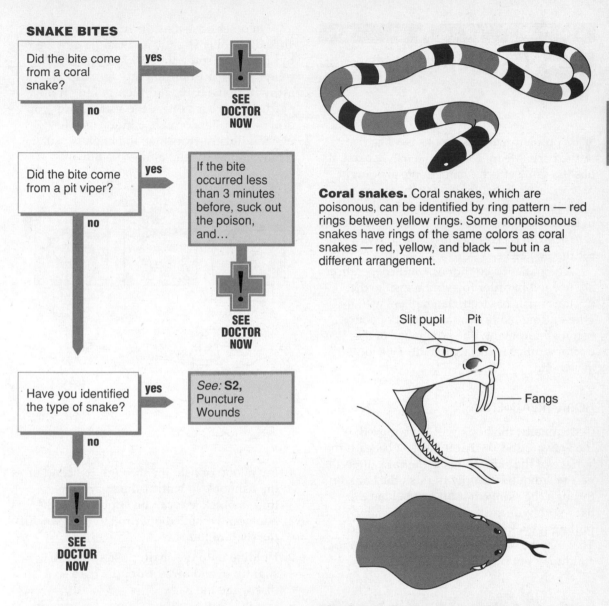

Coral snakes. Coral snakes, which are poisonous, can be identified by ring pattern — red rings between yellow rings. Some nonpoisonous snakes have rings of the same colors as coral snakes — red, yellow, and black — but in a different arrangement.

Slit pupil   Pit

Fangs

Pit vipers. *Top:* The pit viper's "pits" are small depressions located between the eye and nostril on either side of the snake's head. *Bottom:* Venom glands on either side of the head (inside the mouth) create the distinctive triangular head shape the pit viper has when viewed from above.

15 Fishhooks

The problem with fishhooks is, of course, the barb. Meant to keep the fish hooked, it has the same effect when people are caught. Nevertheless, a fishhook usually can be removed without a doctor's help, unless it is in someone's eye. *Never try to remove hooks that have actually penetrated the eyeball*; this is a job for the doctor.

The patient's confidence and cooperation are needed in order to avoid a visit to the doctor. A pair of electrician's pliers with a wire-cutting blade should be part of your fishing equipment. The advantage of the doctor's office is the availability of a local anesthetic.

HOME TREATMENT

Occasionally, the hook will have moved all the way around so that it lies just beneath the surface of the skin. If this is the case, often the best technique is simply to push the hook on through the skin, cut it off just behind the barb with wire cutters, and remove it by pulling it back through the way it entered. This may be somewhat painful; the average child may not be able to tolerate it.

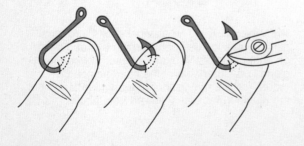

On other occasions the hook will be embedded only slightly and can be removed by simply grasping the shank of the hook (pliers help), pushing slightly forward and away from the barb, and then pulling it out.

If the barb isn't near the surface or if you don't have pliers or wire cutters, use the method illustrated below; the hook is usually removed quickly and almost painlessly.

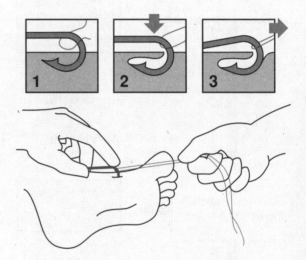

1. Put a loop of fish line through the bend of the fishhook so that, at the appropriate time, a quick jerk can be applied and the hook can be pulled out directly in line with the shaft of the hook.

2. Holding onto the shaft, push the hook slightly in and away from the barb so as to disengage the barb.

3. Holding this pressure constant to keep the barb disengaged, give a quick jerk on the fish line and the hook will pop out.

If you aren't successful, push the hook all the way through and out so that the barb can be cut off with wire cutters.

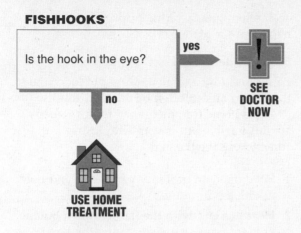

FISHHOOKS

Is the hook in the eye?

yes → **SEE DOCTOR NOW**

no ↓ **USE HOME TREATMENT**

A **splinter** under the skin can often be pulled out with tweezers. If some material remains, you can usually dislodge it by picking away at the overlying skin with a clean needle. Sterilize the needle first by dipping it in rubbing alcohol or holding it in a match flame. Another option is to soak the area of skin twice a day in a cup of very warm, but not hot, water mixed with one tablespoon (15 ml) of baking soda **(M2);** the splinter will probably come out by itself in a day or two. Don't let a splinter wound become infected.

Be sure that the person's tetanus shots are up to date **(S5).** Treat the wound as in the home treatment section for Puncture Wounds **(S2).** If all else fails, a visit to the doctor should solve the problem.

WHAT TO EXPECT AT THE DOCTOR'S OFFICE

The doctor will use one of the three methods above to remove the hook. If necessary, the area around the hook can be numbed with a local anesthetic before the hook is removed. Often, however, injecting a local anesthetic is more painful than just removing the hook without the anesthetic.

If the hook is in the eye, it's likely that the doctor will recommend the help of an eye specialist (ophthalmologist), and it may be necessary to remove the hook in the operating room.

SYMPTOM   S16

16 Smashed Fingers

Smashing fingers in car doors or desk drawers, or with hammers or baseballs, is all too common. If the injury involves only the end segment of the finger (the terminal phalanx) and doesn't involve a significant cut, the help of a doctor is seldom needed. Blood under the fingernail (subungual hematoma) is a painful problem that you can treat.

Joint Fractures

Fractures of the bone in the end segment of the finger aren't treated unless they involve the joint. Many doctors feel that it is unwise to splint the finger even if there is a fracture of the joint. Although the splint will decrease pain, it may also increase the stiffness of the joint after healing. However, if the fracture isn't splinted, the pain may persist longer, and you may end up with a stiff joint anyway. Discuss the advantages and disadvantages of splinting with your doctor.

Dislocated Nails

Fingernails are often dislocated in these injuries. It isn't necessary to have the entire fingernail removed. The nail that is detached should be clipped off to avoid catching it on other objects. Nails will take from four to six weeks to grow back.

HOME TREATMENT

If the injury doesn't involve other parts of the finger and if the finger can be moved easily, apply an ice pack for swelling and use acetaminophen, aspirin, ibuprofen, or naproxen for pain **(M4).**

Blood Under a Nail

Pain caused by a large amount of blood under the fingernail can often be relieved simply.

This home (or emergency room) remedy sounds terrible but is very simple and can sometimes save the nail.

1. Bend open an ordinary paper clip and hold it with a pair of pliers.
2. Heat one end with the flame from a butane lighter or gas stove, steadying the hand holding the pliers with the opposite hand.
3. When the tip is very hot, touch it to the nail; it will melt its way through the fingernail, leaving a clean, small, painless hole. There is no need to press down hard. Take your time, lifting the paper clip to see if you are through the nail; usually the blood will spurt a little when you are through. Reheat the paper clip if necessary.

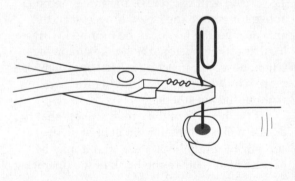

The blood trapped beneath the nail can now escape through the small hole, and the pain will be relieved as the pressure is released. If the hole closes and the blood reaccumulates, the procedure can be repeated using the same hole once again.

SMASHED FINGERS

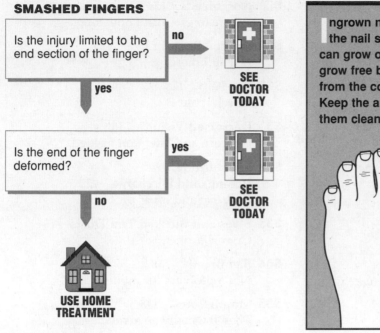

Is the injury limited to the end section of the finger? — **no** → **SEE DOCTOR TODAY**

yes ↓

Is the end of the finger deformed? — **yes** → **SEE DOCTOR TODAY**

no ↓

USE HOME TREATMENT

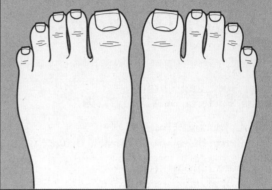

Ingrown nails can be treated at home. Cut the nail straight across so that its corner can grow outside the skin. Let the nail grow free by firmly pushing the skin back from the corner with a Q-tip twice a day. Keep the area clean. For **hangnails,** keep them clean. Don't chew on them.

WHAT TO EXPECT AT THE DOCTOR'S OFFICE

The doctor will examine the finger. An X-ray is likely if it appears that more than the end segment is involved. If there is a fracture involving the last joint on the finger, you should expect a discussion of the advantages and disadvantages of splinting the finger. Often the injured finger is splinted by bandaging it together with an adjacent finger. If the finger is splinted, exercise it periodically to keep it mobile. Severe finger injuries may occasionally require surgery.

CHAPTER 4

Ears, Nose, Throat, Eyes, and Mouth Problems

EARS, NOSE, AND THROAT: VIRUS, BACTERIA, OR ALLERGY?

The first part of this chapter discusses upper respiratory problems, including colds and flu, sore throats, ear pain or stuffiness, runny nose, cough, hoarseness, swollen glands, and nosebleeds. A central question is important to each of these complaints: Is it caused by a virus, bacteria, or an allergic reaction? In general, the doctor has more effective treatment than is available at home only for bacterial infections. Viral infections and allergies don't improve with treatment by penicillin or other antibiotics. To demand a "penicillin shot" for a cold or allergy is to ask for a drug reaction, risk a more serious "superinfection," and waste time and money.

Among common problems well treated at home are:

- The common cold, often termed "viral URI (Upper Respiratory Infection)" by doctors
- The flu, when uncomplicated
- Hay fever
- Mononucleosis — infectious mononucleosis or "mono"

Medical treatment is commonly required for:

- Strep throat
- Ear infection

How can you tell these conditions apart? Table 6 and the decision charts for the symptoms discussed in this chapter will usually suffice. Here are some brief descriptions that may also help.

Viral Syndromes

Viruses usually involve several portions of the body and cause many different symptoms.

Three basic patterns (or syndromes) are common in viral illnesses; however, overlap among these three syndromes is not unusual. Your illness may have features of each.

Viral URI. This is the "common cold." It includes some combination of the following: sore throat, runny nose, stuffy or congested ears, hoarseness, swollen glands, and fever. One symptom usually precedes the others, and another symptom (usually hoarseness or cough) may remain after the others have disappeared.

The Flu. Fever may be quite high. Headache can be excruciating, muscle aches and pain (especially in the lower back and eye muscles) are equally troublesome.

Viral Gastroenteritis. This is "stomach flu" with nausea, vomiting, diarrhea, and crampy abdominal pain. It may be incapacitating and can mimic a variety of other more serious conditions, including appendicitis.

Hay Fever

Allergic rhinitis is commonly called "hay fever" even though it's not a fever and not caused by hay. It is, however, the most common problem caused by allergies. A stuffy, runny nose, watering itchy eyes, headache, and sneezing are all common symptoms. Hay fever seems to run in families. Patients usually diagnose this condition accurately themselves.

As with viruses, hay fever is treated simply to relieve symptoms. Given enough time, the condition runs its course without doing any permanent harm. Avoiding the offending allergen is often the best preventive action. The cause in infants is often dust or food; in adults, it's dust or pollens.

TABLE 6   *Virus, Bacteria, or Allergy?*

	Virus	Bacteria	Allergy
Runny nose?	Often	Rare	Often
Aching muscles?	Usual	Rare	Never
Headache (non-sinus)?	Often	Rare	Never
Dizzy?	Often	Rare	Rare
Fever?	Often	Often	Never
Cough?	Often	Sometimes	Rare
Dry cough?	Often	Rare	Sometimes
Raising sputum?	Rare	Often	Rare
Hoarseness?	Often	Rare	Sometimes
Recurs at a particular season?	No	No	Often
Only a single complaint? (sore throat, earache, sinus pain, or cough)	Unusual	Usual	Unusual
Do antibiotics help?	No	Yes	No
Can the doctor help?	Seldom	Yes	Sometimes

Remember, viral infections and allergies **do not** *improve with treatment by penicillin or other antibiotics.*

Antihistamines block the action of histamine, a substance released during allergic reactions. They also have a drying effect on the runny nose and alleviate nasal stuffiness. Some antihistamines are available over-the-counter. Their most common side effect is drowsiness, and this may interfere with work or school. Decongestants (pseudoephedrine, etc.) can be added to antihistamine medication. They may help with the runny nose as well as combat the sleepiness **(M8).**

Sinusitis

Inflammation of the sinuses is often associated with hay fever and asthma. Symptoms include a sense of heaviness behind the nose and eyes, often resulting in a "sinus headache." If the sinuses are infected, there may be fever and nasal discharge. Antihistamines and decongestants **(M8)** may be helpful in cases of sinusitis that accompany colds or hay fever. Don't use nasal sprays **(M9)** for more than three days. For recurring sinusitis, consult a doctor to determine the precise cause and treatment; a course of antibiotics is frequently prescribed.

Strep Throat

Bacterial infections tend to localize at a single point. Involvement of the respiratory tract by strep is usually limited to the throat. However, symptoms outside the respiratory tract can occur, most commonly fever and swollen lymph glands (from draining the infection) in the neck. A scarlet fever rash sometimes may help to distinguish a streptococcal (strep) from a viral infection. In children, abdominal pain may be associated with a strep throat. This disorder must be diagnosed and treated because serious heart and kidney complications can follow if adequate antibiotic therapy isn't given.

Other Conditions

Factors other than diseases may cause or contribute to upper respiratory symptoms. Smoking is probably the largest single cause of coughs and sore throats. Pollution (smog) can produce the same problems. Tumors and other frightening conditions account for only a very small number. Complaints lasting beyond two weeks without one of the common diseases as the obvious cause aren't alarming but should be investigated by the doctor.

17 Colds and Flu

Most doctors believe that colds and the flu account for more unnecessary visits than any other group of problems. Because these are viral illnesses, they can't be cured by antibiotics or any other drugs. However, there are nonprescription drugs — pain relievers, decongestants, antihistamines — that may decrease symptoms while these problems cure themselves.

There seem to be three main reasons why colds and flu result in unnecessary doctor visits:

- A few patients aren't sure that their illness is a cold or the flu.

- Many come seeking a cure, though there is none.

- Many patients feel so sick that they believe the doctor must be able to do *something*. Faced with this expectation, doctors sometimes try too hard, giving an antibiotic, performing tests, or taking X-rays that aren't really needed.

Of course, complications from colds and flu do lead to necessary visits as well, most often to treat bacterial ear infections and bacterial pneumonia. In very young children viral infections of the lung may lead to complications. The questions in the decision chart will help you look for complications.

HOME TREATMENT

Take two aspirin and call me in the morning. This familiar phrase doesn't indicate neglect or lack of sympathy. Acetaminophen, aspirin, ibuprofen, and naproxen are effective remedies for the fever and muscular aches of the common cold. The fever, aches, and exhaustion are most pronounced in the afternoon and evening, so take medications regularly over this period. Because of the rare but serious problem of the brain and liver known as Reye's syndrome, give children and teenagers acetaminophen instead of aspirin **(M4).**

You may buy a patent cold formula but remember that the formulas are simply combinations of drugs available singly without a prescription. The combination you buy may not be right for your symptoms and may cost more than a more effective single drug **(M10).**

Drink a lot of liquid. This is insurance. The body requires more fluid when you have a fever. Be sure you get enough. Fluids help to keep the mucus more liquid and help prevent complications such as bronchitis and ear infection. A vaporizer (particularly in the winter) will help liquefy secretions.

Rest. How you feel is an indication of your need to rest. If you feel like being up and about, go ahead. It won't prolong your illness, and your friends and family were exposed during the incubation period, the three days or so before you had symptoms.

For relief of particular symptoms, see the appropriate sections of this book: Runny Nose **(S22),** Ear Pain and Stuffiness **(S19),** Sore Throat **(S18),** Cough **(S23),** Nausea and Vomiting **(S85),** Diarrhea **(S86),** and so on.

If symptoms persist beyond two weeks, call the doctor.

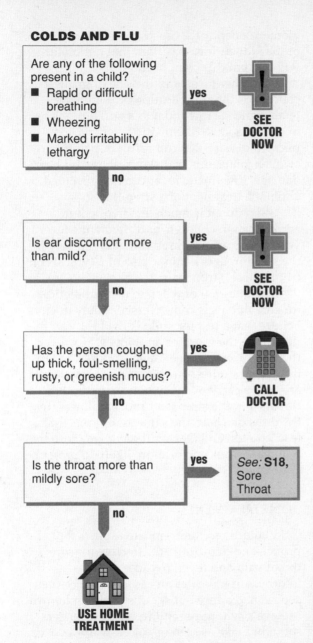

COLDS AND FLU

Are any of the following present in a child?
- Rapid or difficult breathing
- Wheezing
- Marked irritability or lethargy

yes → SEE DOCTOR NOW

no ↓

Is ear discomfort more than mild?

yes → SEE DOCTOR NOW

no ↓

Has the person coughed up thick, foul-smelling, rusty, or greenish mucus?

yes → CALL DOCTOR

no ↓

Is the throat more than mildly sore?

yes → *See:* S18, Sore Throat

no ↓

USE HOME TREATMENT

WHAT TO EXPECT AT THE DOCTOR'S OFFICE

The ears, nose, throat, and chest will be examined, and the abdomen may be examined. If a bacterial pneumonia is suspected, a chest X-ray may be done, but X-rays rarely help. If a bacterial infection is present, antibiotics will be prescribed.

If the cold or flu is uncomplicated, the doctor should explain this and prescribe home treatment. Unnecessary use of antibiotics invites unnecessary complications, such as reaction to the antibiotics and superinfections by bacteria that are resistant to antibiotics.

A word about chicken soup: People with colds often feel dizzy when standing up, and this condition is helped by drinking salty liquids. Bouillon and chicken soup are excellent.

18 Sore Throat

Sore throats can be caused by viruses or bacteria. Especially in the winter, breathing through the mouth can dry and irritate the throat. This type of irritation subsides quickly after the throat becomes moist again.

Sore Throat Viruses

Viral sore throats, like other viral infections, can't be treated successfully with antibiotics; they must run their course. Pain relievers are often helpful.

Older children and adolescents may develop a viral sore throat known as infectious mononucleosis or "mono." Mononucleosis is also called the "kissing disease" because the virus is spread through saliva. The mono sore throat is often severe and lasts more than a week. The person may feel particularly weak, but complications seldom occur. Resting is important. There is no antibiotic cure for this virus.

Strep Throat

Sore throats due to the streptococcal bacteria are commonly referred to as "strep throat." A strep throat should be treated with an antibiotic because of two types of complications. First, an abscess may form in the throat. This is an extremely rare complication but should be suspected if a child shows great difficulty in swallowing or opening the mouth, or excessive drooling.

The second and more significant type of complication occurs from one to four weeks after the throat pain disappears and takes one of two forms. One form, called acute glomerulonephritis, causes an inflammation of the kidney. It isn't certain that antibiotics will prevent this complication.

The other form, and the one of greatest concern, is the complication of rheumatic fever, which is rare today but still a problem in some regions. Rheumatic fever is a complicated disease that can result in painful, swollen joints; unusual skin rashes; and heart damage. Rheumatic fever can be prevented by antibiotic treatment of a strep throat.

Strep throat is much less frequent in adults than in children, and rheumatic fever is very rare in adults. Strep throat is unlikely if the sore throat is a minor part of a typical cold (runny nose, stuffy ears, cough, and so on).

The question of when to use antibiotics for sore throats is controversial. Many doctors believe that a test for strep is the best way to determine the need for antibiotics. However, the test's accuracy has ranged from 31 to 98% in various studies. Furthermore, many people are "strep carriers": they have strep in their throats, but the strep isn't causing illness. In the decision chart, the same symptoms that lead you to "Call Doctor Today" are those that will make your doctor more likely to prescribe antibiotics.

HOME TREATMENT

Cold liquids, acetaminophen, aspirin, ibuprofen, and naproxen are effective for sore throat pain and fever. Because recent information indicates an association between aspirin and a rare but serious problem known as Reye's syndrome, children and teenagers shouldn't take aspirin or cold remedies containing it. Home remedies that may help include saltwater gargles and tea with honey or lemon. Time is the most important healer for pain. A vaporizer makes the waiting more comfortable for some.

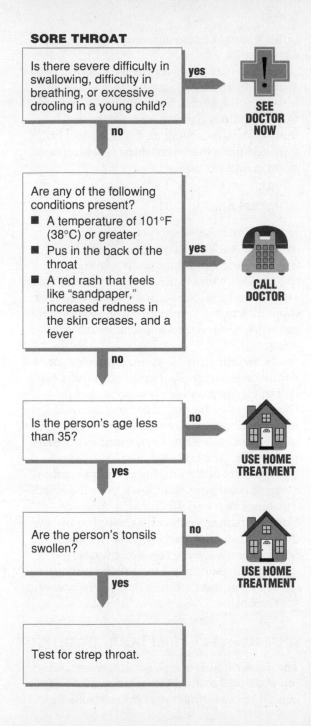

SORE THROAT

Is there severe difficulty in swallowing, difficulty in breathing, or excessive drooling in a young child?

yes → **SEE DOCTOR NOW**

no ↓

Are any of the following conditions present?
- A temperature of 101°F (38°C) or greater
- Pus in the back of the throat
- A red rash that feels like "sandpaper," increased redness in the skin creases, and a fever

yes → **CALL DOCTOR**

no ↓

Is the person's age less than 35?

no → **USE HOME TREATMENT**

yes ↓

Are the person's tonsils swollen?

no → **USE HOME TREATMENT**

yes ↓

Test for strep throat.

WHAT TO EXPECT AT THE DOCTOR'S OFFICE

The doctor may perform one of the tests for strep, such as a throat culture. Many doctors will delay treating a sore throat until the test results are known. Delaying treatment, even by one or two days, doesn't seem to increase the risk of developing rheumatic fever. Furthermore, antibiotic treatment reduces only the complications, not the discomfort, of a sore throat. Because the majority of sore throats are due to viruses, treating all sore throats with antibiotics will expose many patients without strep to the risk of allergic reactions to the drugs. Doctors often will begin treatment with antibiotics immediately if there is a family history of rheumatic fever, if the patient has scarlet fever (the rash described in the decision chart), or if rheumatic fever is commonly occurring in the community at the time.

If one child has a strep throat, the chances are very good that any family members with a sore throat will also have strep. However, brothers and sisters without symptoms usually should not be tested for strep.

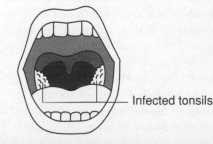

Infected tonsils

Children between the ages of five and ten commonly have sore throats. There is no evidence that removing the tonsils lowers their frequency. Doctors now agree that children very seldom need the tonsillectomy operation.

19 Ear Pain and Stuffiness

Ear pain often is caused by a buildup of fluid and pressure in the middle ear (the portion of the ear behind the eardrum). Under normal circumstances, the middle ear is drained by a short narrow tube, the eustachian tube, into the nasal passages. Often during a cold or allergy, the mucous membranes lining the eustachian tube will swell, closing off the tube; this occurs most easily in small children in whom the tube is smaller. When the tube closes, the normal flow of fluid from the middle ear is prevented, and the fluid begins to accumulate. This causes stuffiness and decreased hearing.

The stagnant fluid provides a good place for the start of a bacterial infection. A bacterial infection usually results in pain and fever, often in one ear only.

Ear pain and ear stuffiness may occur when going from low to high altitudes, as when going up in an airplane. Here again the mechanism for the stuffiness or pain is a clog in the eustachian tube. Swallowing will frequently relieve this pressure. Closing the mouth and holding the nose closed while pretending to blow your nose is another way to open the eustachian tube. Using a decongestant may help prevent this problem.

Ear Infection in Children

The symptoms of an ear infection in children may include fever, ear pain, fussiness, increased crying, irritability, or pulling at the ears. Because infants can't tell you that their ears hurt, increased irritability or ear pulling should make a parent suspicious of ear infection.

Parents are often concerned about whether their children will lose hearing after ear infections. Most children will have a temporary and minor hearing loss during and immediately following an ear infection, but with adequate treatment there is seldom any permanent hearing loss.

HOME TREATMENT

Antihistamines, decongestants, and nose drops are used to decrease the amount of fluid flowing from the middle ear and shrink the mucous membranes in order to open the eustachian tube. See sections **M8** and **M9** for more information on these drugs. Fluid in the ear will often respond to home treatment alone.

Acetaminophen, aspirin, ibuprofen, or naproxen will provide partial pain relief **(M4).** Although ear pain isn't usually a part of chicken pox or the flu, avoid the use of aspirin in teenagers or children because of the association with Reye's syndrome, a serious problem of the brain and liver.

Moisture and humidity are important in keeping the mucus that flows from the middle ear thin. Use a vaporizer if you have one. Curious maneuvers (such as hopping up and down in a steamy shower while shaking the head and swallowing) are sometimes dramatically successful in clearing out mucus.

If symptoms continue beyond two weeks, see the doctor.

WHAT TO EXPECT AT THE DOCTOR'S OFFICE

The doctor will examine the ear, nose, and throat as well as the bony portion of the skull behind the ears, known as the mastoid. Pain,

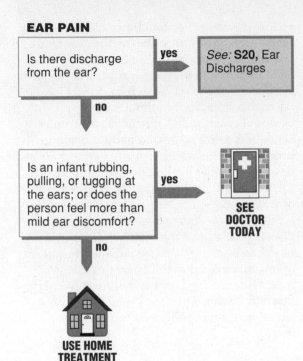

EAR PAIN

Is there discharge from the ear? — **yes** → *See:* **S20**, Ear Discharges

no ↓

Is an infant rubbing, pulling, or tugging at the ears; or does the person feel more than mild ear discomfort? — **yes** → **SEE DOCTOR TODAY**

no ↓

USE HOME TREATMENT

insertion of ear tubes in order to reestablish proper functioning of the middle ear. Placing ear tubes sounds frightening, but this is actually a simple and very effective procedure.

tenderness, or redness of the mastoid means a serious infection.

Therapy will generally consist of an antibiotic and an attempt to open the eustachian tube by medication. Nose drops, decongestants, and antihistamines can be used for this purpose. Antibiotic therapy generally will be prescribed for at least a week, while other treatments will usually be given for a shorter period. Be sure to take all of the antibiotic prescribed, and on schedule.

Occasionally fluid in the middle ear will persist for a long period without infection. In this case there may be a slight decrease in hearing. This condition, known as "serous otitis media," is usually treated by trying to open the eustachian tube to allow the fluids to drain; it isn't treated with antibiotics. If this condition persists the doctor may resort to

20 Ear Discharges

Ear discharges are usually just wax but may be caused by minor irritation or infection. Ear wax is almost never a problem unless attempts are made to "clean" the ear canal, the opening that leads from the external part of the ear to the internal parts. Ear wax functions as a protective lining for the ear canal. Taking warm showers or washing the external ears with a washcloth dipped in warm water usually provides enough vapor to prevent the buildup of wax. Children often like to push things in their ear canals, and they may pack the wax tightly. Adults armed with a cotton swab on a stick (for example, a Q-tip) often accomplish the same awkward result.

Swimmer's Ear

In the summertime ear discharges are commonly caused by swimmer's ear, an irritation of the ear canal and not a problem of the inner ear or eardrum. A tug on the ear that causes pain can be a helpful clue to an inflammation of the outer ear and canal, such as swimmer's ear. Children with such inflammation will often complain that their ears are itchy. The urge to scratch inside the ear is very tempting but must be resisted. We especially caution against the use of hairpins or other instruments because injury to the eardrum can result.

Ruptured Eardrum

In a child who has been complaining of ear pain, relief of pain accompanied by a white or yellow discharge — sometimes bloody — may be the sign of a ruptured eardrum. Sometimes parents will find dry crusted material on the child's pillow; here again, a ruptured eardrum should be suspected. The child should be taken to a doctor for antibiotic therapy. Don't be unduly alarmed. A ruptured eardrum is actually the first stage of a natural healing process that the antibiotics will help. Children have remarkable healing powers, and most eardrums will heal completely within a matter of weeks.

A very rare, but very serious, cause of ear discharge is a head injury **(S10).** If a person has clear discharge that began after a head injury, there is a possibility that a serious injury has occurred and spinal fluid is leaking through the ear. Treat the possibility of this situation as an urgent need for the doctor's help.

HOME TREATMENT

Packed-down ear wax can be removed by using warm water flushed in gently with a syringe available at drugstores. A water jet (Water Pik, etc.) that is set at the lowest setting can also be useful, but it can be frightening to young children and is dangerous at higher settings. We don't advise that parents try to remove impacted ear wax unless they are dealing with an older child and can see the impacted, blackened ear wax.

Wax softeners such as ordinary olive oil, Debrox, or Cerumenex are useful; however, all commercial products may be irritating, especially if not used properly. Cerumenex, for example, must be flushed out of the ear within 30 minutes using warm water.

Two warnings:

- The water must be as close to body temperature as possible; the use of cold

EAR DISCHARGES

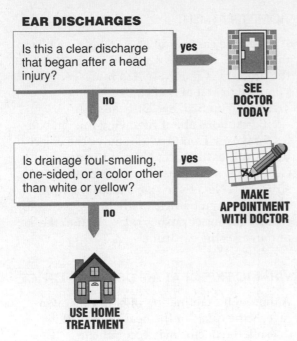

Is this a clear discharge that began after a head injury?

yes → SEE DOCTOR TODAY

no ↓

Is drainage foul-smelling, one-sided, or a color other than white or yellow?

yes → MAKE APPOINTMENT WITH DOCTOR

no ↓

USE HOME TREATMENT

particularly severe or itching cases or persistence beyond five days, a doctor's visit is advisable.

WHAT TO EXPECT AT THE DOCTOR'S OFFICE

A thorough examination of the ear will be performed. In severe cases, a culture for bacteria may be taken. Corticosteroid and antibiotic preparations that are placed in the ear canal may be prescribed, or one of the regimens described above under "Home Treatment" may be advised. Oral antibiotics will usually be given if a perforated eardrum is causing the discharge.

water may result in dizziness and vomiting.

- Washing should never be tried if there is any question about the condition of the eardrum; it must be intact and undamaged.

Although swimmer's ear (or other causes of similar "otitis externa") is often caused by a bacterial infection, the infection is very shallow and doesn't often require antibiotic treatment. The infection can be effectively treated by placing a cotton wick soaked in Burow's solution in the ear canal overnight, followed by a brief washing out with 3% hydrogen peroxide and then warm water. Success has also been reported with Merthiolate mixed with mineral oil (enough to make it pink), followed by the hydrogen peroxide and warm water rinse. For

21 Hearing Loss

Problems with hearing may be divided into two broad categories: sudden and slow. When a child of age five or older complains of a difficulty in hearing that has developed over a short period, the problem is usually a blockage in the ear. On the outside of the eardrum, such blockage may be due to the accumulation of wax, a foreign object that the child has put in the ear canal, or an infection of the ear canal. On the inside of the eardrum, blockage may occur when fluid accumulates because of an ear infection or allergy.

Hearing problems in children may be present from birth. Hearing can now be tested in a child of any age through the use of computers that analyze changes in brain waves in response to sounds. More simply, an infant with normal hearing will react to a noise such as a hand clap, horn, or whistle. Normal speech development relies on hearing. A child whose speech is developing slowly or not at all may, in fact, have hearing problems.

Some decrease in hearing, especially of the higher frequencies, is normal after the age of 20. If this decrease becomes a problem in later life, it is time to visit the doctor. Occasionally, hearing problems will mimic problems with thinking or understanding, so people will wrongly suspect senility, Alzheimer's disease, or other neurological problems.

HOME TREATMENT

An accurate ear examination requires a trip to the doctor. However, if you know for sure that the problem is caused by too much ear wax, you may treat it at home. (See "Home Treatment" in S20, Ear Discharges.)

Be cautious about removing foreign bodies from ears. Don't try to remove the object unless it is easily accessible and removing it clearly poses no threat of damage to ear structures. Never use sharp instruments to remove foreign bodies. Many times, trying to remove an object pushes it farther into the ear or damages the eardrum.

WHAT TO EXPECT AT THE DOCTOR'S OFFICE

A thorough examination of both ears often reveals the cause of the hearing loss. If it doesn't, the doctor may recommend audiometry (an electronic hearing test) or other tests. Hearing can often be improved by a variety of methods, including hearing aids.

HEARING LOSS

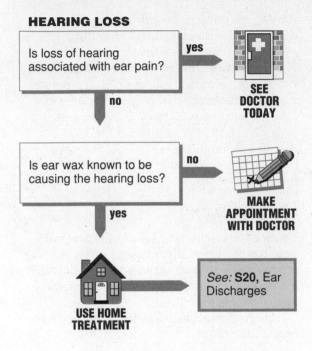

Is loss of hearing associated with ear pain? — **yes** → **SEE DOCTOR TODAY**

no ↓

Is ear wax known to be causing the hearing loss? — **no** → **MAKE APPOINTMENT WITH DOCTOR**

yes ↓

USE HOME TREATMENT

See: **S20**, Ear Discharges

22 Runny Nose

The hallmark of the common cold is a runny nose. It's intended by nature to help the body fight the virus infection. Nasal secretions contain antibodies which act against viruses. A runny nose means these secretions are carrying the virus outside the body.

Allergy is also a common cause of runny noses. People whose runny noses are due to an allergy have allergic rhinitis, better known as hay fever. The nasal secretions in this instance are often clear and very thin. People with hay fever will often have other symptoms, including sneezing and itching, and watery eyes. This problem lasts longer than a viral infection, often for weeks or months, and occurs most commonly during the spring and fall when pollen particles or other allergens are in the air. A great many other substances may aggravate allergic rhinitis, including house dust, mold, and animal dander.

Another common cause of runny noses as well as stuffy noses is prolonged use of nose drops. This problem of too much medication is known as "rhinitis medicamentosum." Nose drops containing substances like ephedrine should never be used for longer than three days. This problem can be avoided by switching to saline nose drops for a few days (M9).

Complications from a runny nose are due to the excess mucus. The mucus can run into the throat (postnasal drip) and cause a sore throat or a cough that is most obvious at night. The mucus drip may plug the eustachian tube between the nasal passages and the ear, resulting in ear infection and pain. It may plug the sinus passages, resulting in secondary sinus infection and sinus pain.

A very rare, but very serious, cause of a runny nose is a head injury (S10). If a person has clear discharge that began after a head injury, there is a possibility that a serious injury has occurred and spinal fluid is draining through the nose. Treat the possibility of this situation as an urgent need for the doctor's help.

HOME TREATMENT

Using handkerchiefs or tissues to blow your nose has the great advantage of safely moving mucus, virus particles, and allergens outside the body. A facial tissue has no side effects and costs less than drugs.

If drugs must be used, there are two basic types:

- **Decongestants** such as pseudoephedrine and ephedrine shrink the mucous membranes and open the nasal passages.

- **Antihistamines** block allergic reactions and decrease the amount of secretion.

Decongestants make some children overly active. Antihistamines may cause drowsiness and interfere with sleep (M8).

If you choose to treat a runny nose with medication, nose drops are suitable. Saline nose drops are fine for young children. Older children and adults may use drops containing decongestants (M9).

Complications such as ear and sinus infections may often be prevented by ensuring that the mucus is thin rather than thick and sticky. This helps prevent plugging of the nasal passages. Increasing the humidity in the air with a vaporizer or humidifier helps liquefy the mucus. Heated air inside a house is often very dry; cooler air contains more

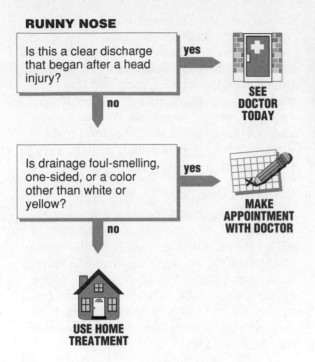

RUNNY NOSE

Is this a clear discharge that began after a head injury?
— **yes** → **SEE DOCTOR TODAY**
— **no** ↓

Is drainage foul-smelling, one-sided, or a color other than white or yellow?
— **yes** → **MAKE APPOINTMENT WITH DOCTOR**
— **no** ↓

USE HOME TREATMENT

Sneezes are healthy, removing germs, allergens, or dust from the nose. The only danger is infecting other people with the germ or virus that makes you sneeze. Cover your nose and mouth with a tissue or handkerchief. Wash your hands frequently. And let people say, "Bless you."

moisture. Drinking a large amount of liquid will also help liquefy the secretions. If symptoms persist beyond three weeks, consult your doctor.

WHAT TO EXPECT AT THE DOCTOR'S OFFICE

The doctor will thoroughly examine the ears, nose, and throat and will check for tenderness over the sinuses. Often a swab of the nasal secretions will be taken and examined under a microscope. The presence of certain types of cells, known as eosinophils, will indicate the presence of hay fever (allergic rhinitis). If allergic rhinitis is found, antihistamines may be prescribed, and an avoidance program of dust, mold, dander, and pollen will be explained.

23 Cough

The cough reflex is one of the body's best defense mechanisms. Irritation or obstruction in the breathing tubes triggers this reflex, and the violent rush of air helps clear material from the breathing tubes. If abnormal material, such as pus, is being expelled from the body by coughing, the cough is desirable. Such a cough is termed "productive" and usually shouldn't be suppressed by drugs.

Often a minor irritation or a healing area in a breathing tube will start the cough reflex even though there is no abnormal material to be expelled. At other times, mucus from the nasal passages will drain into breathing tubes at night (postnasal drip) and initiate the cough reflex. Such coughs aren't beneficial and may be decreased with cough suppressants.

Smoker's Cough

The smoker's cough bears testimony to the continual irritation of the breathing tubes. Smoke also poisons the cells lining these tubes so mucus can't be expelled normally. Smoker's cough is a sign of deadly diseases yet to come.

Viruses and Bacteria

Next to smoking, viral infections are the most common causes of coughs. These coughs usually bring up only yellow or white mucus. In contrast, coughs producing mucus that is rusty or green and looks like it contains pus are most likely to be caused by a bacterial infection. Bacterial infections require the doctor's help and antibiotics. Viral infections are not helped by antibiotics and usually run their course within several days.

The term "pneumonia" is most often used to refer to a bacterial infection of the lung but can be used for viral infection and other problems as well. In fact, a "chest cold" is a viral pneumonia, as are "double pneumonia" and "walking pneumonia." So don't panic when you hear "pneumonia"; it isn't a very precise term.

Children's Coughs

In very young infants, coughing is unusual and may indicate a serious lung problem. In older infants, who are prone to swallowing foreign objects, an object may become lodged in the windpipe and cause coughing. Young children also tend to inhale bits of peanut and popcorn, which can produce coughing. If the child's cough sounds like a seal's bark, refer also to Croup (S24).

HOME TREATMENT

When mucus in the breathing tubes is the problem, this may be made thinner and less sticky by several means. Increased humidity in the air will help. A vaporizer and a steamy shower are two ways to increase the humidity. In the severe croup cough of small children, high humidity is absolutely essential. Drinking large quantities of fluids also is helpful for the cough. Guaifenesin (Robitussin or Naldecon CX, for example) is available without prescription and may help thin the mucus. Liberal use of such common home substances as pepper and garlic does likewise and may help relieve the cough.

Decongestants and/or antihistamines may help if a postnasal drip is causing the cough. Otherwise, avoid drugs that contain antihistamines because they dry the secretions and make them thicker.

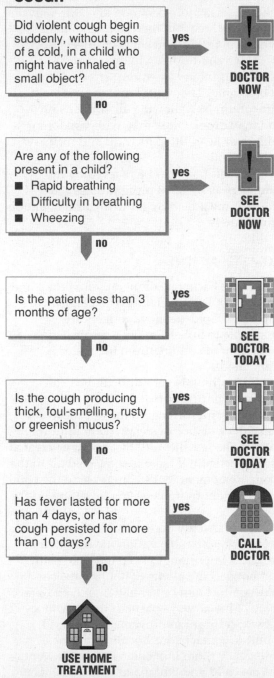

COUGH

Did violent cough begin suddenly, without signs of a cold, in a child who might have inhaled a small object? — **yes** → **SEE DOCTOR NOW**

no

Are any of the following present in a child?
- Rapid breathing
- Difficulty in breathing
- Wheezing

yes → **SEE DOCTOR NOW**

no

Is the patient less than 3 months of age? — **yes** → **SEE DOCTOR TODAY**

no

Is the cough producing thick, foul-smelling, rusty or greenish mucus? — **yes** → **SEE DOCTOR TODAY**

no

Has fever lasted for more than 4 days, or has cough persisted for more than 10 days? — **yes** → **CALL DOCTOR**

no

USE HOME TREATMENT

Dry, tickling coughs are often relieved by cough lozenges or sucking on hard candy. Dextromethorphan (Romilar, Vicks Formula 44, Robitussin-DM, etc.) is an effective cough suppressant. Neither dextromethorphan nor codeine will completely eliminate coughs at any dosage, and side effects of drowsiness or constipation can occur **(M11)**.

WHAT TO EXPECT AT THE DOCTOR'S OFFICE

The doctor will examine the ears, nose, throat, and chest; a chest X-ray may be taken in some instances. Don't expect antibiotics to be prescribed for a routine viral or allergic cough; they don't help.

Hiccups, which are caused by irregular contractions of the diaphragm muscle, may occasionally prove troublesome. Although there have been many home remedies recommended over the years, including drinking large amounts of water and startling the sufferer, research suggests that one-half teaspoon (3 ml) of dry sugar placed on the back of the tongue is the most effective treatment.

SYMPTOM   S24

24 Croup

Croup may be the most frightening of the common illnesses that parents encounter. It generally occurs in children under the age of three or four. In the middle of the night, a child may sit up in bed gasping for air. Often there will be an accompanying cough from the area of the voice box in the neck that sounds like the barking of a seal. The child's symptoms are so frightening that panic is often the response. However, the most severe problems with croup usually can be relieved safely, simply, and efficiently at home.

Croup is caused by one of several viruses. The viral infection causes a swelling and outpouring of secretions in the larynx (voice box), trachea (windpipe), and bronchi (the larger airways going to the lungs). The air passages of the young child are narrowed by the swelling and further aggravated by the secretions, which may become dry and caked, making it difficult to breathe. There may also be a considerable amount of spasm of the airway passages, further complicating the problem. Treatment is aimed at dissolving the dried secretions.

In some children croup is a recurring problem. These children may have three or four bouts of croup. This seldom represents a serious underlying problem, but you should seek a doctor's advice. Croup will be outgrown as the airway passages grow larger; it is unusual after the age of seven.

Epiglottitis

Occasionally a more serious obstruction caused by a bacterial infection and known as epiglottitis can be confused with croup. Epiglottitis is more common in children over the age of three, but there is considerable overlap in the ages of children affected by these two conditions. Children with epiglottitis often have more serious difficulty in breathing. They may have an extremely difficult time swallowing all of their saliva and may drool. Often they will gasp for air with their head tilted forward and their jaw pointed out.

Epiglottitis won't be relieved by the simple measures that bring prompt relief of croup. It must be brought to medical attention immediately.

HOME TREATMENT

Mist is the backbone of therapy for croup and can be supplied efficiently by a cold-steam vaporizer. Cold-steam vaporizers are preferable to hot-steam ones because the possibility of scalding from hot water is eliminated.

If breathing is very difficult you can obtain faster results by taking the child to the bathroom and turning on the hot shower to make thick clouds of steam. (Don't put the child in the hot shower!) Steam can be created more efficiently if there is some cold air in the room. Remember that steam rises, so the child won't benefit from the steam by sitting on the floor.

Relief usually occurs promptly and should be noticeable within the first 15 minutes. It is important to keep the child calm and not become alarmed; holding the child may comfort him or her and may help relieve some of the airway spasm. If the child doesn't show significant improvement within 15 minutes, contact your doctor or the local emergency room immediately. They'll want to see the child and will make arrangements in

CROUP

Are any of the
following present?
- Drooling
- Breathing with chin
jutting out and
mouth open
- Severe difficulty in
breathing

yes → **SEE DOCTOR NOW**

no

Are the following
present?
- Cough sounding
like seal's bark
- Difficulty inhaling

no → *Suspect...* problem other than croup. *See:* **S23,** Cough

yes

Does breathing
improve with steam
after 15 minutes?

no → **CALL DOCTOR NOW**

yes

USE HOME TREATMENT

advance while you are in transit. Unfortunately, few emergency rooms can provide steam as easily as the home shower.

If the child shows significant improvement but the problem persists for more than an hour, call the doctor.

WHAT TO EXPECT AT THE DOCTOR'S OFFICE

If the doctor feels confident that this is croup, further use of mist will be tried. In difficult cases, X-rays of the neck are a reliable way of differentiating croup from epiglottitis. A swollen epiglottis often can be seen in the back of the throat. If epiglottitis is diagnosed, the child will be admitted to the hospital; an airway will be placed in the child's trachea to enable the child to breathe, and intravenous antibiotics directed at curing the bacterial infection will be started. In the case of croup the trip to the doctor often cures the problem that was resistant to steam at home.

25 Wheezing

Wheezing is the high-pitched whistling sound produced by air flowing through narrowed breathing tubes (bronchi and bronchioles). It's most obvious when the person breathes out but may be present when breathing both in and out. Wheezing comes from the breathing tubes deep in the chest, in contrast to the croupy, crowing, or whooping sounds that come from the area of the voice box in the neck (see Croup, **S24)**. Most often, a narrowing of the breathing tubes is due to a viral infection or an allergic reaction, as in asthma.

In infants younger than age two, the smallest air passages can narrow because of a viral infection. Pneumonia can also produce wheezing. Occasionally, a foreign body may be lodged in a breathing tube, causing a localized wheezing that's difficult to hear without a stethoscope.

Wheezing is commonly associated with emphysema (chronic obstructive pulmonary disease or COPD), and asthma often exacerbates this problem. The irritation of smoking by itself is sufficient to cause wheezing, although almost all smokers have some degree of emphysema and bronchitis as well.

Asthma

Asthma is an obstructive lung disease that's most common in children and adolescents. The wheezing in asthma is caused by spasm of the muscles in the walls of the smaller air passages in the lungs. An excess amount of mucus production further narrows the air passages and can aggravate the difficulty in getting the air out.

An asthmatic attack can be triggered by an infection, an emotionally upsetting event, cold air, air pollution, or exposure to an allergen. Common allergens include house dust, pollen, mold, food, and animal dander. Wheezing can follow an insect sting or the use of a medicine; some individuals even wheeze after taking aspirin. Most often, however, there's no clear reason for a particular asthmatic attack.

Wheezing Alongside Fever

In a child with a respiratory infection, wheezing may occur before shortness of breath is obvious. Therefore, when wheezing appears in the presence of a fever — a sign of possible respiratory infection — early consultation with a doctor is advisable, even though the illness seldom turns out to be serious.

Treatment of wheezing is for temporary relief only. There are no drugs that cure viral illnesses or asthma. Home treatment is an important part of this approach. However, the doctor's help is needed so that drugs that widen the breathing passages can be used. Intravenous fluids may be required on some occasions.

HOME TREATMENT

All wheezing in children is potentially serious and should be evaluated by a medical professional, at least for the first few occurrences. Asthma tends to occur in families where other members have either asthma, hay fever, or eczema **(S46)**.

Drinking fluids is very important. It's best to drink water, but fruit juices or soft drinks may be used if the person will swallow more. Hydration (drinking more water) will be part of the therapy that the doctor recommends, so

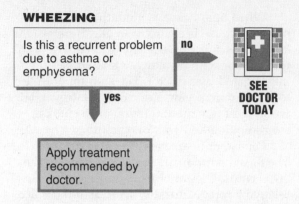

WHEEZING

Is this a recurrent problem due to asthma or emphysema? — no → **SEE DOCTOR TODAY**

yes ↓

Apply treatment recommended by doctor.

you may begin even before you visit the doctor.

The use of a vaporizer, preferably one that produces a cold mist, may sometimes help. Unfortunately it's difficult to get much vapor down to the small breathing tubes deep inside the lungs. If a vaporizer isn't available, you can use the shower to produce a mist.

A relatively clean and dust-free house is healthy for all people but essential for a person whose allergies cause asthma. Regularly vacuum rugs, furniture, drapes, bedspreads, and other items that are particular dust-catchers, especially in an asthmatic's bedroom. Keep toy animals clean; washable ones are best. Avoid products that may be stuffed with animal hair. Finally, don't forget to change heating filters and air conditioner filters regularly.

Asthmatics *can* participate in athletics. Athletes with asthma have won numerous gold medals in Olympic swimming. Swimming appears to be far and away the best exercise and the best sport for the asthmatic.

WHAT TO EXPECT AT THE DOCTOR'S OFFICE

Physical examination will focus on the chest and neck. The doctor will ask questions not only about the current illness but also about a past history of allergies either in the patient or the family. The possibility that a foreign body has been swallowed may also be investigated in small children. Infections can trigger asthma, but the doctor shouldn't give antibiotics unless an infection is definitely present.

Drugs to open the breathing tube, such as epinephrine or theophylline, may be given by injection, by mouth, or by rectal suppository. Occasionally the patient will need to stay in a hospital to receive replacement fluids through a vein and to breathe humidified air. Most important, in a hospital the patient can be closely watched to prevent the condition from getting worse before it gets better.

After the crisis has passed, the doctor will work with you to prevent future asthma attacks. This should include working on environmental and emotional causes. More than half of the children diagnosed with asthma never have an asthmatic attack as an adult, and another 10% will have only occasional attacks during adult life.

Drug Treatments for Asthma

The doctor may prescribe one of a variety of medications that produce symptomatic relief of asthma, including epinephrine, isoproterenol, ephedrine, and theophylline. Try to avoid drugs that combine two or more of these ingredients because of the added side effects. Use corticosteroid drugs, such as prednisone, only after full discussion with your doctor.

Learn to administer inhaled drugs correctly. If you feel the medicine hit your tongue or the back of your throat, it's not going into your airways where it belongs.

Antihistamines aren't useful in the treatment of asthma. In fact, by drying nasal secretions, antihistamines may actually cause airways to plug up.

26 Hoarseness

Hoarseness is usually caused by a problem in the vocal cords.

Children

In infants under three months of age this can be due to a serious problem, such as a birth defect or thyroid disorder. In young children hoarseness is more often due to prolonged or excessive crying, which puts a strain on the vocal cords.

In older children viral infections are the most common cause of hoarseness. If the hoarseness is accompanied by difficulty in breathing or a cough that sounds like a barking seal, the hoarseness is considered a symptom of croup (S24). Croup is characteristic in children under age three or four, while the symptom of hoarseness by itself is more common in older children.

If hoarseness is accompanied by difficulty in breathing or swallowing, drooling, gasping for air, or breathing with the mouth wide open and the chin jutting forward, a doctor must be seen immediately. This is a medical emergency. This problem is known as epiglottitis and is a bacterial infection that affects the entrance to the airway.

Adults

In adults a virus is most often responsible for the development of hoarseness or laryngitis when no other symptoms are present. As with any symptom of an upper respiratory tract infection, hoarseness may linger after other symptoms disappear.

When hoarseness is mild, the most common cause is cigarette smoke. If persistent hoarseness is not associated with either a viral infection or with smoking, it should be investigated by a doctor. The amount of time to wait before seeing a doctor is controversial; we suggest one month. If you are a smoker, stop smoking and wait one month.

Persistent hoarseness has many causes. The most common are cysts or polyps on the vocal cords. Cancer is also a cause but is relatively rare. Naturally, overuse of the voice may result in hoarseness.

HOME TREATMENT

Hoarseness not associated with other symptoms is resistant to medical therapy. Nature must heal the inflamed area. Humidifying the air with a vaporizer or taking in fluids can offer some relief; however, healing may not occur for several days. Resting the vocal cords is sensible; crying or shouting makes the situation worse. For the treatment of hoarseness associated with coughs, see Cough (S23).

WHAT TO EXPECT AT THE DOCTOR'S OFFICE

If a child has severe difficulty in breathing, the first priority is to ensure that the air passage is adequate. This may require the placement of a breathing tube at the emergency room, hospital, or doctor's office. If X-rays of the neck are taken, a doctor should accompany the child at all times in case emergency care is needed.

In uncomplicated hoarseness that has persisted for a long time, a doctor will look at the vocal cords with the aid of a small mirror. Occasionally a more extensive physical examination and blood tests will be performed.

HOARSENESS

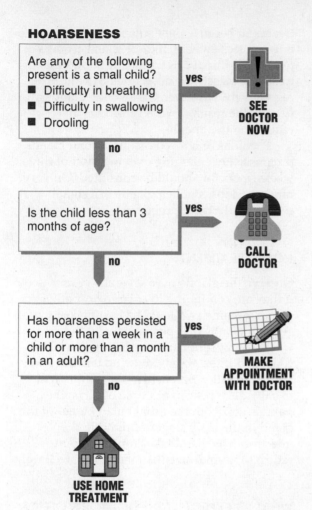

Are any of the following present is a small child?
- Difficulty in breathing
- Difficulty in swallowing
- Drooling

yes → **SEE DOCTOR NOW**

no ↓

Is the child less than 3 months of age?

yes → **CALL DOCTOR**

no ↓

Has hoarseness persisted for more than a week in a child or more than a month in an adult?

yes → **MAKE APPOINTMENT WITH DOCTOR**

no ↓

USE HOME TREATMENT

27 Swollen Glands

The most common types of swollen glands are lymph glands and salivary glands. The biggest salivary glands are located below and in front of the ears. When they swell, the characteristic swollen jaw appearance of mumps is the result **(S59).**

Lymph glands play a part in the body's defense against infection. They may become swollen even if the infection is trivial or not apparent, although you can usually identify the infection that is causing the swelling. The locations of the lymph glands appear on page 89.

- Swollen neck glands frequently accompany sore throats or ear infections. The swelling of a gland simply indicates that it is taking part in the fight against infection.

- Lymph glands in the groin are enlarged when there is infection in the feet, legs, or genital region. These glands are often swollen when no obvious infection can be found.

- Swollen glands behind the ears are often the result of an infection in the scalp. If there is no scalp infection, it is possible that the person currently has or recently had rubella **(S62).** Infectious mononucleosis (mono) can also cause swelling of the glands behind the ears (see Sore Throat, **S18**).

If a swollen gland is red and tender, there may be a bacterial infection within the gland itself that requires antibiotic treatment. Swollen glands otherwise require no treatment because they are merely fighting infections elsewhere. If there is an accompanying sore throat or earache, these should be treated as described in sections **S18** and **S19,** respectively. However, the swollen glands are usually the result of viral infections that require no treatment.

If you have noticed one or several glands progressively enlarging over a period of three weeks, a doctor should be consulted. On very rare occasions, swollen glands can signal serious underlying problems.

HOME TREATMENT

Observe the glands over several weeks to see if they are continuing to enlarge or if other glands become swollen. The vast majority of swollen glands that persist beyond three weeks aren't serious, but a doctor should be consulted if the glands show no tendency to become smaller. Soreness in the glands will usually disappear in a couple of days; the pain results from the rapid enlargement of the gland in the early stages of fighting the infection. The gland takes much longer to return to normal size than it does to swell up.

WHAT TO EXPECT AT THE DOCTOR'S OFFICE

The doctor will examine the glands and search for infections or other causes of the swelling. Other glands that may not have been noticed by the patient will be examined. The doctor will inquire about fever, weight loss, or other symptoms associated with the swelling of the glands. The doctor may decide that blood tests are indicated or may simply observe the glands for a period of time. In rare cases it might be necessary to remove (biopsy) a small piece of the gland for examination under the microscope.

SWOLLEN GLANDS

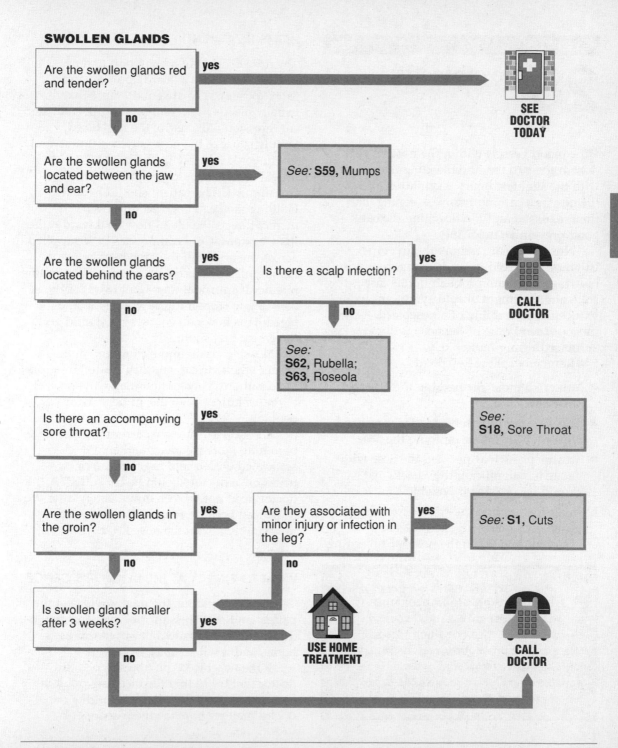

Are the swollen glands red and tender? — **yes** → SEE DOCTOR TODAY

no ↓

Are the swollen glands located between the jaw and ear? — **yes** → *See:* **S59**, Mumps

no ↓

Are the swollen glands located behind the ears? — **yes** → Is there a scalp infection? — **yes** → CALL DOCTOR

no ↓ (scalp infection) → *See:* **S62**, Rubella; **S63**, Roseola

no ↓

Is there an accompanying sore throat? — **yes** → *See:* **S18**, Sore Throat

no ↓

Are the swollen glands in the groin? — **yes** → Are they associated with minor injury or infection in the leg? — **yes** → *See:* **S1**, Cuts

no ↓   no ↓ → USE HOME TREATMENT

Is swollen gland smaller after 3 weeks? — **yes** → USE HOME TREATMENT

no ↓ → CALL DOCTOR

28 Nosebleeds

The blood vessels within the nose lie very near the surface, and bleeding may occur with the slightest injury. In children, picking the nose is a common cause. Keeping their fingernails cut and discouraging the habit are good preventive medicine.

Nosebleeds are frequently due to irritation by a cold virus or to vigorous nose blowing. The main problem in this case is the cold, and treatment of cold symptoms will reduce the probability of a nosebleed. If the mucous membrane of the nose is dry, cracking and bleeding are more likely.

Remember these key points:

- You can almost always stop the bleeding yourself.

- The majority of nosebleeds are associated with colds or minor injury to the nose.

- Treatment such as packing the nose with gauze has significant drawbacks and should be avoided if possible.

- Investigation into the cause of recurrent nosebleeds is not urgent and is best accomplished when the nose isn't bleeding.

Medical opinion is divided about whether **high blood pressure** causes nosebleeds, but most doctors believe that the two conditions are seldom related. As a precaution, an individual with high blood pressure who experiences a nosebleed may want to have his or her blood pressure taken within a few days.

HOME TREATMENT

The nose consists of a bony part and a cartilaginous part: a "hard" portion and a "soft" portion. The area of the nose that usually bleeds lies within the soft portion, and compression will control the nosebleed. Simply squeeze the nose between thumb and forefinger just below the hard portion of the nose. Pressure should be applied for at least five minutes. The patient should be seated. Holding the head back isn't necessary. It merely directs the blood flow backward rather than forward. Cold compresses or ice applied across the bridge of the nose may help. Almost all nosebleeds can be controlled in this manner if sufficient time is allowed for the bleeding to stop. If it just won't stop and bleeding is major, of course you should go to the emergency room.

Nosebleeds are more common in the winter when viruses and dry, heated interiors are common. A cooler house and a vaporizer to return humidity to the air help many people.

If nosebleeds are a recurrent problem, are becoming more frequent, and aren't associated with a cold or other minor irritation, a doctor should be consulted. A doctor need not be seen immediately after the nosebleed because examination at that time may simply restart the nosebleed.

WHAT TO EXPECT AT THE DOCTOR'S OFFICE

To stop the bleeding, the doctor will seat the patient and compress the nostrils. This will be done even if the patient has tried this at home, and it will usually work.

If the nosebleed can't be stopped, the doctor will try to find the bleeding point in the nose. If a bleeding point is visible, the doctor may try to make the blood clot by

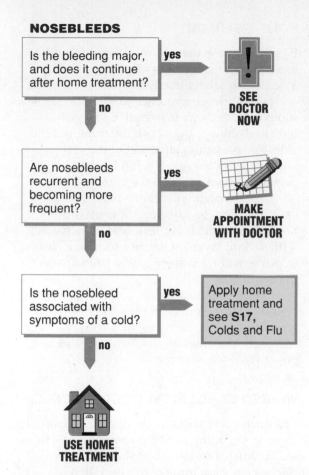

NOSEBLEEDS

Is the bleeding major, and does it continue after home treatment? — **yes** → **SEE DOCTOR NOW**

no ↓

Are nosebleeds recurrent and becoming more frequent? — **yes** → **MAKE APPOINTMENT WITH DOCTOR**

no ↓

Is the nosebleed associated with symptoms of a cold? — **yes** → Apply home treatment and see **S17**, Colds and Flu

no ↓

USE HOME TREATMENT

searing the bleeding point with either electrical or chemical cauterization. If this isn't successful, packing of the nose may be unavoidable. Such packing is uncomfortable and may lead to infection; thus, the patient must be carefully observed.

If a doctor is visited because of recurrent nosebleeds, questions about events preceding the nosebleeds and a careful examination of the nose itself should be expected. Depending on the history and the physical examination, blood-clotting tests may be ordered on rare occasions.

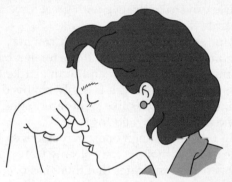

To stop a nosebleed. Sit down and squeeze just below the hard portion of the nose. Hold for five minutes. It isn't necessary to tilt the head back.

29 Foreign Body in Eye

Eye injuries must be taken seriously. If there's any question, visit the doctor. A foreign body in the eye must be removed to avoid the threat of infection and loss of sight. Be particularly careful if the foreign body was caused by metal striking metal; a small metal particle can strike the eye with great force and penetrate the eyeball.

Under certain circumstances, you may treat this problem at home. If the foreign body was minor, such as sand, and didn't strike the eye with great velocity, it is easily removed. Small round particles like sand rarely stick behind the upper eyelid for long.

In fact, the foreign body may not even be in the eye any more; it may simply feel as if it is. This feeling indicates that there has been a scrape or cut on the cornea, the clear membrane that covers the colored portion of the eye. A minor corneal injury will usually heal quickly without problems, but a major one requires medical attention.

Even if you think the injury is minor, run through the decision chart daily. If any symptoms at all are present after 48 hours and aren't clearly resolving, see a doctor. Minor problems will heal within 48 hours; the eye repairs injury quickly.

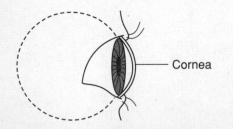

Cornea

HOME TREATMENT

Be gentle. Wash the eye out. Water is good; a weak solution of boric acid is better, if available (follow label directions).

Inspect the eye yourself and have someone else check it as well. Use a good light and shine it from both the front and the side. Pay particular attention to the cornea.

Don't rub the eye; if a foreign body is present, you will scratch the cornea.

An eye patch will relieve pain. Take it off each day to recheck the eye; it is usually needed for 24 hours or less. Make the patch with several layers of gauze and tape it firmly in place; you want some gentle pressure on the eye.

Check vision each day; compare the two eyes by reading different sizes of newspaper type from across the room, first with one eye, then with the other. If you aren't sure all is going well, see a doctor.

WHAT TO EXPECT AT THE DOCTOR'S OFFICE

The doctor will check your vision and inspect the eye, including under the upper lid — this isn't painful. Usually he or she will drop a fluorescent stain into the eye and then examine it under ultraviolet light — this isn't painful or hazardous. An ophthalmologist (surgeon specializing in diseases of the eye) will examine the eye with a microscope.

The doctor will remove any foreign body in the eye. In the office, the doctor may use a cotton swab, an eyewash solution, or a small needle or "eye spud." He or she sometimes applies an antibiotic ointment or provides an eye patch. Eye drops that dilate the pupil may be employed. The doctor may have X-rays taken if a foreign body may be inside the globe of the eye.

FOREIGN BODY IN EYE

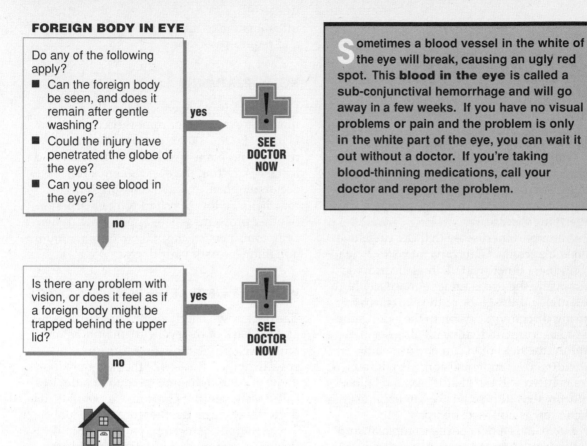

Do any of the following apply?

- Can the foreign body be seen, and does it remain after gentle washing?
- Could the injury have penetrated the globe of the eye?
- Can you see blood in the eye?

yes → SEE DOCTOR NOW

no

Is there any problem with vision, or does it feel as if a foreign body might be trapped behind the upper lid?

yes → SEE DOCTOR NOW

no

USE HOME TREATMENT

Sometimes a blood vessel in the white of the eye will break, causing an ugly red spot. This **blood in the eye** is called a sub-conjunctival hemorrhage and will go away in a few weeks. If you have no visual problems or pain and the problem is only in the white part of the eye, you can wait it out without a doctor. If you're taking blood-thinning medications, call your doctor and report the problem.

30 Eye Pain

Pain in the eye can be an important symptom and can't be safely ignored for long. Fortunately it is an unusual complaint. Itching and burning **(S32)** are more common. Eye pain may be due to injury, infection, or an underlying disease.

An important disease that can cause eye pain is glaucoma. Glaucoma may slowly lead to blindness if not treated. In glaucoma, the fluid inside the eye is under abnormally high pressure, and the globe of the eye is tense, causing discomfort. Vision to the sides is the first to be lost. Gradually and almost imperceptibly, the field of vision narrows until the individual has "tunnel vision." In addition, a person often will see "halos" around lights. Unfortunately, this sequence can occur even when there is no associated pain.

Eye pain is a nonspecific complaint, and questions relating to the pain are often better answered under the more specific headings in this chapter.

A feeling of tiredness in the eyes or some discomfort after a long period of fine work (eyestrain) is generally a minor problem and doesn't really qualify as eye pain. Severe pain behind the eye may result from migraine headaches, and pain either above or below the eye may suggest sinus problems.

Pain in both eyes, particularly upon exposure to bright light, "photophobia," is common with many viral infections such as the flu and will go away as the infection improves. More severe photophobia, particularly when only one eye is involved, may indicate inflammation of the deeper layers of the eye and requires a doctor.

HOME TREATMENT

Except for eye pain associated with a viral illness or eyestrain, or minor discomfort that is more tiredness than pain, we don't recommend home treatment. In these instances, resting the eyes, taking a few acetaminophen, and avoiding bright light may help. Follow the chart to the discussion of other problems where appropriate. When symptoms persist, check them out in a routine appointment with your doctor.

WHAT TO EXPECT AT THE DOCTOR'S OFFICE

The doctor will check vision, eye movements, and the back of the eye with an ophthalmoscope. An ophthalmologist (surgeon specializing in diseases of the eye) may look at the eye through a microscope or a device called a slit lamp. If glaucoma is possible, the doctor may check the pressure of the globe. This is simple, quick, and painless. (Many doctors commonly refer patients with eye symptoms to an ophthalmologist. You may wish to go directly to an ophthalmologist if you have a major concern.)

EYE PAIN

Is the pain related to a significant injury, or is a foreign body present? — **yes** → *See:* **S29,** Foreign Body in Eye

no ↓

Is the pain an itching or burning sensation, or are the eyes runny? — **yes** → *See:* **S32,** Eye Burning, Itching, and Discharge

no ↓

Is there any decrease in vision? — **yes** → *See:* **S31,** Decreased Vision

no ↓

Is the pain severe or prolonged beyond 48 hours? — **yes** → **SEE DOCTOR TODAY**

no ↓

Is the pain more of a feeling of tiredness in the eyes, or are flu-like symptoms present? — **yes** → **MAKE APPOINTMENT WITH DOCTOR**

no ↓

USE HOME TREATMENT

Staring at a **computer screen** for a long time can cause eyestrain, irritation, blurred vision, and headaches. However, several studies conclude that these problems are temporary. To make them less likely:

- Blink often, rest your eyes with momentary glances away from the screen, and use eye drops if necessary. Staring at the screen tends to reduce your blinking and thus dry out your eyes.

- Avoid glare from the screen by using indirect lighting, repositioning the screen, or using an antiglare filter over it.

- Make sure your monitor produces sharp, crisp images. Fuzzy screen images increase eyestrain.

- Get special glasses for your computer work if necessary. If you wear bifocals, you may be tilting your head at an uncomfortable angle to see the screen through the lower portion of your glasses.

For more information about working at your computer, see Wrist Pain (**S71**).

31 Decreased Vision

Few people need urging to protect their sight. Decreased vision is a major threat to the quality of life. Usually, professional help is needed.

A few situations don't require a visit to a health professional. When small, single "floaters" drift across the eye from time to time and don't affect vision, they aren't a matter for concern. Slight, reversible blurring of vision may occur after outdoor exposure or with overall fatigue. In young people, sudden blindness in both eyes is commonly a hysterical reaction and isn't a permanent threat to sight; such patients need a doctor but not necessarily an eye doctor.

Usually the question is not whether to see a health professional but, rather, which one to see. Opticians dispense glasses; they aren't medical doctors and don't diagnose eye problems.

The optometrist evaluates the need for glasses, screens for eye diseases, and determines what prescription lens gives the best vision. Conditions usually treated by an optometrist are nearsightedness (myopia), farsightedness (hyperopia), and crooked-sightedness (astigmatism). Although optometrists aren't medical doctors, in some states they can prescribe medicine.

If another problem is suspected, the optometrist may refer you to an ophthalmologist, who is a medical doctor and a surgical specialist. The ophthalmologist is the final authority on eye diseases. Sometimes an eye problem is part of a general health problem; in these cases, the primary physician may be appropriate.

Try to find the right health professional on the first attempt; this will save you time and money. The following examples may help you in your decision making:

- **School nurse detects decreased vision in child:** Visit ophthalmologist or optometrist — possible myopia (nearsightedness)

- **Sudden blindness in one eye in an elderly person:** Visit ophthalmologist or internist — possible stroke or temporal arteritis

- **Halos around lights and eye pain:** Visit ophthalmologist — possible acute glaucoma (increased pressure in the eye)

- **Gradual decrease in vision in an adult who wears glasses:** Visit ophthalmologist or optometrist — change in refraction of the eye

- **Sudden blindness in both eyes in a healthy young person:** Visit internist or ophthalmologist — possible hysterical reaction

- **Gradual blurring of vision in an older person,** with no improvement by moving closer or farther away: Visit ophthalmologist — possible cataract (scar tissue forming in the lens of the eye)

- **Older person who sees far objects best:** Visit optometrist or ophthalmologist — possible presbyopia (condition that diminishes the eye's ability to focus on near objects)

- **Visual change while taking a medicine:** Call the prescribing doctor — the drug may be responsible

- **Decreased vision in one eye,** with a "shadow" or "flap" in the visual field: Visit ophthalmologist — possible retinal detachment

DECREASED VISION

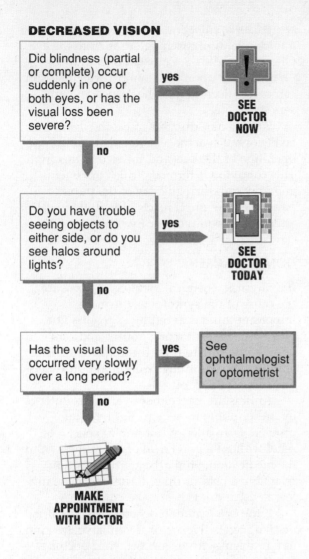

Did blindness (partial or complete) occur suddenly in one or both eyes, or has the visual loss been severe? — **yes** → **SEE DOCTOR NOW**

no ↓

Do you have trouble seeing objects to either side, or do you see halos around lights? — **yes** → **SEE DOCTOR TODAY**

no ↓

Has the visual loss occurred very slowly over a long period? — **yes** → See ophthalmologist or optometrist

no ↓

MAKE APPOINTMENT WITH DOCTOR

WHAT TO EXPECT AT THE DOCTOR'S OFFICE

The doctor will check vision, eye movements, pupils, back of the eye, and eye pressure when appropriate; a slit-lamp examination may be done. A general medical evaluation will be done as required. Testing for eyeglasses may be needed; busy ophthalmologists will sometimes refer this procedure to an optometrist. Surgery may be recommended for some conditions.

32 Eye Burning, Itching, and Discharge

These symptoms usually mean conjunctivitis, or "pink eye," with inflammation of the membrane that lines the eye and the inner surface of the eyelids. The inflammation may be due to an irritant in the air, an allergy to something in the air, a viral infection, or a bacterial infection. The bacterial infections and some of the viral infections (particularly herpes) are potentially serious but are least common.

Chemicals and particles in smog can produce burning and itching that sometimes seem as severe as the symptoms experienced in a teargas attack. These symptoms represent a chemical conjunctivitis and affect anyone exposed to enough of the chemical. The smoke-filled room, the chlorinated swimming pool, the desert sandstorm, sun glare on a ski slope, or exposure to a welder's arc can provoke similar physical or chemical irritation.

In contrast, allergic conjunctivitis affects only those people who have allergies. Almost always the allergen (what causes the body's reaction) is in the air. This problem may occur in spring, summer, or fall, depending on the offending pollen, and usually lasts two to three weeks. Grass pollens are probably the most frequent offender.

A minor conjunctivitis frequently accompanies a viral cold, triggering the well-known symptoms and lasting only a few days. Some viruses, such as herpes, cause deep ulcers in the cornea and interfere with vision.

Bacterial infections cause pus to form, and a thick, plentiful discharge runs from the eye. Often the eyelids are crusted over and "glued" shut upon wakening. These infections can cause ulceration of the cornea and are serious.

Some major diseases affect the deeper layers of the eye, those layers that control the operation of the lens and the size of the pupil. This condition is termed "iritis" or "uveitis" and may cause irregularity of the pupil or pain when the pupil reacts to light. Medical attention is required. For Eye Pain, see **S30.**

HOME TREATMENT

If a physical, chemical, or allergic exposure is the cause of the symptoms, the most important thing is avoiding exposure. Dark glasses, goggles at work, houses and cars with air-conditioning to filter the air, avoidance of chlorinated swimming pools, and other such measures are appropriate.

Antihistamines, either over-the-counter or by prescription, may help slightly if the problem is an allergy, but don't expect total relief without a good deal of drowsiness from the medication. Similarly, a viral infection related to a cold or flu will run its course in a few days, and it is best to be patient.

If the eye irritation doesn't clear up, if the discharge gets thicker, or if you have eye pain or a problem with vision, see your doctor. Don't expect a fever with a bacterial infection of the eye; it may be absent. Because the infection is superficial, washing the eye gently with a boric acid solution (follow directions on the label) will help remove some of the bacteria, but you should still see a doctor. Eye drops (Murine, Visine, etc.) may soothe minor conjunctivitis but won't cure it **(M15).**

Burning eyes may be a call to social action. If the smoking of others around you is

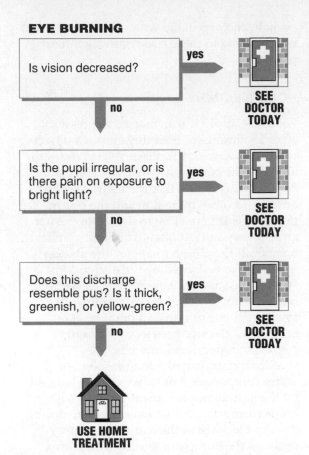

EYE BURNING

Is vision decreased?

yes → **SEE DOCTOR TODAY**

no ↓

Is the pupil irregular, or is there pain on exposure to bright light?

yes → **SEE DOCTOR TODAY**

no ↓

Does this discharge resemble pus? Is it thick, greenish, or yellow-green?

yes → **SEE DOCTOR TODAY**

no ↓

USE HOME TREATMENT

frequently given. Cortisone-like eye ointments should be prescribed infrequently; certain infections (herpes) may get worse with these medicines. If herpes is diagnosed — usually by an ophthalmologist — special eye drops and other medicines will be needed.

annoying, say so. If an industrial plant in your area is polluting, get the company to clean up its act.

WHAT TO EXPECT AT THE DOCTOR'S OFFICE

The doctor will check vision, eye motion, eyelids, and the reaction of the pupil to light. An ophthalmologist (surgeon specializing in eye diseases) may perform a slit-lamp examination. Antihistamines may be prescribed, and general advice may be given. Antibiotic eye drops or ointments are

33 Styes and Blocked Tear Ducts

We might have called this problem "bumps around the eyes" because that is how they appear.

Styes are infections (usually with staphylococcal bacteria) of the tiny glands in the eyelids. They are really small abscesses, and the bumps are red and tender. They grow to full size over a day or so.

Another type of bump in the eyelid, called a chalazion, appears over many days or even weeks and isn't red or tender. A chalazion often requires drainage by a doctor, whereas most styes will respond to home treatment. However, there is no urgency in the treatment of a chalazion.

Tear Ducts

Tears are the lubricating system of the eye. They are continually produced by the tear glands and then drained away into the nose by the tear ducts. These tear ducts are often incompletely developed at birth so that the drainage of tears is blocked. When this happens, the tears may collect in the tear duct and cause it to swell, appearing as a bump along the side of the nose just below the inner corner of the eye. This bump isn't red or tender unless it has become infected. Most blocked tear ducts will open by themselves in the first month of life, and most of the remainder will respond to home treatment. Tears running down the cheek are seldom noted in the first month of life because the infant produces only a small volume of tears.

The eyeball itself isn't involved in a stye or a blocked tear duct. Problems with the eyeball, and especially with vision, should not be attributed to these two relatively minor problems.

HOME TREATMENT

For styes, apply warm, moist compresses for 10 to 15 minutes at least three times a day. As with all abscesses, the objective is to drain the abscess. The compresses help the abscess to "point." This means that the tissue over the abscess becomes quite thin and the pus in the abscess is very close to the surface. After an abscess points, it often will drain spontaneously. If this doesn't happen, the abscess may need to be lanced by the doctor. Most styes will drain spontaneously even without home treatment. They may drain inward toward the eye or outward onto the skin. Sometimes the stye goes away without coming to a point and draining.

Chalazions usually don't respond to warm compresses, but they won't be harmed by them. If no improvement is noted with home treatment after 48 hours, see the doctor.

For blockage of the tear ducts, simply massage the bump downward with warm, moist compresses several times a day. If the bump is not red and tender (indicating infection), this may be continued for up to several months. If the problem exists for this long, discuss it with your doctor. If the bump becomes red and swollen, antibiotic drops will be needed.

WHAT TO EXPECT AT THE DOCTOR'S OFFICE

If the stye is pointing and ready to be drained, the doctor will open it with a small needle. If it isn't pointing, compresses will usually be advised, and antibiotic eye drops sometimes will be added. Trying to drain a stye that isn't pointing is usually not very satisfactory.

STYES, ETC.

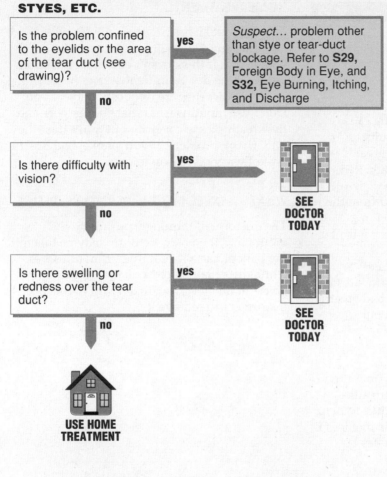

Is the problem confined to the eyelids or the area of the tear duct (see drawing)?

yes → *Suspect...* problem other than stye or tear-duct blockage. Refer to **S29,** Foreign Body in Eye, and **S32,** Eye Burning, Itching, and Discharge

no ↓

Is there difficulty with vision?

yes → **SEE DOCTOR TODAY**

no ↓

Is there swelling or redness over the tear duct?

yes → **SEE DOCTOR TODAY**

no ↓

USE HOME TREATMENT

A chalazion may be removed with minor surgery. Whether to have the surgery will be up to you. Chalazions aren't dangerous and usually don't require removal.

If a child is over six months of age and is still having problems with blocked tear ducts, the ducts can be opened in almost all cases with a very fine probe. This probing is successful on the first try in about 75% of all cases and on subsequent attempts in the remainder. Only rarely is a surgical procedure necessary to open a tear duct. For red and swollen ducts, antibiotic drops as well as warm compresses will usually be recommended.

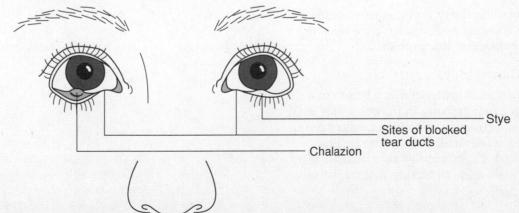

Stye

Sites of blocked tear ducts

Chalazion

34 Bad Breath

Poor dental hygiene and smoking cause most cases of bad breath in adults. Infections of the mouth and sore throat infections may also cause bad breath. Recently it has been suggested that bad breath is occasionally due to gases absorbed from the intestine and released through the lungs. Unfortunately, even if this is correct, it isn't clear what can be done about it.

Finally, unusual problems such as abscesses of the lung or heavy worm infestations have been reported to cause bad breath, although we haven't seen these in our practices.

Smoker's Breath

The bad breath of smoking comes from the lungs as well as the mouth. Thus, mouthwashes and breath fresheners do little to help smoker's breath. Getting rid of this problem is another benefit of giving up cigarettes.

Morning Breath

Bad breath in the morning is very common in adults. Flossing and regular tooth brushing should eliminate this problem.

In Children

A rare cause of prolonged bad breath in a child is a foreign body in the nose. This is especially common in toddlers, who have inserted some small object that remains unnoticed. Often, but not always, there is a white, yellowish, or bloody discharge from one nostril.

HOME TREATMENT

Proper dental hygiene, especially flossing, and avoiding smoking will prevent most cases of bad breath. If this doesn't eliminate the odor, a visit to the doctor or dentist may be helpful.

Mouthwashes are of questionable value. Don't use mouthwashes that simply perfume the breath. These cover up but don't treat the underlying problem. If you smoke, bad breath is another good reason to quit.

WHAT TO EXPECT AT THE DOCTOR'S OFFICE

The doctor will thoroughly examine the mouth and the nose. A culture may be taken if the patient has a sore throat or mouth sores. Antibiotics may be prescribed. If there is an object in the nose, the doctor will use a special instrument to remove it.

BAD BREATH

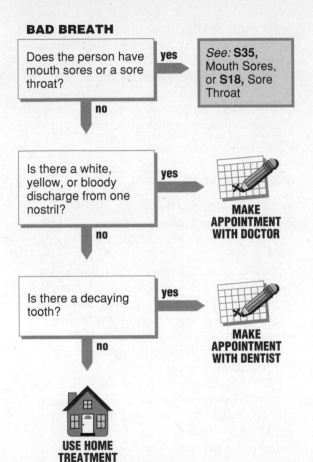

Does the person have mouth sores or a sore throat?

yes → *See:* **S35,** Mouth Sores, or **S18,** Sore Throat

no ↓

Is there a white, yellow, or bloody discharge from one nostril?

yes → **MAKE APPOINTMENT WITH DOCTOR**

no ↓

Is there a decaying tooth?

yes → **MAKE APPOINTMENT WITH DENTIST**

no ↓

USE HOME TREATMENT

35 Mouth Sores

Fever blisters or cold sores are a familiar problem caused by the herpes virus **(S112)**. They are usually found on the lips, although they can sometimes appear inside the mouth. Often the blisters have ruptured and only the remaining sore is seen. Fever is usually but not always present. Herpes viruses often live in the body for years, causing trouble only when another illness causes a rise in body temperature. Generally, fever blisters heal by themselves several days after the fever diminishes.

A canker sore is a painful ulcer that often follows an injury, such as accidentally biting the inside of the lip or the tongue, or it may appear without obvious cause. Eventually, it heals by itself.

In Children

Large white spots on the roof of the mouth are a sign of thrush, a yeast infection. It often disappears without treatment.

A virus that can cause mouth lesions in children is the Coxsackie virus. These lesions are often accompanied by spots on the hands and feet — hence the name "hand-foot-mouth syndrome." The child feels well and there is no fever. Again, this problem will go away by itself.

Other Causes

Drugs sometimes cause mouth ulcers. In such cases a skin rash may be present on other parts of the body as well, and a doctor must be contacted.

A cancer of the lip or gum is rare, except for smokers. It must be treated but is not an emergency. Syphilis transmitted by oral sexual contact may produce a mouth sore. Both of these problems are usually painless. Other conditions that may cause mouth ulcers also cause problems with eyes, joints, or other organs.

HOME TREATMENT

Mouth sores caused by viruses heal by themselves. The goal of treatment is to reduce fever, relieve pain, and maintain adequate fluid intake.

Children will seldom want to eat when they have painful mouth lesions. Although children can go several days without taking solid foods, it is very important that they maintain an adequate liquid diet. Cold liquids are the most soothing, and Popsicles or iced frozen juices are often helpful.

For sores inside the lip and on the gums, a nonprescription preparation called Orabase may be applied for protection. For canker sores and fever blisters, one of the phenol and camphor preparations (Blistex, Campho-Phenique, etc.) may provide relief, especially if applied early. If one of these preparations appears to cause further irritation, discontinue its use.

Mouth sores usually resolve in one to two weeks. Any sore that persists beyond three weeks should be examined by the doctor.

WHAT TO EXPECT AT THE DOCTOR'S OFFICE

A thorough examination of the mouth will be carried out. A prescription will usually be given for thrush. For viral infections, doctors have no more to offer than home remedies. We caution against the use of oral anesthetics,

MOUTH SORES

Could this problem be due to medication?

yes →

CALL DOCTOR →

...before taking another dose.

no ↓

Are there large white patches on the roof of the mouth or on the tongue?

yes →

CALL DOCTOR →

...suspect thrush.

no ↓

Do the lesions start as blisters and then change to small spots with white ulcerous centers surrounded by redness?

yes →

Suspect...herpes cold sores or canker sores. *See:* **S94,** Fever, and...

→ **USE HOME TREATMENT**

no ↓

Are the lesions accompanied by spots on hands and feet in a child who feels well?

yes →

Suspect... "hand-foot-mouth" syndrome and...

→ **USE HOME TREATMENT**

no ↓

USE HOME TREATMENT

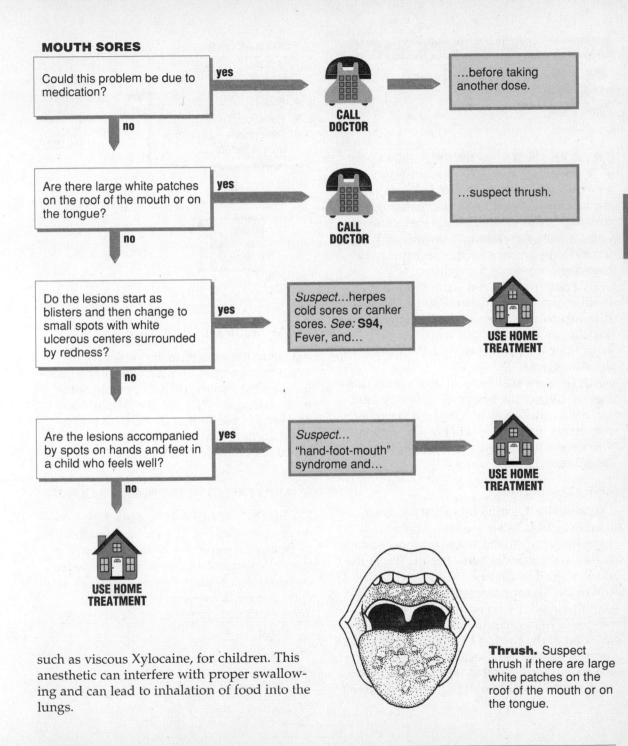

such as viscous Xylocaine, for children. This anesthetic can interfere with proper swallowing and can lead to inhalation of food into the lungs.

Thrush. Suspect thrush if there are large white patches on the roof of the mouth or on the tongue.

36 Toothaches

A toothache is often the sad result of poor dental hygiene. Although resistance to tooth decay is partly inherited, the majority of dental problems are preventable through flossing, brushing with a fluoride toothpaste, and professional cleaning. Sealants and fluoride applications by the dentist may be especially important for children.

Certainly, if you can see a decayed tooth or an area of redness surrounding a tooth, a diseased tooth is most likely the cause of pain. Tapping an infected tooth will often accentuate the pain, even though the tooth appears normal.

If the person appears ill, has a fever, and has swelling of the jaw or redness surrounding the tooth, a tooth abscess — a pocket of pus inside the gum — is likely. The person will need antibiotics in addition to proper dental care.

Other Possibilities

Occasionally it is difficult to distinguish a toothache from other sources of pain. Earaches, sore throats, mumps, sinusitis, and injury to the joint that attaches the jaw to the skull may all be confused with a toothache. A call to the doctor may clarify the situation.

If pain occurs every time the patient opens his or her mouth widely, it is likely that the joint of the jaw has been injured. This can occur from a blow or just by trying to eat too big a sandwich. A call to the doctor will help you decide what, if anything, should be done.

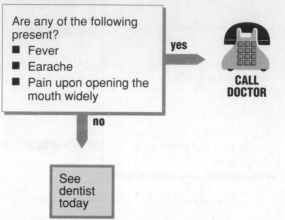

TOOTHACHES

Are any of the following present?
- Fever
- Earache
- Pain upon opening the mouth widely

yes → **CALL DOCTOR**

no ↓

See dentist today

HOME TREATMENT

Acetaminophen, aspirin, ibuprofen, or naproxen may be used for pain when a toothache is suspected and the dental appointment is being arranged. They are also helpful for problems in the joint of the jaw. We recommend acetaminophen for children and teenagers.

WHAT TO EXPECT AT THE DENTIST'S OFFICE

The dentist will fill cavities, extract teeth, or do other procedures. For problems with baby teeth, an extraction will be the most likely course. Root canals are generally performed on permanent teeth if the problem is severe. If there is fever or swelling of the jaw, the dentist will usually prescribe an antibiotic.

CHAPTER 5

Skin Problems and Childhood Diseases

IDENTIFYING SKIN SYMPTOMS

Skin problems must be approached somewhat differently from other medical problems. Decision charts that proceed from complaints such as "red bumps" are complicated and somewhat unsatisfactory, because most people, including doctors, identify skin diseases by recognizing a particular pattern. This pattern is composed of not only what the skin problem looks like at a particular time but also how it began, where it spread, and whether it is associated with other symptoms such as itching or fever. Also important are elements of the medical history that may suggest an illness to which the patient has been exposed.

Fortunately, many times the patient already has a good idea how the problem developed, and it is possible to proceed immediately with the question of whether this is poison ivy, ringworm, or something else.

The decision chart for each section in this chapter begins with the question of whether the problem follows the pattern for the skin disease being discussed. (A longer description of the pattern is given in the text that accompanies each decision chart.) If it doesn't, the chart often directs you to reconsider the problem and to consult the table on pages 144–145.

Most cases of a particular skin disease do not look exactly as a textbook says they should. We have tried to allow for a reasonable amount of variation in the descriptions. Don't be afraid to ask for other opinions. Grandparents and others have seen a lot of skin problems over the years and know what they look like. We have listed some of the more common problems, but by no means all. If your problem doesn't seem to fit any of the descriptions and you think the problem could be serious, call the doctor.

Finally, because every case is at least a little bit different, even the best doctors won't be able to identify all skin problems immediately. Simple office laboratory methods can help sort out the possibilities. Fortunately, the vast majority of skin problems are minor, get better by themselves, and pose no major threat to health. Usually it is reasonable for you to wait quite some time to see if the problem goes away by itself.

If you are confused about where to start, we have provided a decision chart on the facing page to help point you in the right direction. This chart and the table on pages 144–145 allow you to quickly review the major symptoms of common skin problems.

SKIN PROBLEMS

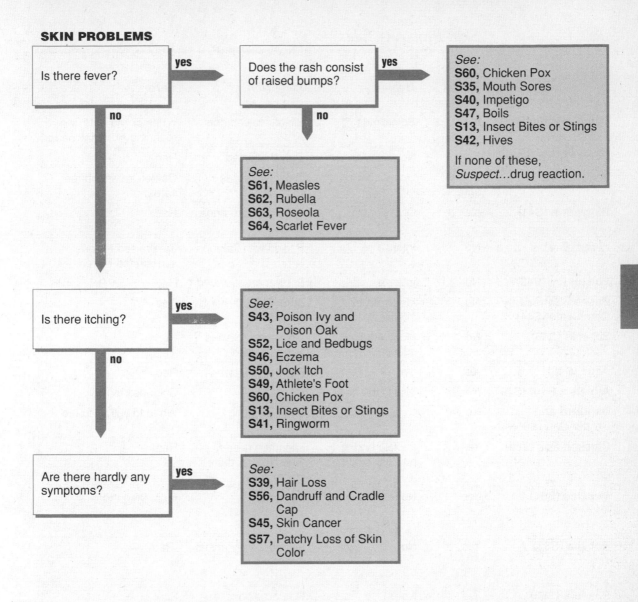

Is there fever? — **yes** → Does the rash consist of raised bumps? — **yes** →

See:
S60, Chicken Pox
S35, Mouth Sores
S40, Impetigo
S47, Boils
S13, Insect Bites or Stings
S42, Hives

If none of these,
*Suspect...*drug reaction.

Does the rash consist of raised bumps? — **no** →

See:
S61, Measles
S62, Rubella
S63, Roseola
S64, Scarlet Fever

Is there fever? — **no** →

Is there itching? — **yes** →

See:
S43, Poison Ivy and Poison Oak
S52, Lice and Bedbugs
S46, Eczema
S50, Jock Itch
S49, Athlete's Foot
S60, Chicken Pox
S13, Insect Bites or Stings
S41, Ringworm

Is there itching? — **no** →

Are there hardly any symptoms? — **yes** →

See:
S39, Hair Loss
S56, Dandruff and Cradle Cap
S45, Skin Cancer
S57, Patchy Loss of Skin Color

TABLE 7   *Skin Problems Table*

	Fever	*Itching*	*Elevation*	*Color*
Baby Rashes (S37)	No	Sometimes	Slightly raised dots	White or red dots; surrounding skin may be red
Diaper Rash (S38)	No	No	Only if infected	Red
Impetigo (S40)	Sometimes	Occasionally	Crusts on sores	Golden crusts on red sores
Ringworm (S41)	No	Occasionally	Slightly raised rings	Red
Hives (S42)	No	Intense	Raised with flat tops	Pale raised lesions surrounded by red
Poison Ivy (S43)	No	Intense	Blisters are elevated	Red
Rashes Caused by Chemicals (S44)	No	Moderate to intense	Sometimes blisters	Red
Eczema (S46)	No	Moderate to intense	Occasional blisters when infected	Red
Acne (S48)	No	No	Pimples, cysts	Red
Athlete's Foot (S49)	No	Mild to intense	No	Colorless to red
Dandruff and Cradle Cap (S56)	No	Occasionally	Some crusting	White to yellow to red
Chicken Pox (S60)	Yes	Intense during pustular stage	Flat, then raised, then blisters, then crusts	Red
Measles (S61)	Yes	None to mild	Flat	Pink, then red
Rubella (S62)	Yes	No	Flat or slightly raised	Red
Roseola (S63)	Yes	No	Flat, occasionally with a few bumps	Pink
Scarlet Fever (S64)	Yes	No	Flat, feels like sandpaper	Red
Fifth Disease (S65)	No	No	Flat, lacy appearance	Red

TABLE 7 *Skin Problems Table*

	Location	Duration of Problem	Other Symptoms
Baby Rashes (S37)	Trunk, neck, skin folds on arms and legs	Until controlled	
Diaper Rash (S38)	Under diaper	Until controlled	
Impetigo (S40)	Arms, legs, face first, then most of body	Until controlled	
Ringworm (S41)	Anywhere, including scalp and nails	Until controlled	Flaking or scaling
Hives (S42)	Anywhere	Minutes to days	
Poison Ivy (S43)	Exposed areas	7 to 14 days	Oozing; some swelling
Rashes Caused by Chemicals (S44)	Areas exposed to chemicals	Until exposure to chemical stopped	Some oozing and/or swelling
Eczema (S46)	Elbows, wrists, knees, cheeks	Until controlled	Moist; oozing
Acne (S48)	Face, back, chest	Until controlled	Blackheads
Athlete's Foot (S49)	Between toes	Until controlled	Cracks; scaling; oozing blisters
Dandruff and Cradle Cap (S56)	Scalp, eyebrows, behind ears, groin	Until controlled	Fine, oily scales
Chicken Pox (S60)	May start anywhere; most prominent on trunk and face	4 to 10 days	Lesions progress from flat to tiny blisters, then become crusted
Measles (S61)	First face, then chest and abdomen, then arms and legs	4 to 7 days	Preceded by fever, cough, red eyes
Rubella (S62)	First face, then trunk, then extremities	2 to 4 days	Swollen glands behind ears; occasional joint pains in older children and adults
Roseola (S63)	First trunk, then arms and neck; very little on face and legs	1 to 2 days	High fever for 3 days that disappears with rash
Scarlet Fever (S64)	First face, then elbows; spreads rapidly to entire body in 24 hours	5 to 7 days	Sore throat; skin peeling afterwards, especially palms
Fifth Disease (S65)	First face, then arms and legs, then rest of body	3 to 7 days	"Slapped-cheek" appearance, rash comes and goes

37 Baby Rashes

The skin of the newborn child may exhibit a wide variety of bumps and blotches. Fortunately almost all of these are harmless and clear up by themselves. Only one, heat rash, requires any treatment. If the baby was delivered in a hospital, many of these conditions may occur before discharge so that advice will be readily available from nurses or doctors.

Heat Rash

Heat rash is caused by blockage of the pores that lead to the sweat glands. It actually can occur at any age but is most common in the very young child whose sweat glands are still developing. When heat and humidity rise, these glands attempt to secrete sweat as they would normally. But because of the blockage, sweat is held within the skin and forms little red bumps. It is also known as "prickly heat" or "miliaria."

Milia

The little white bumps of milia appear when too many normal skin cells accumulate in spots. As many as 40% of children have these bumps at birth. Eventually the bumps break open, the trapped material escapes, and the bumps disappear without treatment.

Erythema Toxicum

Erythema toxicum is an unnecessarily long and frightening term for the flat red splotches that appear in up to 50% of all babies. These seldom appear after five days of age and usually disappear by seven days. Children who exhibit these splotches are otherwise normal.

Acne

Because the baby is exposed to the mother's adult hormones, a mild case of acne may develop. (The little white dots often seen on a newborn's nose represent "sebaceous gland hyperplasia," an excess amount of normal skin oil that has been produced by the hormones.) Acne usually becomes evident at between two and four weeks of age and clears up within six months to a year. It virtually never requires treatment.

HOME TREATMENT

Heat Rash

Heat rash is effectively treated simply by providing a cooler and less humid environment. Powders carefully applied do no harm but are unlikely to help. Avoid ointments and creams because they tend to keep the skin warmer and block the pores.

Milia, Erythema Toxicum, and Acne

Milia and erythema toxicum should require no treatment and will go away by themselves.

Acne in babies should not be treated with the medicines used by adolescents and adults. Normal washing is usually all that is required.

These problems are not associated with fever and, with the exception of minor discomfort in heat rash, should be painless. If any questions arise about these conditions, a telephone call to the doctor's office will often provide answers.

WHAT TO EXPECT AT THE DOCTOR'S OFFICE

Discussion of these problems can usually wait until the regularly scheduled well-baby visit. The doctor then can confirm your diagnosis.

BABY RASHES

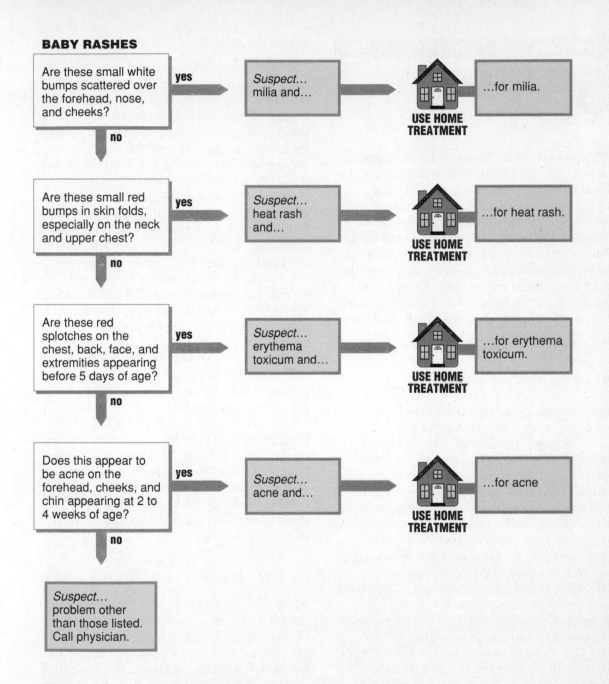

Are these small white bumps scattered over the forehead, nose, and cheeks?

yes → *Suspect...* milia and... → **USE HOME TREATMENT** → ...for milia.

no ↓

Are these small red bumps in skin folds, especially on the neck and upper chest?

yes → *Suspect...* heat rash and... → **USE HOME TREATMENT** → ...for heat rash.

no ↓

Are these red splotches on the chest, back, face, and extremities appearing before 5 days of age?

yes → *Suspect...* erythema toxicum and... → **USE HOME TREATMENT** → ...for erythema toxicum.

no ↓

Does this appear to be acne on the forehead, cheeks, and chin appearing at 2 to 4 weeks of age?

yes → *Suspect...* acne and... → **USE HOME TREATMENT** → ...for acne

no ↓

Suspect... problem other than those listed. Call physician.

38 Diaper Rash

The only children who never have diaper rash are those who never wear diapers. An infant's skin is particularly sensitive and likely to develop diaper rash. Diaper rash is basically an irritation caused by dampness and the interaction of urine, feces, and skin. An additional factor is thought to be the ammonia produced from urine, and often its odor is unmistakably present. Factors that tend to keep the baby's skin wet and exposed to the irritant promote diaper rash. These are:

- Constantly wet or infrequently changed diapers
- Using plastic pants

For the most part, treatment consists of reversing these factors.

The irritation of simple diaper rash may become complicated by an infection due to yeast (Candida) or bacteria. When yeast is the culprit, small red spots may be seen. Also, small patches of the rash may appear outside the area covered by the diaper, as far away as the chest. Infection with bacteria leads to development of large fluid-filled blisters. If the rash is worse in the skin creases (a condition called intertrigo), a mild underlying skin problem known as seborrhea may be present. This skin condition is also responsible for dandruff and cradle cap (S56).

Occasionally parents may notice blood or what appears to be blood spots when boys have diaper rash. This is due to a rash at the urinary opening at the end of the penis. This problem will clear up with the diaper rash.

HOME TREATMENT

Treatment of diaper rash is aimed at keeping the skin dry and exposed to air. As implied above, the first things to do are change the diapers frequently and stop using plastic pants. Leaving diapers off altogether for as long as possible will also help. Cloth diapers should be washed in a mild soap and rinsed thoroughly. Occasionally the soap residues left in diapers will act as an irritant. Adding a half-cup (120 ml) of vinegar to the last rinse cycle may help counter the irritating ammonia.

While the rash will take at least several days to completely clear, you should see definite improvement within the first 48 to 72 hours. If the rash does not start clearing up by that time or if it is extraordinarily severe, consult your doctor.

To prevent diaper rash, some parents use zinc oxide ointments, petroleum jelly, or other protective ointments. Others use baby powders. (**Caution:** Talc dust can injure babies' lungs if they breathe it in.) Always place powder in your hand first and then pat on the baby's bottom. Caldesene powder is helpful in preventing seborrhea and monilial rashes. We do not feel that all babies need powders and creams. If a rash has begun, avoid ointments and creams because they may delay healing.

WHAT TO EXPECT AT THE DOCTOR'S OFFICE

All of the baby's skin should be inspected to determine the true extent of the rash. Occasionally a scraping from the involved skin will be examined under the microscope. If a yeast (monilial) infection has complicated a simple diaper rash, the doctor will prescribe home treatment plus a medication to kill the yeast. If a bacterial infection has occurred,

DIAPER RASH

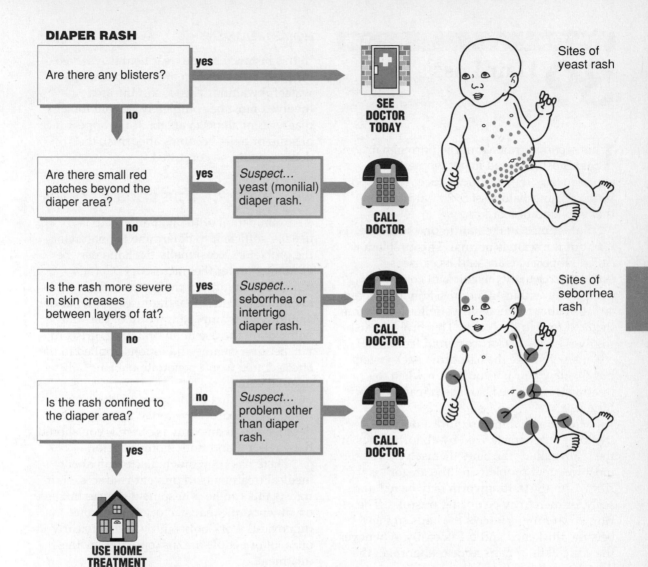

Are there any blisters? — **yes** → **SEE DOCTOR TODAY**

no ↓

Are there small red patches beyond the diaper area? — **yes** → *Suspect...* yeast (monilial) diaper rash. → **CALL DOCTOR**

no ↓

Is the rash more severe in skin creases between layers of fat? — **yes** → *Suspect...* seborrhea or intertrigo diaper rash. → **CALL DOCTOR**

no ↓

Is the rash confined to the diaper area? — **no** → *Suspect...* problem other than diaper rash. → **CALL DOCTOR**

yes ↓

USE HOME TREATMENT

Sites of yeast rash

Sites of seborrhea rash

then an antibiotic to be taken orally will be recommended. If the rash is very severe or seborrhea is suspected, then a steroid cream (usually stronger than the 1% hydrocortisone available without prescription) may be advised. In any case, home therapy may be safely started before seeing the doctor.

39 Hair Loss

This section is not about the normal hair loss that most men and many women experience as they get older. (See Aging Spots, Wrinkles, and Baldness, **S58**.) Baldness isn't the only kind of hair loss.

Sometimes all the hair in one small area is lost, but the scalp is normal. This problem is called alopecia areata, and its cause is unknown. Usually the hair will come back completely within 12 months, although about 40% of patients will have a similar loss within the next four to five years. This problem also resolves by itself. Corticosteroid (cortisone) creams will make the hair grow back faster, but the new hair falls out again when the treatment is stopped, so these creams are of little use.

Hair loss that may require a doctor's treatment is characterized by abnormalities in the scalp skin or the hairs themselves. The most frequent problem in this category is ringworm **(S41)**. Ringworm may be red and scaly, or there may be oozing pustules. The ringworm fungus infects the hairs so they become thickened and break easily. Whenever the scalp skin or hairs appear abnormal, the doctor may be able to help.

Hair pulling by children is often responsible for hair loss. Tight braids or ponytails may also cause some hair loss. If a child constantly pulls out his or her hair, you should discuss the problem with a doctor.

HOME TREATMENT

In this instance, home treatment is reserved for presumed alopecia areata and consists of watchful waiting. The skin in the area involved must be completely normal for a diagnosis of alopecia areata. If the appearance of scalp or hairs becomes abnormal, the doctor should be consulted.

WHAT TO EXPECT AT THE DOCTOR'S OFFICE

An examination of the hair and scalp is usually sufficient to determine the nature of the problem. Occasionally the hairs may be examined under the microscope. Certain types of ringworm of the scalp can be identified because they fluoresce (glow) under an ultraviolet lamp. Ringworm of the scalp will require the use of an oral drug, griseofulvin, because creams and lotions applied to the affected area won't penetrate the hair follicles to kill the fungus.

We hope that no doctor would recommend the use of X-rays today as some did decades ago. If an X-ray is offered, you should flatly reject it and find another doctor.

There has been much discussion about medical treatments to prevent baldness. Hair transplants can help in some instances but are usually not fully satisfactory. The creams (minoxidil) work only a little and only early on; a lot of people are disappointed by this treatment.

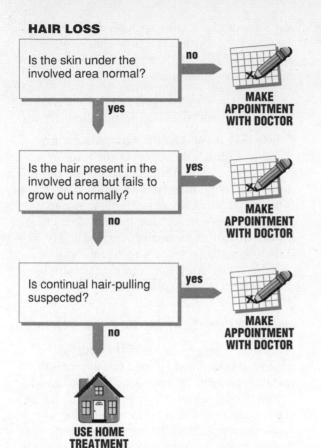

HAIR LOSS

Is the skin under the involved area normal?

no → MAKE APPOINTMENT WITH DOCTOR

yes

Is the hair present in the involved area but fails to grow out normally?

yes → MAKE APPOINTMENT WITH DOCTOR

no

Is continual hair-pulling suspected?

yes → MAKE APPOINTMENT WITH DOCTOR

no

USE HOME TREATMENT

40 Impetigo

Impetigo can be recognized by the characteristic rash that begins as small red spots and progresses to tiny blisters that eventually rupture, producing an oozing, sticky, honey-colored crust. This rash usually spreads very quickly with scratching and is particularly troublesome in the summer, especially in warm, moist climates.

Impetigo is a skin infection caused by streptococcal bacteria; occasionally other bacteria may also be found. If it spreads, impetigo can be a very uncomfortable problem. There is usually a great deal of itching. After the sores heal, there may be a slight decrease in skin color at the site. Skin color usually returns to normal, so this need not concern you.

Complication in the Kidneys

Of greatest concern is a rare reaction to streptococcal infection, a kidney problem known as glomerulonephritis. Glomerulonephritis will cause the urine to turn a dark brown (cola) color and is often accompanied by headache and elevated blood pressure. Although this complication has a formidable name it is short-lived and heals completely in most people.

Unfortunately, antibiotics won't prevent glomerulonephritis but may help prevent the impetigo from spreading to other people, thus protecting them from both conditions. Antibiotics are effective in healing the impetigo.

Although there is some debate on this matter, many doctors believe that if only one or two lesions are present and the lesions are not progressing, home treatment may be used for impetigo. The exception to this rule is if an epidemic of glomerulonephritis is occurring within your community.

HOME TREATMENT

Crusts may be soaked off with either warm water or Burow's solution (Domeboro, Bluboro, etc.). Antibiotic ointments are no more effective than soap and water. The lesions should be scrubbed with soap and water after the crusts have been soaked off. If lesions do not show prompt improvement or if they seem to be spreading, see the doctor without delay. Antibiotic ointments may be used, but their value is debatable.

WHAT TO EXPECT AT THE DOCTOR'S OFFICE

After examining the sores and taking an appropriate medical history, the doctor will usually prescribe an antibiotic to be taken by mouth. The drug of choice is penicillin unless there is penicillin allergy, in which case erythromycin is usually prescribed. Some doctors may check the blood pressure or urine in order to look for early signs of glomerulonephritis.

IMPETIGO

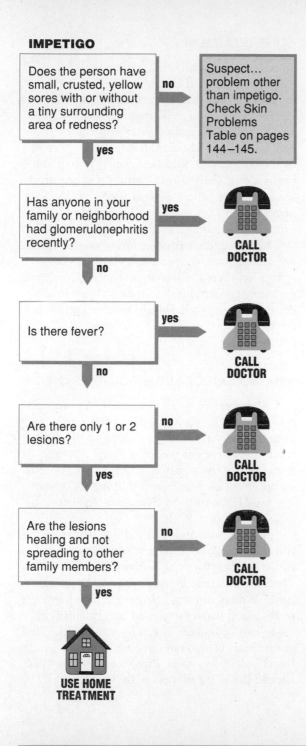

Does the person have small, crusted, yellow sores with or without a tiny surrounding area of redness?

no → Suspect... problem other than impetigo. Check Skin Problems Table on pages 144–145.

yes ↓

Has anyone in your family or neighborhood had glomerulonephritis recently?

yes → CALL DOCTOR

no ↓

Is there fever?

yes → CALL DOCTOR

no ↓

Are there only 1 or 2 lesions?

no → CALL DOCTOR

yes ↓

Are the lesions healing and not spreading to other family members?

no → CALL DOCTOR

yes ↓

USE HOME TREATMENT

41 Ringworm

Worms have nothing whatsoever to do with this condition. Ringworm is a shallow fungus infection of the skin. The designation "ringworm" is derived from the characteristic red ring that appears on the skin.

Ringworm can generally be recognized by its pattern of development. The lesions begin as small, round, red spots and get progressively larger. When they are about the size of a pea, the center begins to clear. When the lesions are about the size of a dime, they will have the appearance of a ring. The border will be red, elevated, and scaly. Often there are groups of infections so close to one another that it is difficult to recognize them as individual rings.

Ringworm may also affect the scalp or nails. These infections are more difficult to treat but, fortunately, are not seen very often. Ringworm epidemics of the scalp were common many years ago.

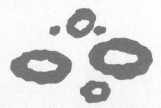

Ringworm. Lesions begin as small, round, red spots. When they are about the size of a dime, they will have the appearance of a ring.

HOME TREATMENT

Tolnaftate (Tinactin, etc.), miconazole (Micatin, etc.), and clotrimazole (Lotrimin, etc.) applied to the skin are effective treatments for ringworm. They are available in cream, solution, and powder and can be purchased over-the-counter. Either the cream or the solution should be applied two or three times a day. Only a small amount is required for each application. Selsun Blue shampoo, applied as a cream several times a day, will often do the job and is less expensive **(M17).**

Resolving this problem may take several weeks, but you should see improvement within one week. Ringworm that either shows no improvement after a week of therapy or continues to spread should be checked by a doctor.

WHAT TO EXPECT AT THE DOCTOR'S OFFICE

The diagnosis of ringworm can be confirmed by scraping the scales, soaking them in a potassium hydroxide solution, and viewing them under the microscope. Some doctors may culture the scrapings. One of two agents usually will be prescribed if home treatment has failed: haloprogin (Halotex, etc.) or ciclopirox (Loprox, etc.).

In infections involving the scalp, an ultraviolet light (called a Wood's lamp) will cause affected hairs to become fluorescent. The Wood's lamp is used to make the diagnosis; it does not treat ringworm. Ringworm of the scalp must be treated by griseofulvin, taken orally, usually for at least a month. This medication is also effective for fungal infections of the nails. Ringworm of the scalp should never be treated with X-rays.

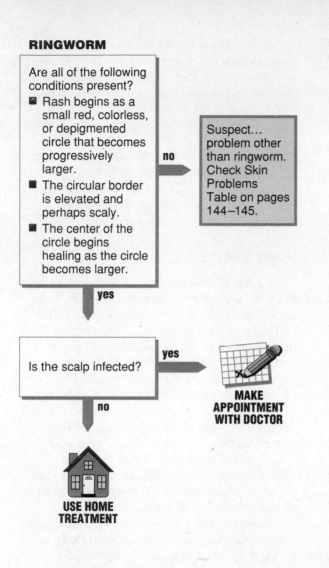

RINGWORM

Are all of the following conditions present?

- Rash begins as a small red, colorless, or depigmented circle that becomes progressively larger.
- The circular border is elevated and perhaps scaly.
- The center of the circle begins healing as the circle becomes larger.

no → Suspect… problem other than ringworm. Check Skin Problems Table on pages 144–145.

yes

Is the scalp infected?

yes → **MAKE APPOINTMENT WITH DOCTOR**

no → **USE HOME TREATMENT**

42 Hives

Hives, also called urticaria, are an allergic reaction. Unfortunately, the reaction can be to almost anything, including cold, heat, and even emotional tension. Unless you already have a good idea what is causing the hives or you have just taken a new drug, the doctor is unlikely to be able to determine the cause. Most often, searching for a cause is fruitless.

Here is a list of some of the things that are frequently mentioned as causes:

- Drugs
- Eggs
- Milk
- Wheat
- Pork
- Shellfish
- Freshwater fish
- Berries
- Cheese
- Nuts
- Pollens
- Animal dander
- Insect bites

The only sure way to know whether one of these is the culprit is to expose the patient to it. The problem with this approach is that if an allergy does exist, the allergic reaction may include not only hives but also a general reaction causing difficulty with breathing or circulation.

As indicated by the decision chart, a systemic reaction is a potentially dangerous situation, and a doctor should be consulted immediately. Avoid exposure to a suspected cause to see if the attacks cease. Such a test is difficult to interpret because attacks of hives are often separated by long periods of time. Actually, most people suffer only one attack, lasting from a period of minutes to weeks.

Finally, an occasional single hive on the arm or trunk is so common that it's considered normal and of no significance.

HOME TREATMENT

Determine whether there has been any pattern to the appearance of the hives. Do they appear after meals? After exposure to cold? During a particular season of the year? If there seem to be likely causes, eliminate them and see what happens.

If the reactions seem to be related to foods, an alternative is available. Lamb and rice virtually never cause allergic reactions. The person with hives may be placed on a diet consisting only of lamb and rice until completely free of hives. Foods are then added back to the diet one at a time, and the person is observed for a recurrence of hives. This is referred to as an elimination diet.

Itching may be relieved by applying cold compresses, taking acetaminophen **(M4),** or trying antihistamines such as diphenhydramine or chlorpheniramine **(M8).**

WHAT TO EXPECT AT THE DOCTOR'S OFFICE

If the patient is suffering a systemic reaction with difficulty breathing or dizziness, injections of adrenalin and other drugs may be given. In the more usual case of hives alone, the doctor may do two things. First, the doctor may prescribe an antihistamine or use

HIVES

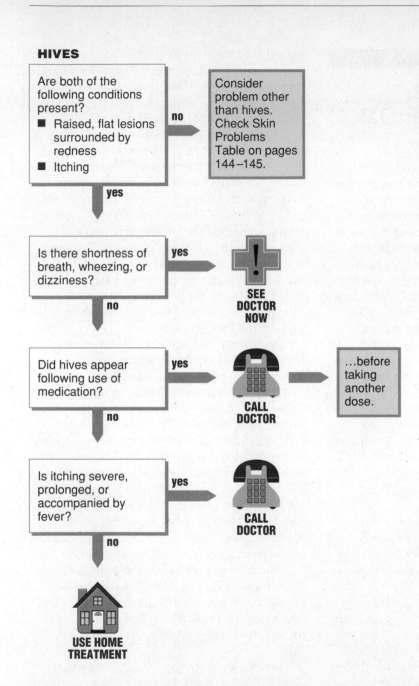

Are both of the following conditions present?

- Raised, flat lesions surrounded by redness
- Itching

no → Consider problem other than hives. Check Skin Problems Table on pages 144–145.

yes ↓

Is there shortness of breath, wheezing, or dizziness?

yes → SEE DOCTOR NOW

no ↓

Did hives appear following use of medication?

yes → CALL DOCTOR **→** ...before taking another dose.

no ↓

Is itching severe, prolonged, or accompanied by fever?

yes → CALL DOCTOR

no ↓

USE HOME TREATMENT

adrenalin injections to relieve swelling and itching. Second, the doctor can review the history of the reaction to try to find an offending agent and advise home treatment. Remember that most often the cause of hives goes undetected, and they stop occurring without any therapy.

43 Poison Ivy and Poison Oak

Poison ivy and poison oak need little introduction. The itching skin lesions that follow contact with the plant oil of these and other members of the *Rhus* plant category are the most common example of a larger category of skin problems known as contact dermatitis. Contact dermatitis simply means that something that has touched the skin has caused the skin to react. An initial exposure is necessary to "sensitize" the person; a subsequent exposure will result in an allergic reaction if the plant oil remains in contact with skin for several hours. The resulting rash begins after a delay of 12 to 48 hours and persists for about two weeks.

You do not have to come into direct contact with plants to get poison ivy. The plant oil may be spread by pets, contaminated clothing, or the smoke from burning *Rhus* plants. It can occur during any season.

HOME TREATMENT

The best approach is learning to recognize and avoid these plants, which are hazardous even in the winter when they have dropped their leaves.

Next best is to remove the plant oil from the skin as soon as possible. If the oil has been on the skin for less than six hours, thorough cleansing with ordinary soap, repeated three times, will often prevent a reaction. Alcohol-based cleansing tissues, available in prepackaged form (such as Alco-wipe), are much more effective. Rubbing alcohol on a washcloth is even better and is our favorite remedy.

Recently a new solvent (Tecnu) has been shown to be effective in removing the oil and preventing the rash. Rubbing alcohol is a lot less expensive, however.

To relieve itching, many doctors recommend cool compresses of Burow's solution (Domeboro, BurVeen, Bluboro) or baths with Aveeno or oatmeal (one cup to a tub full of water). Acetaminophen, aspirin, ibuprofen, and naproxen are also effective in reducing itching. The old standby, calamine lotion, sometimes helps for early lesions but may spread the plant oil. **(Caution:** Caladryl and Ziradryl are reported to cause allergic reactions in some people. Plain calamine lotion may be best.) Be sure to cleanse the skin, as above, even if you are too late to prevent the rash entirely.

Another method of obtaining symptomatic relief is a hot bath or shower. Heat releases histamine, the substance in skin cells that causes the intense itching. A hot shower or bath will cause intense itching as the histamine is released. The heat should be gradually increased to the maximum tolerable and continued until the itching has subsided. This process will deplete the cells of histamine, and the person will obtain up to eight hours of relief from the itching. This method has the advantage of not requiring frequent applications of ointments to the lesions and is a good way to get some sleep at night.

The itching may be treated with either an antihistamine (Benadryl or Vistaril, for example) or acetaminophen, aspirin, ibuprofen, and naproxen **(M4).** The antihistamines may cause drowsiness and interfere with sleep **(M8).**

One-half percent hydrocortisone creams (Cortaid or Lanacort, for example) are available without prescription. They will decrease inflammation and itching, but relief is not immediate. The cream must be applied

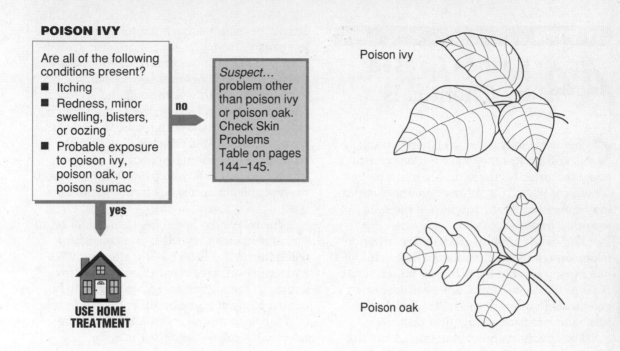

POISON IVY

Are all of the following conditions present?
- Itching
- Redness, minor swelling, blisters, or oozing
- Probable exposure to poison ivy, poison oak, or poison sumac

no →

Suspect... problem other than poison ivy or poison oak. Check Skin Problems Table on pages 144–145.

yes ↓

USE HOME TREATMENT

Poison ivy

Poison oak

often (four to six times a day). Do not use these creams for long periods **(M18).**

Poison ivy and poison oak will persist for the same length of time with or without medication. If secondary bacterial infection occurs, healing will be delayed; hence, scratching is not helpful. (Just in case you can't avoid the urge to scratch, cut your nails to avoid damage to the skin.)

Poison ivy is not contagious. It can't be spread once the oil has been either absorbed by the skin or removed.

If the lesions are too extensive to be easily treated, if home treatment is ineffective, or if the itching is so severe that it can't be tolerated, a call to the doctor may be necessary.

WHAT TO EXPECT AT THE DOCTOR'S OFFICE

After a history and physical examination, the doctor may prescribe a corticosteroid cream stronger than 0.5% hydrocortisone to be applied to the lesions four to six times a day. This often helps only moderately. An alternative is to give a steroid (such as prednisone) by mouth for a short period. A rather large dose is given the first day, and the dose is then gradually reduced. We don't recommend oral steroids except when there have been previous severe reactions or extensive exposure to poison ivy or poison oak.

44 Rashes Caused by Chemicals

Chemicals may cause a rash in two ways. The chemical may have a direct caustic effect that irritates the skin — a minor "chemical burn." Or, more often, the chemical may cause an allergic reaction of the skin, resulting in a rash.

The most common allergic skin irritation is poison ivy **(S43)**. If you see a rash that looks like poison ivy, but contact with poison ivy or poison oak seems impossible, consider other chemicals that might cause "contact dermatitis" and produce an identical rash.

The chemicals most frequently found to cause contact dermatitis are dyes and other chemicals found in clothing, chemicals used in elastic and rubber products, cosmetics, and deodorants (including "feminine" deodorants).

Usually the tip-off to the cause of the rash is its location and shape. Sometimes this is very striking, as when the rash leaves a perfect outline of a bra or the elastic bands of underwear or some other article of clothing. More often the rash is not so distinct, but its location suggests the possible cause.

HOME TREATMENT

If you have had difficulty with particular types of clothing, cosmetics, deodorants, and so on, then avoiding contact is the best way to avoid a problem. Changing brands may also help. For example, some cosmetics are manufactured so that they are less likely to cause an allergic reaction (hypoallergenic products). Rashes caused by deodorants are often relieved by using a milder preparation less often.

Once the rash has occurred, eliminating contact with the chemical is essential. Washing thoroughly with soap and water may remove chemicals on the skin and is especially important with materials such as cement dust. Oily substances may best be removed with rubbing alcohol, or use paint thinner quickly followed by soap and water to prevent contact dermatitis from the thinner itself.

The rest of the home treatment is identical to that for poison ivy **(S43)** and consists of using Burow's solution, hot water, and 0.5% hydrocortisone cream to achieve relief from itching. If the lesions are too extensive to be treated easily, if home treatment is ineffective, or if the itching is so severe that it can't be tolerated, a call to the doctor may be necessary.

WHAT TO EXPECT AT THE DOCTOR'S OFFICE

The doctor will examine the rash. A review of the patient's history will focus on possible exposure to substances such as those mentioned above. A corticosteroid cream stronger than 0.5% hydrocortisone may be prescribed. Another alternative is to give a corticosteroid (such as prednisone) for a short time; a rather large dose is given the first day, and the dose is then gradually reduced.

Itching may be treated with either an antihistamine (Benadryl, Vistaril, etc. — see **M8**) and/or pain relievers (acetaminophen, aspirin, ibuprofen, or naproxen — see **M4**). Antihistamines may cause drowsiness or interfere with sleep.

RASHES CAUSED BY CHEMICALS

Is this a red rash (sometimes with bumps or blisters and usually itchy or burning) that by its shape and location suggests contact with articles of clothing, cosmetics, deodorant, or other chemicals?

no →

Suspect... problem other than contact dermatitis. Check Skin Problems Table on pages 144–145.

yes

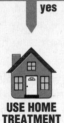

USE HOME TREATMENT

45 Skin Cancer

Irregular borders — Asymmetrical shape

Diameter of greater than ¼ inch

Color variations: tans, browns, blacks, red, white, blue

Characteristics of skin cancer. Look for changes in size, color, surface, or border. It is not necessary for all of these characteristics to be present for a spot to be regarded as suspicious.

There is no easy, sure way to identify skin cancer. The guidelines here are those that doctors use in confronting this dilemma. When in doubt, they will remove the lesion for testing (biopsy). You can do no better, so when in doubt, see a doctor.

Decisions will be easier if you are familiar with common noncancerous skin lesions:

- Plain old freckles (flat, uniform, tan to dark brown color, regular border, usually less than one-quarter inch, or 6 mm, in diameter)

- Warts (skin-colored, raised, rounded, rough or flat surface)

- Skin tags (wobbly tags of skin on a stalk)

- Seborrheic keratoses (greasy, dirty tan to brown, raised, flat lesions that first appear in midlife on face, chest, and back and increase in number with the passing years)

Types of Skin Cancer

The vast majority of skin cancers fall into three categories.

Malignant Melanoma. Malignant melanoma is by far the most dangerous. Though described as moles that have undergone cancerous change, melanomas often do not look like moles — they may be flat.

Doctors look for three characteristics in judging the likelihood of a melanoma:

- Changes in size, color, surface, shape, or border appear. The more rapid, unusual,

and irregular these changes are, the higher suspicion is raised.

- Variation in color (tans, browns, or blacks) is unusual for a benign lesion. Hues of red, white, and blue may signal melanomas.

- An irregular border suggests the spread of abnormal cells; a benign lesion usually has a regular border.

Squamous Cell Cancers. Squamous cell cancers are raised, usually somewhat bumpy lesions with rough, scaly surfaces on a reddish base, and they often bleed. The border is usually irregular. These lesions grow slowly and usually do not spread to other parts of the body. Most often they are recognized as sores that don't heal. Solar keratoses appear similar to squamous cell carcinoma, but they are not bumps and rarely bleed. Although solar keratoses are not malignant, they are considered to be a precursor of cancer and are often treated to avoid the development of cancer.

Basal Cell Cancers. Basal cell cancers appear as pearly or waxy nodules with central depressions or craters. As this cancer enlarges, the center usually becomes more ulcerated,

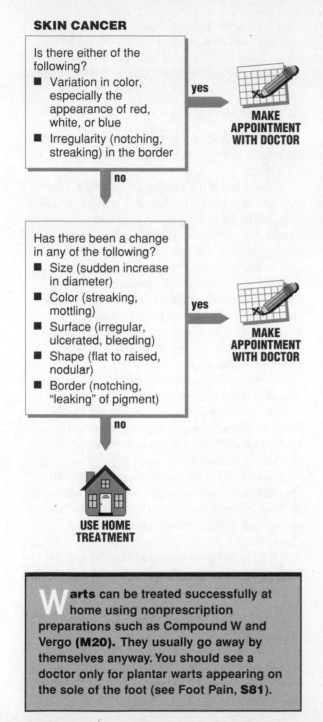

SKIN CANCER

Is there either of the following?
- Variation in color, especially the appearance of red, white, or blue
- Irregularity (notching, streaking) in the border

yes → **MAKE APPOINTMENT WITH DOCTOR**

no ↓

Has there been a change in any of the following?
- Size (sudden increase in diameter)
- Color (streaking, mottling)
- Surface (irregular, ulcerated, bleeding)
- Shape (flat to raised, nodular)
- Border (notching, "leaking" of pigment)

yes → **MAKE APPOINTMENT WITH DOCTOR**

no ↓

USE HOME TREATMENT

Warts can be treated successfully at home using nonprescription preparations such as Compound W and Vergo **(M20).** They usually go away by themselves anyway. You should see a doctor only for plantar warts appearing on the sole of the foot (see Foot Pain, **S81**).

giving it the appearance of having been gnawed. Hence, the term "rodent ulcer" is sometimes applied. This type of cancer grows slowly and only by direct extension so that it never spreads (metastasizes) to other organs of the body.

All these cancers are related to sun exposure. Squamous cell and basal cell cancers appear almost exclusively on the areas of skin most exposed to sun (head, neck, hands). Melanoma is also common in these areas but may appear on the chest or back. Melanoma is most common in people who have had one or more severe blistering sunburns before the age of 18.

HOME TREATMENT

Home treatment consists of watchful waiting and prevention. If the lesion has none of the characteristics that raise suspicion, then closely watching for change makes sense. But if you are in doubt, see the doctor or ask questions at your next visit.

Let's face it, sun is no good for your skin. Sunscreens, hats with wide brims, long sleeves, and pants will lower the risk of skin cancer and keep your skin younger looking.

WHAT TO EXPECT AT THE DOCTOR'S OFFICE

Dermatologists (skin specialists) can usually offer the best advice about skin lesions. Successful treatment can be done on the initial visit and often doesn't require surgery.

A reminder: If you get one of these cancers, you are likely to get another. So, once you've had the first one cured, it is a good idea to have regular examinations to make sure that nothing new has developed. Avoid further damage to the skin from the sun.

46 Eczema

Eczema, or atopic dermatitis, is commonly found in people with a family history of eczema, hay fever, or asthma. As with asthma, a variety of conditions can aggravate eczema: infection, emotional stress, food allergy, and sweating.

The underlying problem is the inability of the skin to retain adequate amounts of water. The skin of people with eczema is consequently very dry, which causes the skin to itch. Most of the manifestations of eczema are a result of scratching. The scratching produces weeping, infected skin. Dried weepings lead to crusting. Sufficient scratching will produce a thickened, rough skin, which is characteristic of long-standing atopic dermatitis.

In young infants who can't scratch, the most common manifestation is red, dry, mildly scaling cheeks, caused when the child rubs them against the sheets. In infants eczema may also be found in the area where plastic pants meet the skin. The tightness of the elastic produces the characteristic red, scaling lesion. In older children it's very common for eczema to involve the area behind the knees and inside the elbows. Adults often have problems with their hands, especially if they're in frequent contact with water.

If there's a large amount of weeping or crusting, the eczema may be infected with bacteria, and a call to the doctor will most likely be required.

The course of eczema is quite variable. Some people will have only a brief, mild problem; others have mild-to-severe manifestations throughout life. Bouts of eczema are often related to emotional factors; identifying and dealing with such emotional triggers may be the key to successful therapy.

HOME TREATMENT

Therapy is based on good skin care and, if the eczema is allergic in nature, avoiding allergens.

Try to keep the skin from becoming too dry. Frequent bathing actually makes the skin drier. Although the person will feel comfortable in the bath, the itching will become more intense afterward. Avoid bathing with soap and water because these tend to dry the skin. Instead use "non-lipid" cleansers, such as those with cetyl alcohol (Cetaphil, etc.). Use rubber gloves to protect the hands when washing dishes or the car. Freshwater or pool swimming can aggravate eczema, but ocean swimming doesn't.

Sweating aggravates eczema. Avoid overdressing. Light night clothing is important. Cotton clothing is suggested; contact with wool and silk seems to aggravate eczema and should be avoided. Avoid synthetic fabrics that don't "breathe."

Avoid all oil or grease preparations; they clog the skin, increasing sweat retention and itching. Keep nails trimmed short to minimize the effects of scratching, especially with children.

Itching is often worse at bedtime. Acetaminophen, aspirin, ibuprofen, and naproxen are effective and inexpensive medications that reduce itching **(M4).** Antihistamines also reduce itching but should be used only if necessary **(M8).**

Avoiding cow's milk is often suggested, particularly for children. Make sure this really works for your child before permanently changing to more expensive foods. When

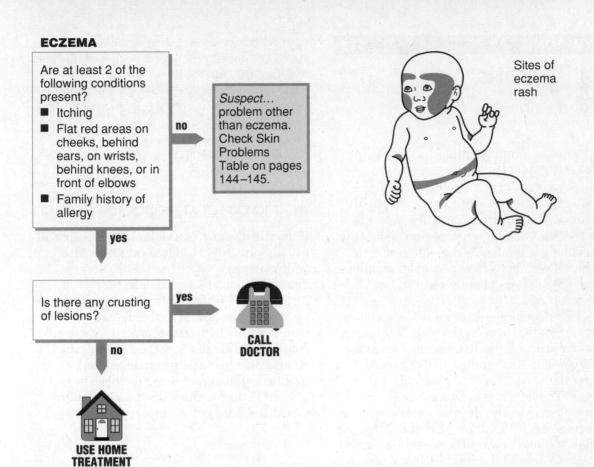

ECZEMA

Are at least 2 of the following conditions present?

- Itching
- Flat red areas on cheeks, behind ears, on wrists, behind knees, or in front of elbows
- Family history of allergy

no →

Suspect... problem other than eczema. Check Skin Problems Table on pages 144–145.

yes ↓

Is there any crusting of lesions?

yes → **CALL DOCTOR**

no ↓

USE HOME TREATMENT

Sites of eczema rash

---

trying any milk-avoidance diet, make no other changes in food or other care for a full two weeks unless absolutely necessary.

WHAT TO EXPECT AT THE DOCTOR'S OFFICE

By gathering the patient's history and examination of the lesions, the doctor can determine whether the problem is eczema. If crusted or weeping lesions are present, bacterial infection is likely and an oral antibiotic will be prescribed. There has been no benefit demonstrated from either skin testing or hyposensitization (allergy shots).

If home treatment hasn't improved the problem, the doctor may prescribe corticosteroid creams and lotions. While these are effective, they aren't curative; eczema is characterized by repeated occurrences. Furthermore, because of their potential side effects, corticosteroid creams should be used only for a short period.

47 Boils

A familiar term, "painful as a boil," emphasizes the severe discomfort that can arise
from this common skin problem. A boil is a
localized infection, usually due to staphylococcus bacteria. Often a particularly savage
strain of the bacteria is responsible. When this
particular germ inhabits the skin, recurrent
problems with boils may persist for months or
years. Often several family members will be
affected at about the same time.

Boils may be single or multiple, and they
may occur anywhere on the body. They range
from the size of a pea to the size of a walnut
or larger. The surrounding red, thickened, and
tender tissue increases the problem even
further. The infection begins in the tissues
beneath the skin and develops into an abscess
— a pocket filled with pus. Eventually the pus
pocket "points" toward the skin surface and
finally ruptures and drains. Then it heals.

Boils often begin as infections around hair
follicles; hence the term folliculitis for minor
infections. Areas under pressure (such as the
buttocks) are often likely spots for boils to
begin. A boil that extends into the deeper
layers of the skin is called a carbuncle.

Special consideration should be given to
boils on the face because they are more likely
to lead to serious complicating infections.

HOME TREATMENT

The goal of treatment is to let it all out — the
pus, that is. Boils are handled gently, because
rough treatment can force the infection deeper
inside the body. Warm, moist compresses are
applied gently several times each day to
speed the development of a pocket of pus and
to soften the skin for the eventual rupture and
drainage. Once drainage begins, the compresses will help keep the opening in the skin
clear. The more drainage, the better. Frequent,
thorough soaping of the entire skin helps
prevent reinfection. Ignore all temptation to
squeeze the boil.

WHAT TO EXPECT AT THE DOCTOR'S OFFICE

If there is fever or a facial boil, the doctor will
usually prescribe an antibiotic. Otherwise
antibiotics may not be used. They are of
limited help in abscesslike infections.

If the boil feels as if fluid is contained in a
pocket but has not yet drained, the doctor
may lance the boil. In this procedure a small
incision is made to allow the pus to drain.
After drainage the pain is reduced, and
healing is quite prompt. While this is not a
complicated procedure, it is tricky enough
that you should not attempt it yourself.

BOILS

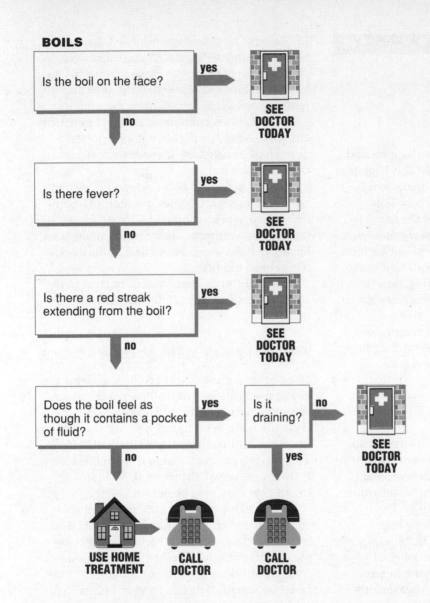

Is the boil on the face?

yes → SEE DOCTOR TODAY

no ↓

Is there fever?

yes → SEE DOCTOR TODAY

no ↓

Is there a red streak extending from the boil?

yes → SEE DOCTOR TODAY

no ↓

Does the boil feel as though it contains a pocket of fluid?

yes → Is it draining?

no → SEE DOCTOR TODAY

no ↓ USE HOME TREATMENT

CALL DOCTOR

yes ↓ CALL DOCTOR

48 Acne

Acne is a superficial skin eruption caused by a combination of factors. It is triggered by the hormonal changes of puberty and is most common in children with oily skin. When oil plugs the openings of the hair follicles and oil glands, increased skin oils accumulate and bacteria grow. These bacteria cause changes in the oil secretions that make them irritating to the surrounding skin. The result is usually a pimple or sometimes a cyst, a larger pocket of secretions.

Blackheads are formed when air causes a chemical change — oxidation — of the plugs, called keratin plugs. Blackheads cause minimal skin irritation.

HOME TREATMENT

While excessive dirt will certainly aggravate acne, careful cleaning won't always prevent it. Nevertheless, the face should be scrubbed several times daily with a warm washcloth to remove skin oils and keratin plugs. The rubbing and heat of the washcloth help dislodge keratin plugs. Soap will help remove skin oil and will decrease the number of bacteria living on the skin. If there are pimples on the back, a backbrush or washcloth should be used. Greases and creams on the skin may aggravate the problem.

Diet isn't an important factor in most cases, but if certain foods tend to aggravate the problem, avoid them. There is little evidence that chocolate aggravates acne, despite popular belief.

Several further steps may be taken at home. An abrasive soap (Pernox, Brasivol, etc.) may be used one to three times daily to further reduce the oiliness of the skin and to remove the keratin plugs from the follicles.

Medications containing benzoyl peroxide are now widely available without prescription. Used as directed, these are effective in mild cases.

Steam may help open clogged pores, so hot compresses are sometimes helpful. Some dermatologists recommend Vlemasque as a hot drying compress. A drying agent such as Fostex may be used, but irritation may occur if it is used too often.

Should these measures fail to control the problem, make an appointment with the doctor.

WHAT TO EXPECT AT THE DOCTOR'S OFFICE

The doctor will advise about hygiene and the use of medications. Topical preparations such as retinoic acid (Retin-A) and benzoyl peroxide have been found helpful; they act by fostering skin peeling or eliminating bacteria. The peeling isn't noticeable if the medication is used properly. Ultraviolet (UV) light treatments may also be helpful.

In resistant cases an antibiotic (tetracycline or erythromycin) may be prescribed to be taken by mouth. Some doctors prescribe these antibiotics for application to the skin as well. Isotretinoin (Accutane) is another drug taken by mouth that can be very helpful in severe cases of acne, but it is a powerful drug that can cause serious side effects. If taken by a pregnant woman, there is a very high risk that the baby will be harmed. Women who might be pregnant shouldn't take isotretinoin.

"Acne surgery" is a term generally applied to the doctor's removal of blackheads

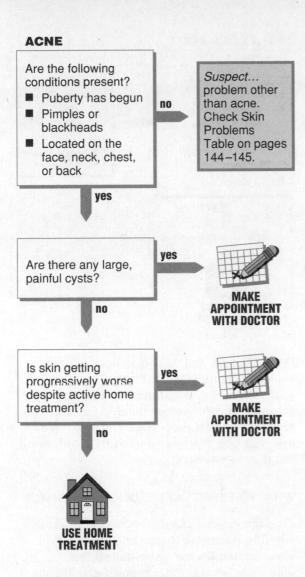

ACNE

Are the following conditions present?
- Puberty has begun
- Pimples or blackheads
- Located on the face, neck, chest, or back

no →

Suspect... problem other than acne. Check Skin Problems Table on pages 144–145.

yes ↓

Are there any large, painful cysts?

yes → **MAKE APPOINTMENT WITH DOCTOR**

no ↓

Is skin getting progressively worse despite active home treatment?

yes → **MAKE APPOINTMENT WITH DOCTOR**

no ↓

USE HOME TREATMENT

with a suction device and an eyedropper. Large developing cysts are sometimes arrested with the injection of corticosteroids. Such procedures should be required only in severe cases and are more often performed on the back than on the face.

49 Athlete's Foot

A thlete's foot is very common during and after adolescence, and relatively uncommon before. It is the most common of the fungal infections and is often persistent. When it involves toenails, it can be difficult to treat.

Moisture contributes significantly to the development of this problem. Some doctors believe bacteria and moisture cause most of the problem and that the fungus is responsible only for keeping things going. When many people share locker room and shower facilities, exposure to this fungus is impossible to prevent; infection is the rule rather than the exception. But you don't have to participate in sports to contract this fungus; it's all around.

HOME TREATMENT

Scrupulous hygiene, without resorting to drugs, is often effective. Twice a day, wash the space between the toes with soap, water, and a cloth. Dry the entire area carefully with a towel, particularly between the toes (despite the pain) and put on clean socks.

Use shoes that allow evaporation of moisture. Avoid shoes with plastic linings. Sandals or canvas sneakers are best. Changing shoes every other day to allow them to dry out is a good idea.

Keeping the feet dry with the use of a powder is helpful in preventing reinfection. Over-the-counter drugs such as Desenex powder or cream may be used. The powder has the virtue of helping keep the toes dry. Tolnaftate (Tinactin, etc.), miconazole

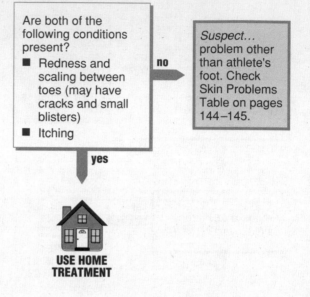

ATHLETE'S FOOT

Are both of the following conditions present?
- Redness and scaling between toes (may have cracks and small blisters)
- Itching

no → *Suspect...* problem other than athlete's foot. Check Skin Problems Table on pages 144–145.

yes ↓

USE HOME TREATMENT

(Micatin, etc.), and clotrimazole (Lotrimin, etc.) are effective **(M17).** The twice-daily application of a 30% aluminum chloride solution has been recommended for its drying and antibacterial properties. You will have to ask your pharmacist to make up the solution, but it is inexpensive.

WHAT TO EXPECT AT THE DOCTOR'S OFFICE

Through history, physical examination, and, possibly, microscopic examination of a skin scraping, the doctor will establish the diagnosis. Several other problems, notably a condition called dyshydrosis, may mimic athlete's foot. Haloprogin (Halotex) and ciclopirox (Loprox) are prescription creams and ointments that work against fungal infections of the skin but not against fungal infections of nails (ciclopirox seems to work on nails occasionally). An oral drug, griseofulvin, may be used for the nails but isn't recommended otherwise.

50 Jock Itch

We might wish for a less picturesque name for this condition, but the medical term, *tinea cruris*, is understood by few. Jock itch is a fungus infection of the pubic region. It is aggravated by friction and moisture. It usually doesn't involve the scrotum or penis, nor does it spread beyond the groin area. (For the most part, this is a male disease.) Frequently the fungus grows in an athletic supporter turned old and moldy in a locker room far from a washing machine. The preventive measure for such a problem is obvious.

HOME TREATMENT

The problem should be treated by removing the contributing factors: friction and moisture. This is done by wearing boxer shorts rather than closer-fitting shorts or jockey briefs, by applying a powder to dry the area after bathing, and by frequently changing soiled or sweaty underclothes. It may take up to two weeks to completely clear the problem, and it may recur. The "powder-air-and-clean-shorts" treatment will usually be successful without any medication. Tolnaftate (Tinactin, etc.), miconazole (Micatin, etc.), or clotrimazole (Lotrimin, etc.) will usually eliminate the fungus if the problem persists **(M17).**

WHAT TO EXPECT AT THE DOCTOR'S OFFICE

Occasionally a yeast infection will mimic jock itch. By examining the area and asking questions, the doctor will try to establish the

JOCK ITCH

Are all of the following conditions present?
- Involves only the groin and thighs
- Redness, oozing, or some peripheral scaling
- Itching

no → *Suspect...* problem other than jock itch. Check Skin Problems Table on pages 144–145.

yes ↓

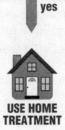

USE HOME TREATMENT

diagnosis and may also make a scraping in order to identify yeast. Medicines for this problem are virtually always applied to the affected skin; oral drugs or injections are rarely used. Haloprogin (Halotex) and ciclopirox (Loprox) are prescription creams and lotions that are effective against both fungi and certain yeast infections.

51 Sunburn

Sunburn is common, painful, and avoidable. It is better prevented than treated. Effective sunscreens are available in a wide variety of strengths, as indicated by their sun protection factor or SPF. An SPF of 4 offers little protection, whereas 15 or above offers substantial protection.

Regardless of what you have heard, there are no sun rays that tan but don't burn. Tanning salons can fry you just as surely as the sun can.

The pain of sunburn is worst between 6 and 48 hours after sun exposure. Peeling of injured layers of skin occurs later — between 3 and 10 days after the burn.

Very rarely, people with sunburn have difficulty with vision. If so, they should see a doctor. Otherwise a visit to the doctor is unnecessary unless the pain is extraordinarily severe or extensive blistering (not peeling) has occurred. Blistering indicates a second-degree burn and rarely follows sun exposure.

HOME TREATMENT

Cool compresses or cool oatmeal baths (Aveeno, etc.) may be useful. Ordinary baking soda (one-half cup to a tub) is nearly as effective. Lubricants such as Vaseline feel good to some people, but they retain heat and shouldn't be used the first day. Avoid products that contain benzocaine. These may give temporary relief but can irritate the skin and may actually delay healing. Pain-relieving medication such as acetaminophen may ease pain and thus help the person sleep **(M4)**.

WHAT TO EXPECT AT THE DOCTOR'S OFFICE

The doctor will direct the history and physical examination toward determining the extent of the burn and the possibility of other heat-related injuries like sunstroke. If only first-degree burns are found, a prescription corticosteroid lotion may be prescribed. This isn't particularly beneficial. The rare second-degree burns may be treated with antibiotics in addition to analgesics (pain relievers).

SUNBURN

Are any of these conditions present following pro-longed exposure to sun?

- Fever
- Fluid-filled blisters
- Dizziness
- Visual difficulties

yes →

CALL DOCTOR

no ↓

USE HOME TREATMENT

Minor **frostbite** is surprisingly common among skiers and others indulging in winter sports. Prevention is the key. Wear warm clothing. When your torso is warm, the blood flow to the fingers and toes is better. Don't forget a face mask. Use mittens instead of gloves when it is very cold. If there is wind, be sure that you have windproof outer garments.

If your fingers or nose or toes start to hurt despite these precautions, it's a warning to get out of the cold. If they begin to numb, you are starting to get frostbite. It used to be said that you should warm up a frostbitten limb slowly. Not so. Warm it up as quickly as possible with gentle rubbing. As the blood flow resumes, the frostbitten part will begin to hurt, sometimes a lot. This is a good sign, since the tissues are obviously still alive.

You may have leftover numbness for several months after minor frostbite, but this doesn't require medical attention. However, if tissues turn black, see a doctor so that the threatened tissues can be preserved.

52 Lice and Bedbugs

Lice and bedbugs are found in the best of families. Lack of prejudice with respect to social class is as close as these insects come to having a virtue. At best they are a nuisance, and at worst they can cause real disability.

Lice

Lice themselves are very small and are seldom seen without the aid of a magnifying glass. Usually it is easier to find the "nits," which are clusters of louse eggs. Without magnification, nits will appear as tiny white lumps on hair strands.

The louse bite leaves only a pinpoint red spot, but scratching makes things worse. Itching and occasional small, shallow sores at the base of hairs are clues to the disease.

Pubic lice aren't a venereal disease, although they may be spread from person to person during sexual contact. Unlike syphilis and gonorrhea, lice may be spread by toilet seats, infected linen, and other sources. Pubic lice bear some resemblance to crabs. Hence, the term "crabs" is used to indicate a lice infestation of the pubic hair. A different species of louse may inhabit the scalp or other body hair.

Lice like to be close to a warm body all the time and won't stay for long in clothing that isn't being worn, bedding, or other places.

Bedbugs

Although related to lice, bedbugs present a considerably different picture. The adult is flat, wingless, reddish in color, oval in shape, and about one-quarter inch (6 mm) in length. Like lice, they stay alive by sucking blood. Unlike lice, they feed for only 10 or 15 minutes at a time and spend the rest of the time hiding in crevices and crannies.

Bedbugs feed almost entirely at night, because that is when bodies are in bed and because bedbugs strongly dislike light. They have such a keen sense of the nearness of a warm body that the army has used them to detect the approach of an enemy at ranges of several hundred feet! Catching these pests out in the open is very difficult and may require some curious behavior. One technique is to dash into the bedroom at bedtime, flip on the lights and pull back the bedcovers in an effort to catch them anticipating their next meal.

The bite of the bedbug leaves a firm bump. Usually there are two or three bumps clustered together. Occasionally sensitivity develops to these bites, in which case itching may be severe and blisters may form.

HOME TREATMENT

Over-the-counter preparations are effective against lice; these include A200, Cuprex, and RID. RID has the advantage of supplying a fine-tooth comb, a rare item these days. Instructions that come with these drugs must be followed carefully. Linen and clothing must be changed simultaneously. Sexual partners should be treated at the same time.

Because bedbugs don't hide on the body or in clothes, it is the bed and the room that should be treated. Contact your local health department for information and help in doing this. Chemical sprays may be useful, but simply getting the infested bedding outdoors and exposed to sun and air for several days works, too.

LICE AND BEDBUGS

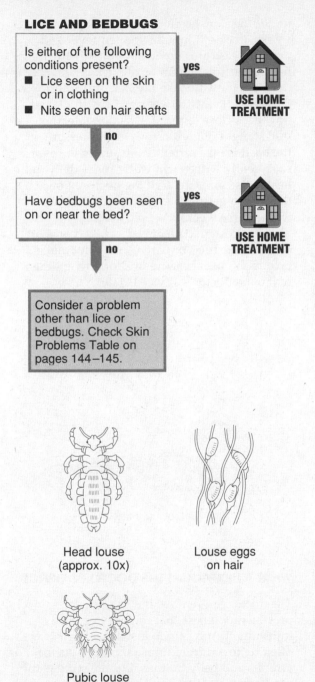

Is either of the following conditions present?
- Lice seen on the skin or in clothing
- Nits seen on hair shafts

yes → USE HOME TREATMENT

no ↓

Have bedbugs been seen on or near the bed?

yes → USE HOME TREATMENT

no ↓

Consider a problem other than lice or bedbugs. Check Skin Problems Table on pages 144–145.

WHAT TO EXPECT AT THE DOCTOR'S OFFICE

If lice are the suspected problem, the doctor will make a careful inspection to find nits or the lice themselves. Doctors almost always use lindane (Kwell, Scabene) for lice. It may be somewhat more effective than the over-the-counter preparations. It is also more expensive, has more side effects, and is too strong to be used more than two times, a week apart.

The doctor will be hard-pressed to make a certain diagnosis of bedbug bites without information from you that bedbugs have been seen in the house. However, the bumps may be suggestive, and initially it may be decided to assume that the problem is bedbugs. If this is the case, treatment with an insecticide as discussed under Home Treatment will be recommended.

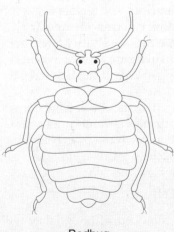

Head louse
(approx. 10x)

Louse eggs
on hair

Pubic louse
(approx. 10x)

Bedbug
(approx. 10x)

Bedbug
(approx. size)

53 Ticks

Outdoor living has its dangers. While bears, mountain lions, and steep cliffs can usually be avoided, shrubs and tall grasses hide tiny insects eager for a blood meal from a passing animal or person. Ticks are the most common of these small hazards.

Ticks are about one-quarter inch (6 mm) long and are easily seen. The creature that made the tick bite can usually be found sticking out of it.

In some areas ticks carry diseases, such as Rocky Mountain spotted fever and Lyme disease. If a fever, rash, joint pains, or headache follow a tick bite by a few days or weeks, a doctor should be consulted.

If a pregnant female tick is allowed to remain feeding for several days, under certain circumstances a peculiar condition called tick paralysis may develop. The female tick secretes a toxin that can cause temporary paralysis, which clears up shortly after the tick is removed. This complication is quite rare and can happen only if the tick stays in place many days.

In tick-infested areas, check yourself, your children, and your pets several times a day. You may be able to catch the ticks before they become embedded.

HOME TREATMENT

Ticks should be removed, although they will eventually "fester out"; complications are unusual. The trick is to get the tick to "let go" and not to squeeze the tick before getting it out. If the mouth parts and the pincers remain under the skin, healing may require several weeks. Rocky Mountain spotted fever and Lyme disease are somewhat more likely if mouth parts are left in or the tick is squeezed during removal. Make the tick uncomfortable. Grasp the tick with tweezers or with gloved fingers as close to the skin as possible, then pull straight out with slow, even pressure. If the head is inadvertently left under the skin, soak gently with warm water twice daily until healing is complete. Call the doctor at once if the person gets a fever, rash, or headache within three weeks.

Corticosteroid creams (Cortaid, Lanacort, etc.) may be tried but are usually not much help; don't use these creams for a long time without a doctor's advice **(M18)**.

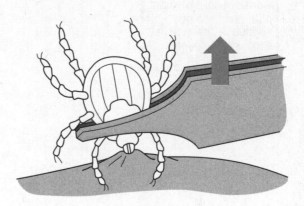

Removing a tick

WHAT TO EXPECT AT THE DOCTOR'S OFFICE

The doctor can remove the tick but can't prevent any illness that might have been transmitted. You can do just as well. Ticks are often removed from unusual places, such as armpits and belly buttons, but the scalp is the most common location. The technique is exactly the same no matter where the tick is.

TICKS

Can tick be seen buried in skin, or is a swollen tick attached to skin?

no → *Suspect...* problem other than ticks. Check Skin Problems Table on pages 144–145.

yes ↓

USE HOME TREATMENT

Deer tick
(approx. 10x)

approx. size

54 Chiggers

Chiggers, like ticks, are a small hazard of nature. Anyone who grew up in areas where they are common can testify to how excruciating the itch from chiggers' bites can be.

Chiggers are small red mites, sometimes called "redbugs," that live on grasses and shrubs. Their bite contains a chemical that eats away at the skin, causing a tremendous itch. Usually the small red sores are around the belt line or other openings in clothes. Careful inspection may reveal the tiny red larvae in the center of the itching sore.

HOME TREATMENT

Chiggers are better avoided than treated. Using insect repellents, wearing appropriate clothing, and bathing after exposure help to cut down on the frequency of bites. Once you get them, they itch, often for several weeks. Keep the sores clean and soak them with warm water twice daily. Cuprex, RID, and A200 applied immediately may help kill the larvae, but the itch will persist.

Corticosteroid creams (Cortaid, Lanacort, etc.) may be tried but are usually not much help; don't use these creams for a long time without a doctor's advice **(M18)**.

Nail polish is said to give relief from itching, but we aren't aware of scientific evaluations of its effect.

WHAT TO EXPECT AT THE DOCTOR'S OFFICE

Doctors will usually prescribe lindane (Kwell, Scabene, etc.), which is perhaps somewhat more effective than A200, RID, or Cuprex but doesn't stop the itching either. Lindane is too strong to be used more than two times, a week apart.

Antihistamines **(M8)** make the patient drowsy and aren't often used unless intense itching persists despite home treatment with pain relievers **(M4),** warm baths, oatmeal soaks (Aveeno, etc.), and calamine lotion.

CHIGGERS

Are any of the
following present?

- Itching red sores
  around the belt line
  or other opening in
  clothes
- Itching red sores
  following contact
  with grass or
  shrubs
- Small red mites
  seen on the skin or
  red spot in center
  of sore

no →

Suspect...
problem other
than chiggers.
Check Skin
Problems
Table on pages
144–145.

yes ↓

**USE HOME
TREATMENT**

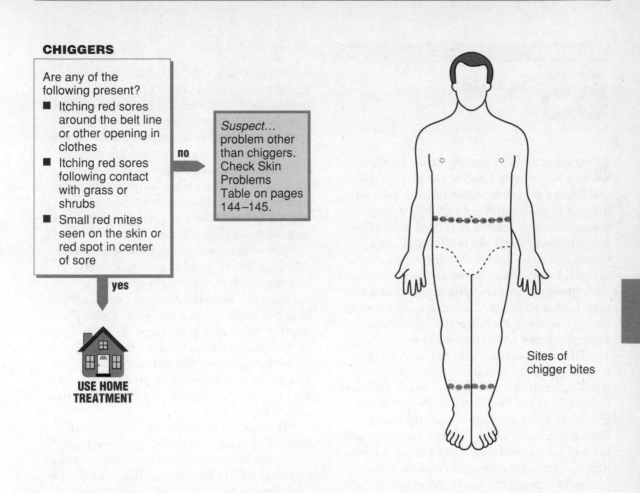

Sites of
chigger bites

55 Scabies

Scabies is an irritation of the skin caused by a tiny mite related to the chigger. No one knows why, but scabies seems to be on the rise in this country. As with lice, it is no longer true that scabies is related to hygiene. It occurs in the best of families and in the cleanest of neighborhoods. The mite easily spreads from person to person or by contact with items such as clothing and bedding that may harbor the mite. Epidemics often spread through schools despite strict precautions against contact with known cases.

The mite burrows into the skin to lay eggs; its favorite locations are given in the decision chart. These burrows may be evident, especially at the beginning of the problem. However, the mite soon causes the skin to have a reaction so that redness, swelling, and blisters follow within a short period. Intense itching causes scratching so that there are plenty of scratch marks. These may become infected from the bacteria on the skin. Thus, the telltale burrows are often obscured by scratch marks, blisters, and secondary infection.

If you can locate something that looks like a burrow, you might be able to see the mite with the aid of a magnifying lens. This is the only way to be absolutely sure that the problem is scabies, but it is often not possible. The diagnosis is most often made based on symptoms and history that are consistent with scabies, as well as the fact that scabies is known to be in the community.

HOME TREATMENT

Benzyl benzoate (25% solution) is effective against scabies and doesn't require a prescription. Unfortunately it isn't widely available. If you are able to find it, apply it once to the entire body except for the face and around the urinary opening of the penis or the vaginal opening. Wash it off 24 hours later. This medicine does have an odor that some find unpleasant. If you can't find benzyl benzoate, you'll have to get a prescription for lindane from your doctor.

For itching, we recommend cool soaks, calamine lotion, and/or pain relievers (acetaminophen, aspirin, ibuprofen, or naproxen — see **M4**). Antihistamines may help but often cause drowsiness **(M8);** follow the directions on the package. As in the case of poison ivy, warmth makes the itching worse by releasing histamine, but if all the histamine is released, relief may be obtained for several hours (see Poison Ivy and Poison Oak, **S43**).

It will take some time before the skin becomes normal, even with effective treat-ment, but at least some improvement should be noted within 72 hours. If this isn't the case, visit the doctor.

WHAT TO EXPECT AT THE DOCTOR'S OFFICE

The doctor should examine the entire skin surface for signs of the problem and may examine an area with a magnifying lens in an attempt to identify the mite. A scraping of a lesion may be taken for examination under the microscope. Most of the time the doctor will be forced to make a decision based on the probability of various kinds of diseases and then treat it much as you would at home. The proof will be whether or not the treatment is successful.

SCABIES

Are all of the following conditions present?

- Intense itching
- Raised red skin in a line (represents a burrow) and possibly blisters or pustules
- Located on the hands, especially between the fingers, elbow crease, armpit, groin crease, or behind the knees
- Exposure to scabies

no →

Consider a problem other than scabies. Check Skin Problems Table on pages 144–145.

yes ↓

USE HOME TREATMENT

Lindane (Kwell, Scabene, etc.) will often be prescribed. Because of the potency of this medication it shouldn't be used more than two times, a week apart.

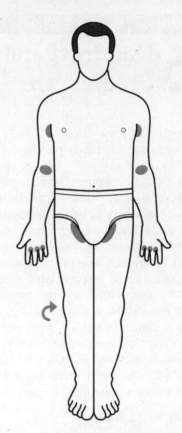

Sites of scabies bites

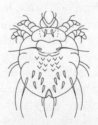

Scabies mite, greatly enlarged (approx. size: ·)

56 Dandruff and Cradle Cap

Although they look different, cradle cap and dandruff are really part of the same problem; its medical term is seborrhea. Oil glands in the skin become stimulated by adult hormones, leading to oiliness and flaking of the scalp. This occurs in infants because of exposure to the mother's hormones and in older children when they begin to make their own adult hormones. The problem also occurs between infancy and puberty, and once a child has the problem, it tends to recur.

Seborrhea itself is a somewhat ugly but relatively harmless condition. However, it may make the skin more susceptible to infection with yeast or bacteria. Children with seborrhea frequently have redness and scaling of the eyebrows and behind the ears as well.

Look-alike Problems

Occasionally this condition is mistaken for ringworm of the scalp. Careful attention to the conditions listed in the decision chart will usually avoid this confusion. Remember also that ringworm would be unusual in the newborn and very young child. See Ringworm **(S41).**

Another potentially confusing problem is psoriasis. This condition resembles seborrhea somewhat but often stops at the hairline. The scales of psoriasis are on top of raised lesions called "plaques," which isn't the case in seborrhea. Home treatment is unlikely to be helpful for psoriasis, so the help of a doctor is needed.

HOME TREATMENT

Many widely available antidandruff shampoos are helpful in mild to moderate cases of dandruff. For severe and more stubborn cases there are some less well-known but effective over-the-counter shampoos that contain selenium sulfide. Selsun (available by prescription only) and Selsun Blue are examples of such shampoos. Over-the-counter preparations, while weaker, are just as good if you apply them more liberally and frequently. When using these shampoos, it is important that you follow directions carefully, because oiliness and yellowish discoloration of the hair may occur. Sebulex, Sebucare, Ionil, and DHS are effective and must be used strictly according to directions also. Unfortunately, none of these shampoos is effective at making it easier to get a date.

Cradle cap is best treated with a soft scrub brush. If it is thick, rub in warm baby oil, cover with a warm towel, and soak for 15 minutes. Use a fine-tooth comb or scrub brush to help remove the scales. Then shampoo with Sebulex or one of the other preparations listed above. Be careful to avoid getting shampoo in the eyes.

No matter what you do, the problem will often return, and you may have to repeat the treatment. If the problem gets worse despite home treatment over several weeks, see the doctor.

WHAT TO EXPECT AT THE DOCTOR'S OFFICE

Severe cases of seborrhea may require more than the medications mentioned above; a cortisone cream is most often prescribed. Usually a trip to the doctor clears up some confusion concerning the diagnosis. The doctor generally makes the diagnosis on the basis of the appearance of the rash.

DANDRUFF

In an infant, are all of the following conditions present?

- Thick, adherent, oily, yellowish scaling or crusting patches
- Located on the scalp, behind the ears, in the eyebrows, or (less frequently) in the skin creases of the groin
- Only mild redness in involved areas

no →

Suspect... problem other than cradle cap. Check Skin Problems Table on pages 144–145.

In an older child (or adult), are all of the following conditions present?

- Fine, white, oily scales
- Confined to scalp and/or eyebrows
- Only mild redness in involved areas

no →

Suspect... problem other than dandruff. Check Skin Problems Table on pages 144–145.

yes ↓

USE HOME TREATMENT

Occasionally scrapings from the involved areas will be looked at under the microscope. Drugs by mouth or by injection aren't indicated for seborrhea unless bacterial infection has complicated the problem.

57 Patchy Loss of Skin Color

Seeing patches of paler skin on yourself or your child can be unnerving. Luckily, this condition is usually temporary and harmless.

Children are constantly getting minor cuts, scrapes, insect bites, and minor skin infections. During the healing process it is common for the skin to lose some of its color. With time, the skin coloring generally returns.

Occasionally ringworm, a fungal infection, will begin as a small round area of scaling with associated loss of skin color **(S41).**

In the summertime, many children have small round spots on the face in which there is little color. The spots have probably been present for some time, but skin doesn't tan in these areas, thus making them visible. This condition is known as pityriasis alba. The cause is unknown, but it is a mild condition of cosmetic concern only. It may take many months to disappear and may recur, but there are virtually never any long-term effects.

If there are slightly scaly, tan, pink, or white patches on the neck or back, the problem is most likely due to a fungal infection known as tinea versicolor. This is a very minor and superficial fungal infection.

HOME TREATMENT

Waiting is the most effective home treatment for loss of skin color. Tinea versicolor can be treated by applying Selsun Blue shampoo to the affected area once every day or so until the lesions are gone.

Tolnaftate (Tinactin, etc.), miconazole (Micatin, etc.), and clotrimazole (Lotrimin, etc.) lotions or creams are also effective **(M17).** Unfortunately, tinea versicolor almost always comes back no matter what type of treatment is used.

WHAT TO EXPECT AT THE DOCTOR'S OFFICE

A history and careful examination of the skin will be performed. Scrapings of the lesions may be taken because tinea versicolor can be identified from them. Pityriasis alba should be distinguished from more severe fungal infections that may occur on the face. Again, scrapings will help to identify the fungus.

PATCHY SKIN COLOR

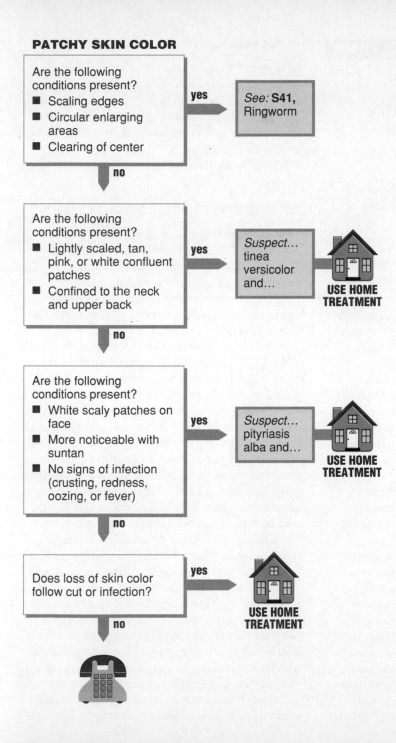

Are the following conditions present?
- Scaling edges
- Circular enlarging areas
- Clearing of center

yes → *See:* **S41,** Ringworm

no ↓

Are the following conditions present?
- Lightly scaled, tan, pink, or white confluent patches
- Confined to the neck and upper back

yes → *Suspect...* tinea versicolor and... **USE HOME TREATMENT**

no ↓

Are the following conditions present?
- White scaly patches on face
- More noticeable with suntan
- No signs of infection (crusting, redness, oozing, or fever)

yes → *Suspect...* pityriasis alba and... **USE HOME TREATMENT**

no ↓

Does loss of skin color follow cut or infection?

yes → **USE HOME TREATMENT**

no ↓

SYMPTOM   S58

58 Aging Spots, Wrinkles, and Baldness

Our aging skin presents a lot of superficial problems. The problems result from a combination of two factors:

- As we age the skin loses its elasticity. It develops more scar tissue and doesn't spring back as quickly into a smooth contour.

- Damage from the sun accumulates over our lifetime and causes additional problems in the sun-exposed areas of our body.

The aging skin lets air leak into the hair follicles so that the hair turns white. Some or all hair follicles lose the ability to produce hairs at all, and the hair thins or disappears. The loss of elasticity means that skin tends to sag, and crinkles in the face turn into deeper, fixed wrinkles.

In general, don't worry about these problems. The aging face is expressive of character. Thinning hair and baldness aren't diseases, nor are aging spots.

Aging spots are pigmentary changes in the skin without any medical significance. Some cells lose the ability to produce the pigment melanin, whereas others produce a bit too much of it. These changes can be thought of as an adult form of freckles. As such, they are flat, uniformly brown or tan in color, and have regular borders. If they are raised, irregular in outline, or have multiple colors in one spot (especially shades of red, white, and blue), then see Skin Cancer (S45).

HOME TREATMENT

Stay out of the sun and use a sunscreen. This is particularly important if you are fair-skinned because such skin is far more prone to sun damage. Outside of these precautions there isn't much you can do at home for these problems except not to worry about them. And that is all that is really needed.

WHAT TO EXPECT AT THE DOCTOR'S OFFICE

There are good medical approaches to these "problems," but they are entirely optional. Many people prefer their natural aging appearance to artificial cosmetic devices. Others, who can afford it, elect to fight the aging stereotype by a variety of measures that preserve a more youthful appearance. Alternatives currently available have low risk but high cost. The choices range all the way from wrinkle creams to an elaborate series of plastic surgical operations.

If you want to go the expensive route, you probably should see a dermatologist first and then, perhaps, a plastic surgeon. The dermatologist is likely to be more familiar with the effective cosmetic interventions than a family physician or internist. The dermatologist is also the key person to take care of any lumps and bumps about which you are concerned.

The most effective approaches to these conditions, among a huge variety of not-so-good treatments, are Retin-A for wrinkles and minoxidil (Rogaine) for hair growth. Retin-A is the first wrinkle cream that actually works, and minoxidil does cause new hair to grow over previously bald spots. Unfortunately, Retin-A doesn't seem to work very well with old, fixed wrinkles, it may cause heat rashes in skin exposed to the sun, and it dries the skin out. The new minoxidil hair isn't usually everything that you would want; it is unusual

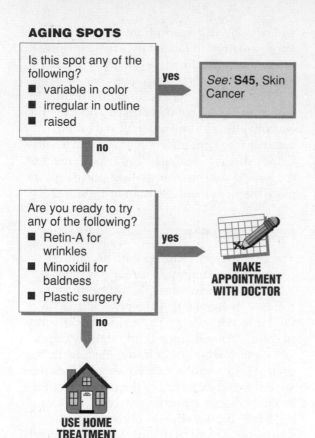

AGING SPOTS

Is this spot any of the following?
- variable in color
- irregular in outline
- raised

yes → *See:* **S45,** Skin Cancer

no ↓

Are you ready to try any of the following?
- Retin-A for wrinkles
- Minoxidil for baldness
- Plastic surgery

yes → **MAKE APPOINTMENT WITH DOCTOR**

no ↓

USE HOME TREATMENT

partially effective in some people. Again, in good hands, done by a surgeon who performs the procedure often, these operations have low risk. However, they are expensive. There is pain and discomfort involved. There is an occasional serious complication. With some of the procedures you won't want to be seen in public for a week or so after the operation.

that very much hair grows back, and the older you are, the less effective this treatment is.

Plastic Surgery

The plastic surgeon can take out wrinkles by removing skin and stretching the remaining skin tighter. Many procedures are available. Wrinkles around the eyes can be taken out, as can bags under the eyes. A full face-lift tightens the skin over the entire face. Sagging breasts can be reduced in size and lifted. Tucks can be taken in the tummy. Liposuction can remove fat, although the result is usually a little lumpy. Hair transplants can be

59 Mumps

Mumps is a viral infection of the salivary glands. The major salivary glands are located directly below and in front of the ear. Before any swelling is noticeable, there may be a low fever, headache, earache, or weakness. Fever is variable. It may be only slightly above normal or as high as 104°F (40°C). After several days of these symptoms, one or both salivary glands (parotid glands) may swell.

It is sometimes difficult to distinguish mumps from swollen lymph glands in the neck **(S27)**. In mumps you won't be able to feel the edge of the jaw that is located beneath the ear. Chewing and swallowing may produce pain behind the ear. Sour substances such as lemons and pickles may make the pain worse. When swelling occurs on both sides, people take on the appearance of chipmunks! Other salivary glands besides the parotid may be involved, including those under the jaw and tongue. The openings of these glands into the mouth may become red and puffy.

Approximately one-third of all patients who have mumps don't demonstrate any swelling of glands whatsoever. Therefore, many people concerned about exposure to mumps will already have had the disease without realizing it.

Mumps is quite contagious during the period from two days before the first symptoms to the complete disappearance of the parotid gland swelling, usually about a week after the swelling has begun. Mumps will develop in a susceptible exposed person approximately 16 to 18 days after exposure to the virus. In children it is generally a mild illness.

The decision chart is directed toward detection of rare complications. These include encephalitis (viral infection of the brain), pancreatitis (viral infection of the pancreas), kidney disease, deafness, and involvement of the testicles or the ovaries. Complications are more frequent in adults than in children.

HOME TREATMENT

The pain may be reduced with acetaminophen, aspirin, ibuprofen, or naproxen **(M4)**. (**Caution:** Aspirin never should be given to children or teenagers if the possibility of a viral infection exists.) There may be difficulty in eating, but adequate fluid intake is important. Sour foods should be avoided, including orange juice. Adults who haven't had mumps should avoid exposure to the patient until the swelling disappears completely.

Many adults who don't recall having mumps as a child may have had an extremely mild case and consequently aren't at risk of developing mumps.

If swelling hasn't gone down within three weeks, call the doctor.

WHAT TO EXPECT AT THE DOCTOR'S OFFICE

If a complication is suspected, a visit to the doctor's office may be necessary. The history and physical examination will be directed at confirming the diagnosis or the presence of a complication. The rare complication of an ovarian mumps infection on the right side may be confused with appendicitis, and blood tests may be required. Because mumps is a viral disease, there is no medicine that will

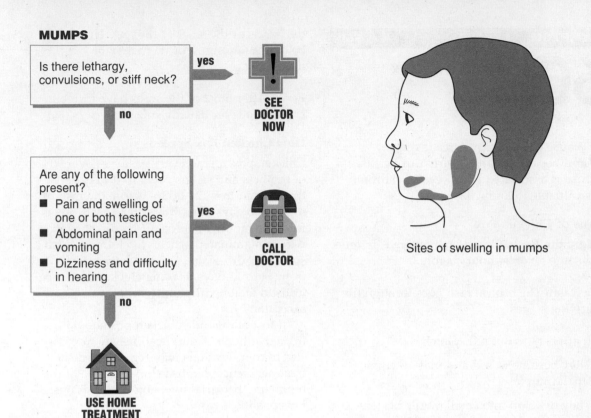

MUMPS

Is there lethargy, convulsions, or stiff neck?

— yes → **SEE DOCTOR NOW**

— no ↓

Are any of the following present?
- Pain and swelling of one or both testicles
- Abdominal pain and vomiting
- Dizziness and difficulty in hearing

— yes → **CALL DOCTOR**

— no ↓

USE HOME TREATMENT

Sites of swelling in mumps

directly kill the virus. Supportive measures may be necessary for some of the complications. Fortunately, complications are rare, and permanent damage to hearing or other functions is unusual. Mumps very rarely produces sterility in men or women even when the testes or ovaries are involved.

60 Chicken Pox

Because chicken pox spreads quickly, and because taking aspirin during this disease is associated with Reye's syndrome, it is valuable to know its signs.

Signs of Chicken Pox

Before the Rash. Occasionally there is fatigue and some fever 24 hours before.

The Rash. The typical rash goes through the following stages:

1. It appears as flat red splotches.

2. They become raised and may resemble small pimples.

3. They develop into small fragile blisters, called vesicles. They may look like drops of water on a red base. The tops are easily scratched off.

4. As the vesicles break, the sores become pustular and form a crust. Itching is often severe. This stage may be reached in the first several hours of the rash.

5. The crust falls away between the ninth and thirteenth day.

The vesicles tend to appear in crops (multiple sores appearing at the same time), with two to four crops appearing within two to six days. The rashes often appear first on the scalp and then spread to the rest of the body, but they may begin anywhere. They are most numerous over the shoulders, chest, and back. They are seldom found on the palms of the hands or the soles of the feet. There may be only a few sores, or there may be hundreds.

Fever. After most of the sores have formed crusts, the fever usually subsides.

How Chicken Pox Spreads

Chicken pox spreads very easily — over 90% of brothers and sisters catch it. It may be transmitted from 24 hours before the rash up to about 6 days after. It is spread by droplets from the mouth or throat or by direct contact with contaminated articles of clothing. It isn't spread by dry scabs. The incubation period is from 14 to 17 days. Having chicken pox once leads to lifelong immunity, with rare exceptions.

Most of the time chicken pox should be treated at home. Complications are rare. Two severe complications may require medical treatment: encephalitis (viral infection of the brain) and bacterial infection of the lesions. Encephalitis is rare.

HOME TREATMENT

The major problems in dealing with chicken pox are control of the intense itching and reduction of the fever. Warm baths containing baking soda (one-half cup to a tubful of water) frequently help. Antihistamines may help **(M8).** Acetaminophen, ibuprofen, and naproxen are effective itch relievers **(M4).**

Caution: Because recent information indicates an association among aspirin, chicken pox, and a rare but serious problem of the liver and brain known as Reye's syndrome, aspirin should never be given to children or teenagers who may have chicken pox or influenza.

Cut the fingernails or use gloves to prevent skin damage from intense scratching.

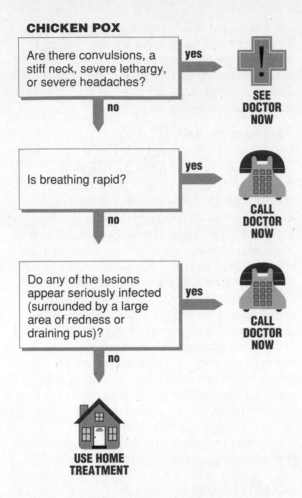

CHICKEN POX

Are there convulsions, a stiff neck, severe lethargy, or severe headaches?

yes → SEE DOCTOR NOW

no ↓

Is breathing rapid?

yes → CALL DOCTOR NOW

no ↓

Do any of the lesions appear seriously infected (surrounded by a large area of redness or draining pus)?

yes → CALL DOCTOR NOW

no ↓

USE HOME TREATMENT

When lesions occur in the mouth, gargling with salt water may help give comfort: add one-half teaspoon (3 ml) salt to an eight-ounce (150 ml) glass of water. Hands should be washed three times a day, and all of the skin should be kept gently but scrupulously clean in order to prevent bacterial infection. Minor bacterial infection will respond to soap and time; if it becomes severe and results in the return of fever, call the doctor. Scratching and infection can result in permanent scars.

If itching can't be controlled or the problem persists beyond three weeks, call the doctor. Using the phone for questions to the doctor will avoid exposing others to the disease.

WHAT TO EXPECT AT THE DOCTOR'S OFFICE

Don't be surprised if the doctor is willing and even anxious to treat the case over the phone. If it is necessary to go to the doctor's office, attempts should be made to keep the patient separate from others. In healthy children chicken pox has few lasting ill effects, but in people with other serious illnesses, it can be a devastating or even fatal disease. A visit to the doctor's office may not be necessary unless a complication seems possible.

The same herpes virus that causes chicken pox also causes shingles, and the individual who has had chicken pox may develop shingles (herpes zoster) later in life. Shingles is usually limited to one side of the body in a broad stripe, representing the skin area of a single nerve. Because it is limited to the nerve in which the virus is living, there is seldom fever although there may be pain. Follow the same treatment as you do for chicken pox.

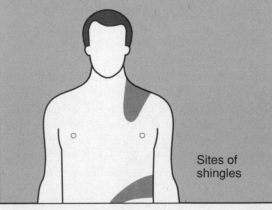

Sites of shingles

61 Measles

This type of measles is also called red measles, seven-day measles, and ten-day measles, as opposed to rubella, also called German or three-day measles (S62). It is a preventable disease but, unlike some of the other childhood illnesses, can be quite severe. It is tragic that decades after the licensing of the measles vaccine thousands of people still contract this disease annually, and some of them die. We would like to be able to eliminate this section in the next edition of this book. Only immunization of everyone can make this possible.

How to Recognize Measles

Early signs. Measles is a viral illness that begins with fever, weakness, a dry "brassy" cough, and inflamed eyes that are itchy, red, and sensitive to light. These symptoms begin three to five days before the appearance of the rash.

Another early sign of measles is the appearance of fine white spots on a red base inside the mouth opposite the molar teeth (Koplik's spots). These fade as the skin rash appears.

The Rash. The rash begins on about the fifth day as a pink, blotchy, flat rash. The rash first appears around the hairline, on the face, on the neck, and behind the ears. The spots, which fade early in the illness when pressure is applied, become somewhat darker and tend to merge into larger red patches as they mature.

The rash spreads from head to chest to abdomen and finally to the arms and legs. It lasts from four to seven days and may be accompanied by mild itching. There may be some light brown coloring to the skin lesions as the illness progresses.

How Measles Spreads

Measles is a highly contagious viral disease. It is spread by droplets from the mouth or throat and by direct contact with articles freshly soiled by nose and throat secretions. It may be spread during the period from three to six days before the appearance of the rash to several days after. Symptoms begin in a susceptible person approximately eight to twelve days after exposure to the virus.

There are a number of complications of measles: sore throats, ear infections, and pneumonia are all common. Many of these complicating infections are due to bacteria and will require antibiotic treatment. The pneumonias can be life-threatening. A very serious problem that can lead to permanent damage is measles encephalitis (infection of the brain); life-support measures and treatment of seizures may be necessary when this rare complication occurs.

HOME TREATMENT

Treatment of symptoms is all that is needed for uncomplicated measles. Acetaminophen (M4) should be used to keep the fever down, and a vaporizer can be used for the cough. Dim lighting in the room is often more comfortable because of the eyes' sensitivity to light. In general, the person feels "measley." The patient should be isolated until the end of the contagious period. All unimmunized people in contact with the patient should be immunized immediately. (People who have had the measles are considered immunized.)

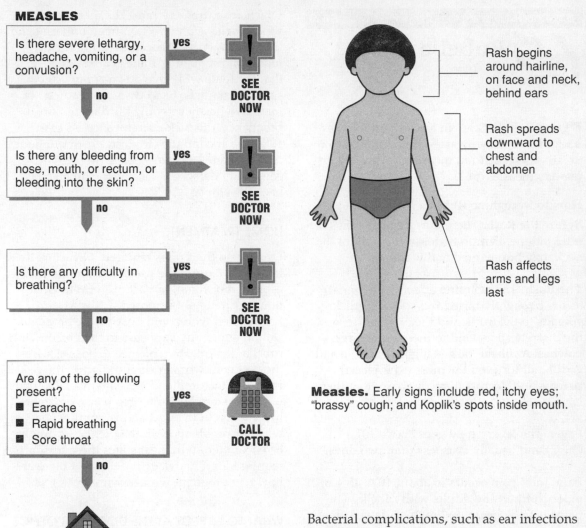

MEASLES

Is there severe lethargy, headache, vomiting, or a convulsion?

yes → **SEE DOCTOR NOW**

no ↓

Is there any bleeding from nose, mouth, or rectum, or bleeding into the skin?

yes → **SEE DOCTOR NOW**

no ↓

Is there any difficulty in breathing?

yes → **SEE DOCTOR NOW**

no ↓

Are any of the following present?
- Earache
- Rapid breathing
- Sore throat

yes → **CALL DOCTOR**

no ↓

USE HOME TREATMENT

Rash begins around hairline, on face and neck, behind ears

Rash spreads downward to chest and abdomen

Rash affects arms and legs last

Measles. Early signs include red, itchy eyes; "brassy" cough; and Koplik's spots inside mouth.

WHAT TO EXPECT AT THE DOCTOR'S OFFICE

The history and physical examination will be directed at determining the diagnosis of measles and the nature of any complications.

Bacterial complications, such as ear infections and pneumonia, can usually be treated with antibiotics. The person with symptoms suggestive of encephalitis (lethargy, stiff neck, convulsions) will be hospitalized, and a spinal tap will be performed. Very rarely, there may be a problem with blood clotting so that bleeding occurs. Usually this is first apparent as dark purple splotches in the skin. It is best, however, to avoid all of the problems through measles immunization.

62 Rubella

Rubella is also known as German measles and three-day measles. It is different from the disease called red measles, seven-day or ten-day measles (S61).

How to Recognize Rubella

Before the Rash. There may be a few days of mild fatigue. Lymph nodes at the back of the neck may be enlarged and tender.

The Rash. The rash first appears on the face as flat or slightly raised red spots. It quickly spreads to the trunk and the extremities, and the discrete spots tend to merge into large patches. A rubella rash is highly variable and is difficult for even the most experienced parents and doctors to recognize. Often there is no rash.

Fever. The fever rarely goes above 101°F (38°C) and usually lasts less than two days.

Pain. Joint pain occurs in about 10 to 15% of older children and adults with rubella. The pains usually begin on the third day of illness.

How Rubella Spreads

Rubella is a mild virus infection that isn't as contagious as measles or chicken pox. It is usually spread by droplets from the mouth or throat. It can be spread from 7 days before the rash appears until 5 days afterwards.

The incubation period is from 12 to 21 days, with an average of 16 days.

The specific questions on the decision chart are addressed to possible complications, which are extremely rare. The main concern with rubella is an infection in an unborn child. If three-day measles occurs during the first month of pregnancy, there is a 50% chance that the fetus will develop an abnormality such as cataracts, heart disease, deafness, or mental deficiency. By the third month of pregnancy, this risk decreases to less than 10%, and it continues to decrease throughout the pregnancy. Because of the problem of congenital defects, a vaccine for rubella has been developed.

HOME TREATMENT

Usually no therapy is required. Occasionally fever will require the use of acetaminophen, aspirin, ibuprofen, or naproxen (M4). Isolation is usually not imposed.

Women who could possibly be pregnant should avoid any exposure to the person with rubella. If a question of such exposure arises, the pregnant woman should discuss the risk with her doctor. Blood tests are available that will indicate whether a pregnant woman has had rubella in the past and is immune, or whether problems with the pregnancy might be encountered. In most states these tests are required for a marriage license, and there are now few pregnant women who are at risk.

WHAT TO EXPECT AT THE DOCTOR'S OFFICE

Visits to the doctor's office are seldom required for uncomplicated rubella. Questions about possible infection of pregnant women are more easily and economically discussed over the telephone. The question of immunization is complex, and we discuss it in detail in our book with Dr. Robert Pantell, *Taking Care of Your Child.*

RUBELLA

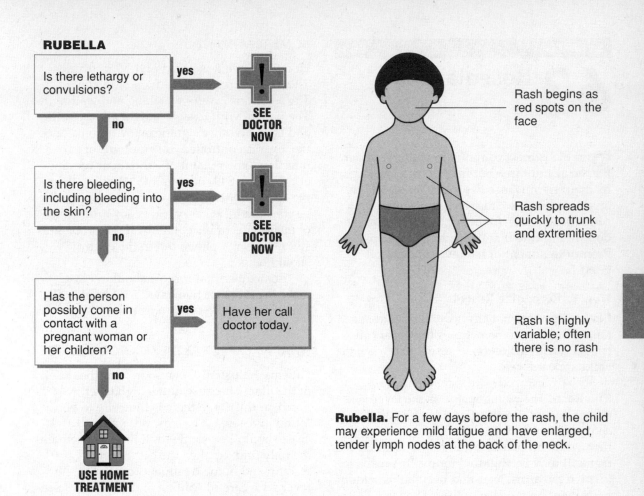

Is there lethargy or convulsions? — yes → **SEE DOCTOR NOW**

no ↓

Is there bleeding, including bleeding into the skin? — yes → **SEE DOCTOR NOW**

no ↓

Has the person possibly come in contact with a pregnant woman or her children? — yes → Have her call doctor today.

no ↓

USE HOME TREATMENT

Rash begins as red spots on the face

Rash spreads quickly to trunk and extremities

Rash is highly variable; often there is no rash

Rubella. For a few days before the rash, the child may experience mild fatigue and have enlarged, tender lymph nodes at the back of the neck.

63 Roseola

Roseola is most common in children under the age of three but may occur at any age. Its main significance lies in the sudden high fever, which may cause a convulsion. Such a convulsion is due to the high temperature and doesn't indicate that the child has epilepsy. Prompt treatment of the fever is essential **(S94).**

How to Recognize Roseola

Fever. There are usually several days of sustained high fever. Sometimes this fever can trigger a convulsion or seizure. Otherwise, the child appears well.

The Rash. The rash appears as the fever is decreasing or shortly after it is gone. It consists of pink, well-defined patches that turn white on pressure and first appear on the trunk. It may be slightly bumpy. It spreads to involve the arms, legs, and neck but is seldom prominent on the face or legs. The rash usually lasts less than 24 hours.

Other Symptoms. Occasionally there is a slight runny nose, red throat, or swollen glands at the back of the head, behind the ears, or in the neck. Most often there are no other symptoms.

This disease is probably caused by a virus and is contagious. Contact with others should be avoided until the fever has passed. The incubation period is from 7 to 17 days.

Encephalitis (infection of the brain) is a very rare complication of roseola. Roseola is basically a mild disease.

HOME TREATMENT

Home treatment is based on two principles. The first is effective treatment of the fever. The second is careful watching and waiting. The patient with roseola should appear well and have no other significant symptoms once the fever is controlled. If symptoms of ear infection (a complaint of ear pain or tugging at the ear — **S19**) or cough **(S23)** occur, then the appropriate sections of this book should be consulted. Lethargy can be a warning sign of meningitis or encephalitis. If the problem is still not clear, a phone call to the doctor should help.

Remember that roseola shouldn't last more than four or five days. You should call your doctor if the symptoms persist.

WHAT TO EXPECT AT THE DOCTOR'S OFFICE

Patients are usually seen soon after the onset of the illness because of the high fever. As noted, at this stage there is little else to be found in roseola. The ears, nose, throat, and chest should be examined. If the fever remains the only finding, then the doctor will recommend home treatment (control of the fever with careful waiting and watching to see if a roseola rash appears). There is no medical treatment for roseola other than that available at home.

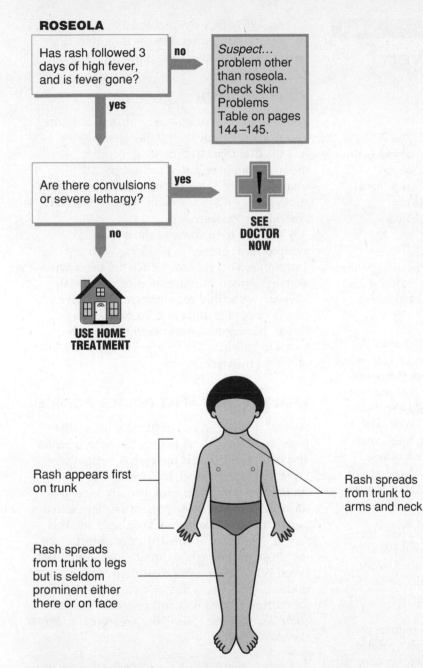

ROSEOLA

Has rash followed 3 days of high fever, and is fever gone?

no → *Suspect...* problem other than roseola. Check Skin Problems Table on pages 144–145.

yes ↓

Are there convulsions or severe lethargy?

yes → **SEE DOCTOR NOW**

no ↓

USE HOME TREATMENT

Rash appears first on trunk

Rash spreads from trunk to arms and neck

Rash spreads from trunk to legs but is seldom prominent either there or on face

Roseola. Several days of sustained high fever may trigger a convulsion or seizure before the onset of the rash.

64 Scarlet Fever

Scarlet fever derived its name over 300 years ago from its characteristic red rash. The illness is caused by a streptococcal infection, usually of the throat. Strep throats are discussed in Sore Throat (S18).

You can recognize the illness by its characteristic features.

1. Fever and weakness are often accompanied by a headache, stomachache, and vomiting. A sore throat is usually but not always present.

2. The rash appears 12 to 48 hours after the illness begins. It begins on the face, trunk, and arms and generally covers the entire body by the end of 24 hours. It is red, very fine, and covers most of the skin surface. The area around the mouth is pale. The rash feels like fine sandpaper. Skin creases, such as in front of the elbow and the armpit, are more deeply red. Pressing on the rash will produce a white spot lasting several seconds.

3. The intense redness of the rash lasts for about five days, although peeling of skin can go on for weeks. It isn't unusual for peeling, especially of the palms, to last for more than a month.

Examination often reveals a red throat, spots on the roof of the mouth (soft palate), and a fuzzy, white tongue that later becomes swollen and red. There may be swollen glands in the neck.

As with other streptococcal infections, the significance of scarlet fever is its connection with rheumatic fever (see Sore Throat, S18).

HOME TREATMENT

You can't treat scarlet fever yourself at home; you must see your doctor. Because scarlet fever is due to a streptococcal infection, a medical visit is required for antibiotic treatment. Streptococcal infections are quite contagious, and other members of the family should also be tested.

You can treat some of the disease's symptoms at home. To go along with the antibiotics, you should reduce the fever with acetaminophen or other medications (M4), keep up with fluid requirements, and give plenty of cold liquids to help soothe the throat. (**Caution:** Aspirin never should be given to children or teenagers if the possibility of a viral infection exists.)

WHAT TO EXPECT AT THE DOCTOR'S OFFICE

Several rashes can be confused with scarlet fever, including those associated with measles and drug reactions. If the rash is sufficiently typical of scarlet fever, the doctor will probably begin antibiotics, usually penicillin (or erythromycin if the patient is allergic to penicillin) and take throat cultures from the rest of the family. If the doctor is uncertain of the cause of the rash, a throat culture may be taken before beginning treatment. Treatment that is delayed by a day or two while waiting for culture results will still prevent the complication that causes the greatest concern, rheumatic fever.

SCARLET FEVER

Are both of the following present?
- Fever
- Fine, red rash on trunk and extremities that feels like sandpaper

no →

Suspect... problem other than scarlet fever. Check Skin Problems Table on pages 144–145.

yes ↓

CALL DOCTOR

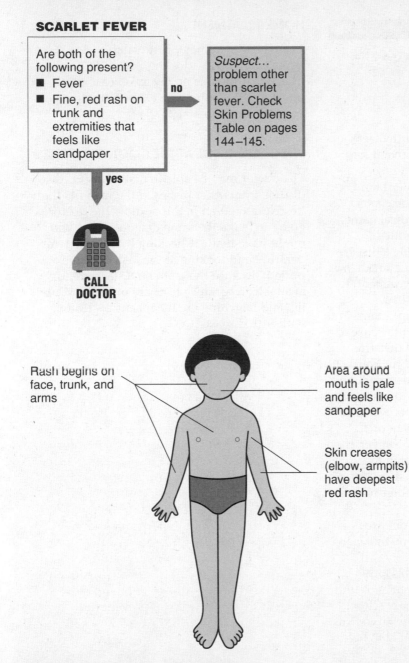

Rash begins on face, trunk, and arms

Area around mouth is pale and feels like sandpaper

Skin creases (elbow, armpits) have deepest red rash

Scarlet fever. Fever and weakness are often accompanied by headache, stomachache, vomiting, and sore throat.

65 Fifth Disease

Consider the strange case of fifth disease, whose only claim to fame is that it might be mistaken for another disease. It is so named because it is always listed last (and least) among the five very common contagious rashes of childhood. Its medical name, *erythema infectiosum*, is easily forgotten.

It comes very close to not being a disease at all. It has no symptoms other than rash, has no complications, and needs no treatment. It can be recognized because it causes a characteristic "slapped cheek" appearance in children. The rash often begins on the cheeks and is later found on the backs of the arms and legs. It often is very fine, lacy, and pink. It tends to come and go and may be present one moment and absent the next. It is prone to recur for days or even weeks, especially as a response to heat (such as warm bath or shower) or irritation. In general, however, the rash around the face will fade within four days of its appearance, and the rash on the rest of the body will fade within three to seven days.

The only significance of fifth disease is that it could worry you or have you make an avoidable trip to the doctor's office.

Its recent resurgence makes this more likely. It is very contagious. Epidemics of fifth disease have resulted in unnecessary school closings. Fifth disease is caused by parvovirus B19; the incubation period is thought to be from 4 to 14 days.

HOME TREATMENT

There is no treatment. Just watch and wait to make sure you are dealing with fifth disease. Check that there is no fever. Fever is very unusual with fifth disease. No restrictions on activities are necessary.

WHAT TO EXPECT AT THE DOCTOR'S OFFICE

The doctor may be able to distinguish fifth disease from other rashes. If the rash fits the description given in this section, the doctor is going to make the same diagnosis that you might have made. Checking the child's temperature and looking at the rash can be expected. Because there are no tests currently available, laboratory tests are unlikely. Waiting and watching are the means of dealing with fifth disease.

FIFTH DISEASE

Are all of the following present?
- No fever
- "Slapped cheek" rash is the first and only symptom
- Palms and soles are not involved

no →

Suspect... problem other than fifth disease. Check Skin Problems Table on pages 144–145.

yes ↓

USE HOME TREATMENT

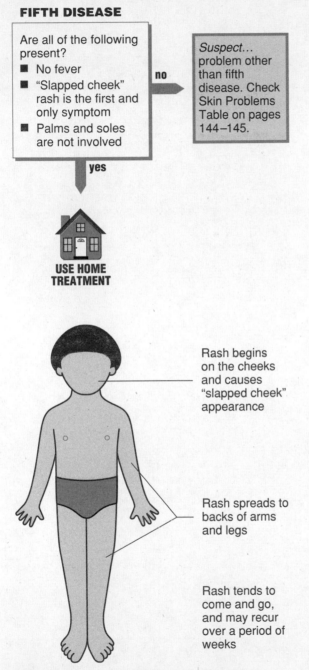

Rash begins on the cheeks and causes "slapped cheek" appearance

Rash spreads to backs of arms and legs

Rash tends to come and go, and may recur over a period of weeks

Fifth disease. Apart from rash, there are no symptoms.

CHAPTER 6

Bones, Muscles, and Joints

66 Arthritis

Most so-called arthritis is not arthritis at all! Misunderstanding comes about because doctors and patients use the term differently. The "arth" part of the word means "joint"—not muscle, tendon, ligament, or bone. The "itis" means "inflamed." Thus, true arthritis means joints that are red, warm, swollen, and painful to move. Pains in the muscles or ligaments are discussed in section **S67**.

Types of Arthritis

There are over 100 types of arthritis. These are the four most common:

- **Osteoarthritis** is usually not serious, occurs in later life, and frequently causes knobby swelling at the most distant joints of the fingers.

- **Rheumatoid arthritis** usually starts in middle life and may cause you to feel sick and stiff all over, in addition to causing joint problems.

- **Gout** occurs mostly in men, with sudden, severe attacks of pain and swelling in one joint at a time, frequently the big toe, the ankle, or the knee.

- **Ankylosing spondylitis** affects the back and joints of the lower back. It may be involved if your back is sore for a long time and particularly stiff in the morning, and if you are unable to touch your toes.

These are described in greater detail in *Arthritis: A Take Care of Yourself Health Guide*, by James Fries.

Lyme Disease

Recently Lyme disease has received much attention as a cause of arthritis. Lyme disease is the result of an infection spread by ticks, usually a small, fairly uncommon type called the deer tick. Three to 20 days following the bite of an infected tick a distinctive oval rash develops in most people, along with fever, headache, stiff neck, and backaches. This is the end of the disease for most people, but others develop arthritis within 1 to 22 weeks. Less often, heart or neurological problems follow the rash.

REASONS TO SEE A DOCTOR

Only rarely does a patient with arthritis need to see a doctor immediately. Urgent problems are:

- Infection
- Nerve damage
- Fractures near a joint
- Gout

In the first three, serious damage may result if the joint is neglected; in the fourth, the pain is so intense that immediate help is needed.

The complications of arthritis occur very slowly and are more easily prevented than corrected. Arthritis results in more lost work-days and sickness than any other chronic disease category—it must be managed correctly and with care.

HOME TREATMENT

Aspirin, ibuprofen (Advil, Nuprin, etc.), and naproxen (Aleve, etc.) can reduce the pain and swelling in the joints. The usual dosage for each is two tablets every four to six hours.

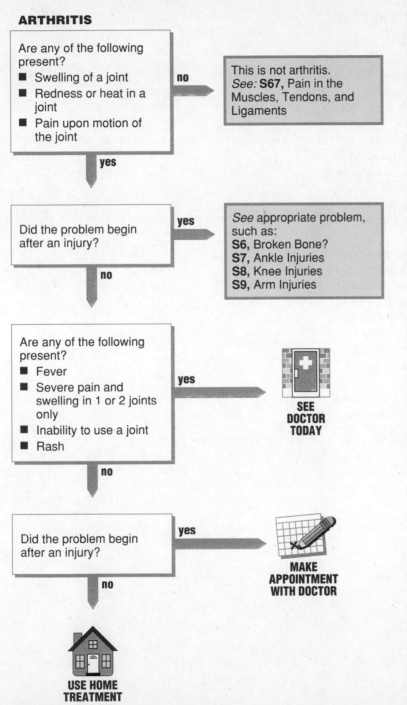

ARTHRITIS

Are any of the following present?
- Swelling of a joint
- Redness or heat in a joint
- Pain upon motion of the joint

no → This is not arthritis. *See:* **S67,** Pain in the Muscles, Tendons, and Ligaments

yes ↓

Did the problem begin after an injury?

yes → *See* appropriate problem, such as:
S6, Broken Bone?
S7, Ankle Injuries
S8, Knee Injuries
S9, Arm Injuries

no ↓

Are any of the following present?
- Fever
- Severe pain and swelling in 1 or 2 joints only
- Inability to use a joint
- Rash

yes → **SEE DOCTOR TODAY**

no ↓

Did the problem begin after an injury?

yes → **MAKE APPOINTMENT WITH DOCTOR**

no ↓

USE HOME TREATMENT

The major concern with each medication is stomach irritation: both may contribute to bleeding and ulcers. Ibuprofen and naproxen are somewhat less likely to cause stomach problems than aspirin but are more expensive. The risk of upset stomach can be reduced by taking the tablets after meals, after an antacid, or by using coated aspirin tablets (Ecotrin, etc.). Warning signs of too much aspirin include ringing ears, dizziness, and hearing problems.

Although acetaminophen may provide some pain relief, it doesn't reduce inflammation and is rarely used in the treatment of arthritis. For more information on aspirin, ibuprofen, and naproxen, see section **M4.**

Resting an inflamed joint can speed healing. Heat may help. Usually a painful joint should be worked through its entire range of motion twice daily to prevent it from becoming stiff and contracted.

If arthritis persists more than six weeks, see a doctor. For more information, consult *Arthritis: A Take Care of Yourself Health Guide,* by James Fries, and *The Arthritis Helpbook,* by Kate Lorig and James Fries.

WHAT TO EXPECT AT THE DOCTOR'S OFFICE

The doctor will examine the joints, obtain blood tests, and may take X-rays. If a single joint is the problem and it contains fluid, this fluid may also be removed and tested.

Most often one of the many nonsteroidal anti-inflammatory drugs (NSAIDs) such as Naprosyn, Feldene, Voltaren, Tolectin, Meclomen, Ansaid, Relafen, or Indocin will be prescribed. Their effects, both good and bad, are essentially the same as those of aspirin, ibuprofen, or naproxen (over-the-counter Naprosyn). The big problem is that they can cause stomach ulcers.

Corticosteroid drugs such as prednisone are very effective in reducing inflammation, but their long-term use causes serious side effects. If they are to be continued for more than a few weeks, we recommend that you consult your doctor first. Occasionally a corticosteroid drug will be injected into a particularly painful joint, but this usually shouldn't be done more than three times.

Rheumatoid arthritis usually requires the use of strong drugs such as methotrexate, gold salts, or hydroxychloroquine.

67 Pain in the Muscles, Tendons, and Ligaments

Here are two lesser-known medical terms: "arthralgia" means pain (without swelling or redness) in the joints, and "myalgia" means pain in the muscles. These pains aren't arthritis but can be very bothersome. Usually they aren't serious and will go away. They can be caused by tension, virus infections, unusual exertion, accidents, or they can have no obvious cause. Seldom do they indicate a serious disease.

In rare cases, thyroid disease, cancer, polymyositis (inflammation of the muscles), or a condition in older patients called polymyalgia rheumatica (aching in the neck, shoulder, and sometimes hip muscles) may cause arthralgias. If there is no fever, weight loss, or severe fatigue, try home treatment for several weeks or even months before seeing a doctor. Pain at the upper neck and base of the skull is almost certainly minor.

Doctors often disagree on terms for diagnosing these problems. Other terms frequently used are nonarticular rheumatism, psychogenic rheumatism, and psychophysiological musculoskeletal pain. These all mean about the same thing: pain in the muscles and joints.

Fibromyalgia, a common condition in this category, is a painful and frequently long-lasting set of pains. Fortunately, fibromyalgia doesn't progress to crippling, but there can be substantial disability from pain and fatigue. People with fibromyalgia syndrome (FMS) have tender points at 18 specific places on the body and usually have sleep problems so that they awaken feeling as though they never had been to sleep at all. They may also have irritable bowel syndrome, morning stiffness, anxiety, and other symptoms, such as memory problems.

HOME TREATMENT

Both rest and exercise are important for musculoskeletal problems. A regular, adequate sleeping pattern seems essential for many people with these problems. Try to relax and gently stretch the involved areas. Warm baths, massage, and stretching exercises should be employed as frequently as possible.

Heat or Cold?

Cold and heat should be applied to painful areas at different times:

- Use cold when you think that damage has just occurred and inflammation is developing.

- Use heat when you think that the initial stages of inflammation are over, in order to improve flexibility and, perhaps, to speed healing.

Cold decreases blood flow, so it's used in the first stage of an injury to reduce the amount of fluid, blood cells, and blood that escapes into joints or muscle tissue. In this way cold may help to reduce the pain, swelling, warmth, and redness.

Heat increases blood vessel size and blood flow, so its use in the first stages of inflammation would likely make things worse. However, heat helps in the final stages of healing when increased blood flow may be useful. Heat has two other important effects on joints and muscles. The flexibility and elasticity of muscles, ligaments, and tendons increases when they are warm. (Ligaments are fibrous bands that extend from bone to bone; tendons are fibrous bands that extend from bone to muscle.) The application of heat may immediately loosen up stiff muscles and joints. Unfortunately, this effect is lost when the heat is removed and the tissue returns to its previous temperature. Heat may also help relieve muscle spasms.

The use of cold and heat is fairly simple when the tissue damage occurs once and is over, as with a sprained ankle. Cold is applied immediately and for as long as the first stages of inflammation may be occurring (usually about 24 hours). After that time heat may be applied to reduce discomfort by loosening up the joint and, perhaps, speeding healing.

The situation isn't so simple when the damage is repeated or constant. For example, some doctors believe that athletes with "bad" knees may damage them whenever they play their sport. These athletes may apply ice immediately before, during, and immediately after playing in an effort to reduce inflammation and then use heat at some later time in an effort to improve healing.

For fibromyalgia syndrome, exercise is crucial. Exercise, slowly increased toward full aerobic cardiovascular conditioning and physical tiredness, is the most important single part of treatment. Start slowly and progress gently. Walking, hiking, swimming, and bicycling are preferred activities; avoid impact exercises such as jogging or tennis. Stretching exercises are important. Pain often gets worse early in an exercise program before it gets better, so you have to persevere. Relief may be months away, and pain can persist in varying degrees of severity for many years.

Preventing the Pain

Sponge-soled shoes may help if you work on hard floors. Better light or a better chair may help if you work at a desk. Regular exercise (slowly increased from very gentle to more vigorous) may help restore proper muscle tone. We recommend walking, bicycling, and swimming. Acetaminophen, aspirin, ibuprofen, or naproxen may help **(M4).**

Since many people feel an improvement after changing their lifestyle, switching jobs, or moving to a new location, stress often seems to be at least part of the problem. If the problem goes away on vacation, you can be relatively certain that everyday stress accounts for it.

If the problem persists beyond three weeks, call your doctor.

WHAT TO EXPECT AT THE DOCTOR'S OFFICE

A physical examination, and often some blood tests, are carried out. X-rays are rarely useful for making a diagnosis. The doctor will probably give advice similar to that above.

In general, pain relievers containing narcotics or codeine aren't useful. Oral corticosteroids such as prednisone should almost never be used unless a specific diagnosis can be made. If a particular spot in the body is causing the pain, a corticosteroid injection into that area may help greatly. Such injections shouldn't be repeated if they don't help, and they should only be repeated one or two times even if they do give prolonged relief.

Fibromyalgia may be managed with regimens such as amitryptyline (Elavil) an hour or so before bedtime and Prozac in the morning. The goal of medication here is to improve the quality of sleep without causing drowsiness during the day.

PAIN IN MUSCLES, TENDONS, LIGAMENTS

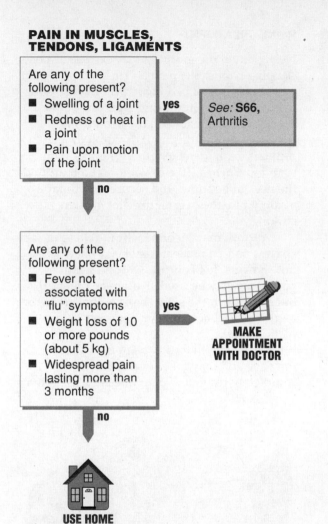

Are any of the following present?
- Swelling of a joint
- Redness or heat in a joint
- Pain upon motion of the joint

yes → *See:* **S66,** Arthritis

no ↓

Are any of the following present?
- Fever not associated with "flu" symptoms
- Weight loss of 10 or more pounds (about 5 kg)
- Widespread pain lasting more than 3 months

yes → **MAKE APPOINTMENT WITH DOCTOR**

no ↓

USE HOME TREATMENT

68 Neck Pain

Most neck pain is due to strain and spasm of the neck muscles. The common crick in the neck upon arising is one example of neck muscle strain. This type of neck pain can be adequately treated at home. Neck pains that require the attention of a doctor include those due to meningitis or a pinched nerve.

Meningitis

With fever and headache, there is a possibility of meningitis. Meningitis may cause intense spasms of the neck muscles and make the neck very stiff. More commonly, though, neck pain is part of a flu syndrome that includes fever, muscle aches, and a headache. When generalized aching throughout the muscles is present, a visit to a doctor is seldom useful. When a stiff neck is due to one of the more common causes of muscle spasm, the sufferer can usually touch the chin to the chest, though perhaps with difficulty. If in doubt, it is better to see the doctor for an ordinary muscle spasm than to attempt to treat meningitis at home.

Pinched Nerve

Arthritis or injury to the neck can result in a pinched nerve. When this is the source of neck pain, the pain may extend down the arm, or there may be numbness or tingling sensations in the arm or hand. This pain is only on one side, and neck stiffness is not prominent.

HOME TREATMENT

Neck pain in the morning may be due to poor sleeping habits. Sleep on a firm surface: a firm mattress is best; a bed board will make a soft mattress firmer. Stop using a pillow, or use special pillows that keep the head from twisting without raising it. If you fold an ordinary bath towel lengthwise into a long strip four inches (10 cm) wide, wrap it around the neck at bedtime, and secure it with tape or a safety pin, the overnight relief is often striking.

Warmth may be of benefit in relieving spasms and pain. Heat may be applied with hot showers, hot compresses, or a heating pad. Heat may be used as often as practical, but don't burn the skin. Aspirin, ibuprofen, or naproxen will help relieve pain and inflammation **(M4)**.

Neck pain, like back pain, is slow to improve and may take several weeks to completely resolve. If pain doesn't lessen in a week, call the doctor.

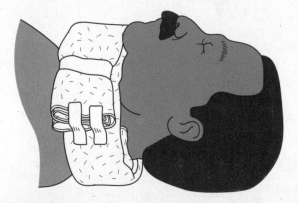

Neck pain relief. An ordinary bath towel, wrapped around the neck at bedtime, may alleviate some neck pain caused by poor sleeping habits.

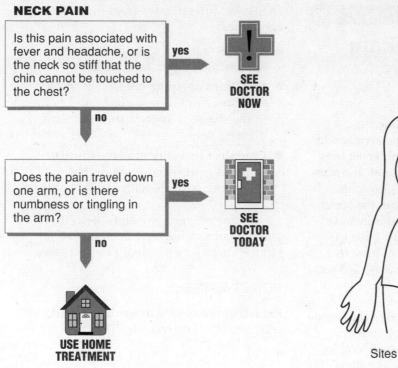

NECK PAIN

Is this pain associated with fever and headache, or is the neck so stiff that the chin cannot be touched to the chest?

yes → **SEE DOCTOR NOW**

no ↓

Does the pain travel down one arm, or is there numbness or tingling in the arm?

yes → **SEE DOCTOR TODAY**

no ↓

USE HOME TREATMENT

Sites of pinched nerve pain

WHAT TO EXPECT AT THE DOCTOR'S OFFICE

If meningitis is suspected, the doctor will perform a spinal tap as well as several blood tests. If a pinched nerve is likely, X-rays of the neck will be taken. A muscle relaxant may be prescribed and perhaps a more powerful pain reliever. Prescription drugs aren't necessarily better than nonprescription aspirin, ibuprofen, or naproxen. Usually you are just as well off with home therapy if no infection or nerve damage is present.

The physician may prescribe a neck collar or, if there is nerve damage, refer you to a neurologist or neurosurgeon for consultation. Today the trend is away from drug treatment for this problem.

69 Shoulder Pain

Pain located around the shoulder is common and almost never poses a serious threat to life. Nonetheless, it can persist for a long time and cause discomfort and disability. Most of the time the pain comes from the soft tissues near the joint and not from the bones or the joint itself. These soft tissues include the ligaments (which connect one bone to another), tendons (which connect bone to muscle), and the bursae (little fluid-filled sacs at the joints).

Bursitis. This is an inflammation of the bursae that starts with an uneasy feeling in the shoulder and may progress to considerable pain within six to twelve hours. There may be swelling at the tip of the shoulder. It is often seen in persons who have been cutting hedges, painting the house, or playing sports.

Rotator Cuff Tendinitis. This is an irritation of the tendons and muscles around the shoulder and is most likely to be seen in baseball pitchers and racquet sports enthusiasts. Unlike bursitis, it is difficult to detect even a small amount of swelling, and the pain seems to occur in only a few positions.

Bicep Tendinitis. Much less common, this occurs in gymnasts and players of baseball and racquet sports. The tenderness and pain are located in the front of the shoulder.

Because these three common problems of the shoulder are treated the same initially, you need not worry about which condition you have. However, there are problems that should be differentiated from these three conditions:

- **Injuries** require a slightly different approach (see Arm Injuries, **S9**).
- **Infections** are quite unusual in the shoulder, but fever, swelling, and redness of the shoulder suggest the need for a doctor's help.
- **Complete inability to move the arm** suggests pain severe enough that consulting with a doctor is reasonable.

If none of these problems seems to fit your situation, give your doctor a call for advice. Often a visit will not be necessary.

HOME TREATMENT

For bursitis, rotator cuff tendinitis, and bicep tendinitis, the key word is RIMS:

- Rest
- Ice
- Maintenance of mobility
- Strengthening

At the first sign of trouble, you should apply ice for 30 minutes, then let the shoulder rewarm for the next 15 minutes. Continue the cycle for the next one to two hours. Be careful not to freeze the skin.

Give the shoulder complete rest for the first 24 to 48 hours. After that time, gently put your arm through a full range of motion several times a day.

Complete immobilization of the arm may result in stiffness and loss of motion in the shoulder (frozen shoulder). Thus, maintenance of the shoulder's range of motion is an important part of the treatment. Wait three to six weeks before returning to the activity that caused the problem, depending on the

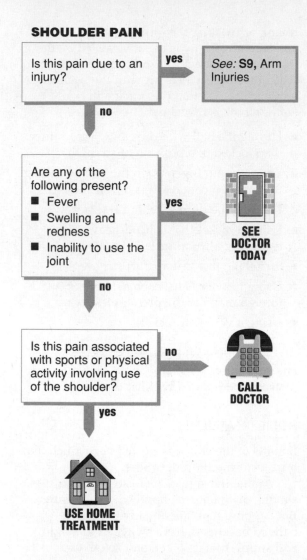

SHOULDER PAIN

Is this pain due to an injury? — **yes** → *See:* **S9**, Arm Injuries

no ↓

Are any of the following present?
- Fever
- Swelling and redness
- Inability to use the joint

yes → **SEE DOCTOR TODAY**

no ↓

Is this pain associated with sports or physical activity involving use of the shoulder? — **no** → **CALL DOCTOR**

yes ↓

USE HOME TREATMENT

motion. Next a small amount of weight (1 to 1.5 pounds, or around half a kilogram) is held in the hand as the exercises are performed. Weight is gradually increased by a half pound (200 g) every ten days. Heat may be applied before the exercise, but ice is recommended after exercise.

Acetaminophen, two tablets every three to four hours, may be taken as needed. Aspirin, ibuprofen, or naproxen may help decrease inflammation **(M4)**.

Call a doctor if the condition persists beyond three weeks.

WHAT TO EXPECT AT THE DOCTOR'S OFFICE

The doctor will examine the shoulder and prescribe a regimen similar to the one above, if one of the common causes of shoulder pain is diagnosed. If the problem is bursitis, a corticosteroid injection may be given on the first visit. Otherwise such injections should be given only if home therapy doesn't work. There should be no more than two or three such injections. Nonsteroidal anti-inflammatory drugs (NSAIDs) may be given. These prescription drugs are similar to aspirin, ibuprofen, and naproxen. They may decrease pain but don't speed the healing process. Expect instruction in rehabilitation exercises.

Surgery is the last resort and is a gamble. Satisfaction isn't guaranteed.

problem's severity. Returning too soon will increase the probability of reinjury.

After the initial rest period, exercises should be started to gradually strengthen the muscles around the shoulder. This is especially important in rotator cuff tendinitis. At first the exercise need consist only of putting the arm through a full range of

Some of the problems related specifically to racquet sports, baseball pitching, or golf are due to poor technique. Coaching from a professional is well worth considering. It is less expensive than going to a doctor, and you will probably improve your game.

70 Elbow Pain

Aside from injuries, the main causes of elbow pain are bursitis and tennis elbow.

Bursitis

The elbow bursa is a fluid-filled sac located right at the tip of the elbow. When it is irritated, the amount of fluid increases, causing a swelling that looks very much like a small egg right at the end of the elbow. The swelling is the cause of discomfort. There should be no fever and only a little redness, if any.

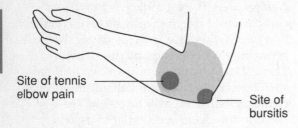

Site of tennis elbow pain

Site of bursitis

Tennis Elbow

Of the cases of tennis elbow that reach the doctor's office, less than half are actually associated with playing tennis. The rest usually result from work that requires a twisting motion of the arm — such as using a screwdriver — or have no obvious cause. The doctor's help is needed only for prolonged cases that don't get better; perhaps one person in 1,000 needs such help.

The diagnosis of tennis elbow doesn't depend on tests or special examinations. Tennis elbow is simply defined as pain in the lateral (outer) portion of the elbow and upper forearm. The pain occurs after repeatedly

rolling or twisting the forearm, wrist, and hand. Tennis elbow is usually caused by the tremendous impact transmitted to the forearm when the tennis ball is hit with the backhand motion. The risk that this force will create tennis elbow is raised by:

- Hitting the ball with the elbow bent rather than locked in a position of strength
- Trying to put top spin on the ball by rolling the wrist on contact (this doesn't work)
- Holding the thumb behind the racket
- Using a racket that is head-heavy, especially a wood racket
- Switching to a faster court surface
- Using heavier balls, such as those of foreign make or the pressureless type
- Using a very stiff racket

According to the experts, the most important preventive measure for tennis players is to use a two-handed backhand stroke.

HOME TREATMENT

Bursitis of the elbow is treated very much like bursitis of the shoulder **(S69).**

At the first sign of tennis elbow, you should, of course, take preventive measures. But suppose that you already use a two-handed backhand, have switched to a light and supple metal racket, and so on. Or suppose your job or favorite hobby requires repeated use of screwdrivers or other tools that aggravate the problem. What now? Resting the arm will surely make it hurt less, but most likely taking two weeks off won't cure it forever. Interestingly, most authorities now think that you can "play with pain" and not cause permanent injury.

We advocate a commonsense approach to tennis elbow: cut down on your playing time.

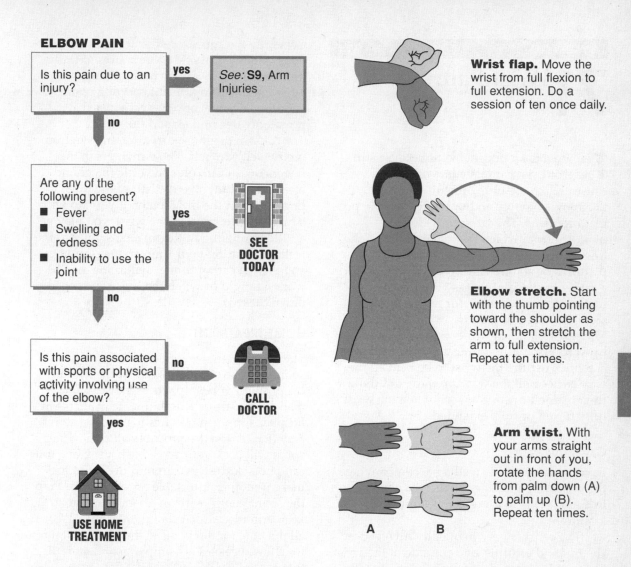

ELBOW PAIN

Is this pain due to an injury? — **yes** → *See:* **S9,** Arm Injuries

no ↓

Are any of the following present?
- Fever
- Swelling and redness
- Inability to use the joint

— **yes** → **SEE DOCTOR TODAY**

no ↓

Is this pain associated with sports or physical activity involving use of the elbow? — **no** → **CALL DOCTOR**

yes ↓

USE HOME TREATMENT

Wrist flap. Move the wrist from full flexion to full extension. Do a session of ten once daily.

Elbow stretch. Start with the thumb pointing toward the shoulder as shown, then stretch the arm to full extension. Repeat ten times.

Arm twist. With your arms straight out in front of you, rotate the hands from palm down (A) to palm up (B). Repeat ten times.

A   **B**

When you do play, warm up slowly and do some stretching exercises of the wrist and elbow before you begin to hit the ball. Using a tennis elbow strap may help. Applying ice after playing may also help.

WHAT TO EXPECT AT THE DOCTOR'S OFFICE

Bursitis of the elbow is treated by the doctor very much like bursitis of the shoulder. If you're the rare person with tennis elbow who has severe persistent pain, the next step is to inject a pain reliever and corticosteroid (cortisonelike drug) into the painful area. Three such injections is the limit. Surgery should be a last resort — an act of desperation. If you get to this point, perhaps it's time to take up another game.

71 Wrist Pain

The wrist is an unusual joint because stiffness or even complete loss of motion causes relatively little difficulty; however, if the joint is wobbly and unstable, this can pose real problems. The wrist provides the platform from which the fine motions of the fingers operate. It is essential that this platform be stable. The eight wrist bones form a rather crude joint that is very limited in motion compared with, for example, the shoulder. But this joint is strong and stable. The wrist platform works best when it is bent upward just a little. Almost no normal human activities require the wrist to be bent all the way back or all the way forward, and the fingers don't operate as well when the wrist is fully flexed or fully extended.

Causes of Pain

Fever and/or rapid swelling accompanying the onset of pain suggests the possibility of an infection. This requires prompt medical attention.

The wrist is very frequently involved in rheumatoid arthritis, and the side of the wrist by the thumb is very commonly involved in osteoarthritis (see Arthritis, **S66**).

Carpal tunnel syndrome can cause pain at the wrist. In addition, this syndrome can cause pains to shoot down into the fingers or up into the forearm. Usually there is a numb feeling in the fingers as if they were asleep. In this syndrome, the median nerve is trapped and squeezed as it passes through the fibrous carpal tunnel in the front of the wrist.

Generally the squeezing results from too much inflamed tissue. Some causes of this inflammation are a blow to the front of the wrist, rheumatoid arthritis, playing tennis, paddling a canoe, or other activities that repeatedly flex and extend the wrist.

You can diagnose carpal tunnel syndrome pretty well yourself. The numbness in the fingers doesn't involve the little finger and often doesn't involve the half of the ring finger nearest the little finger. If you tap with a finger on the front of the wrist, you may get a sudden tingling in the fingers, similar to the feeling of hitting your funny bone. Tingling and pain in carpal tunnel syndrome may be worse at night or when the wrists are cocked down (flexed).

HOME TREATMENT

The key to management of wrist pain is splinting. The strategy is to rest the joint in the position of best function. Wrist splints made of plastic or aluminum are available at hospital supply stores and many drug stores. Any that fit you are probably all right. The splint will cock your wrist back just a bit. You can put a cloth sleeve around the splint to make it more comfortable on your skin. Wrap the splint gently with an elastic bandage to keep it in place. That's all there is to it. Wear it all the time for a few days, then just at night for a few weeks. This simple treatment is all that is required for most wrist flare-ups.

No major pain medication should be necessary. Acetaminophen and similar medications are all right but probably won't help much. If you know what triggered the pain, work out a way to avoid that activity. Common sense means listening to the pain message.

If the problem persists after six weeks of home treatment, see the doctor.

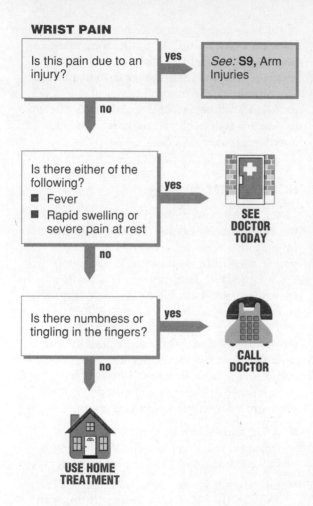

WRIST PAIN

Is this pain due to an injury? — **yes** → *See:* **S9,** Arm Injuries

no ↓

Is there either of the following?
■ Fever
■ Rapid swelling or severe pain at rest
— **yes** → **SEE DOCTOR TODAY**

no ↓

Is there numbness or tingling in the fingers? — **yes** → **CALL DOCTOR**

no ↓

USE HOME TREATMENT

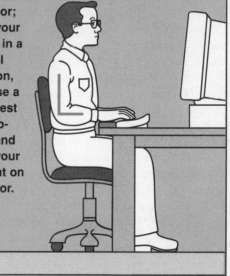

As more people type on computers, there have been more worries about carpal tunnel syndrome. Research continues, but there seem to be two important factors: stress, especially from pressure to type quickly or without interruption, and poor hand positioning. Take brief rests, and consider using a different keyboard to help avoid pain.

For proper typing position: keep your elbows at a 90° angle, with your forearms parallel to the floor; keep your wrists in a neutral position, and use a wrist rest for support; and keep your feet flat on the floor.

WHAT TO EXPECT AT THE DOCTOR'S OFFICE

The wrist will be examined and advice similar to that above will be given. X-rays may be required, but only rarely. Anti-inflammatory drugs may be prescribed. Injection with a corticosteroid medication may be performed on occasion and is likely to help if carpal tunnel syndrome hasn't responded to splinting.

Several different kinds of surgery are available, and one or another procedure may be recommended in difficult cases. Carpal tunnel nerve compression may be released surgically. In rheumatoid arthritis, the synovial tissue that lines the tendon sheaths on the back of the hand may be removed to protect the tendons that run through the inflamed area (synovectomy). The wrist may be casted or the bones fused.

72 Finger Pain

Each hand has 14 finger joints, each like a small hinge. These joints are operated by muscles in the forearm that control them through an intricate system of tendons that run through the wrist and hand. The small size and complex arrangement of these joints and tendons mean that any inflammation or damage to a joint is likely to result in some stiffness and lost motion. Even a small scar may limit motion.

You shouldn't expect that a problem with a small finger joint will resolve completely. Even after healing, some leftover stiffness and occasional twinges of discomfort are likely. Unrealistically high expectations lead to feelings that you did something wrong or that the doctor was no good. In fact, almost all of us have a few fingers that have been injured and remain a bit crooked or stiff.

Osteoarthritis frequently causes knobby swelling of the most distant joints of the fingers as well as swelling of the middle joints. It can also cause problems at the base of the thumb. If we live long enough, all of us get these knobby swellings. They cause most

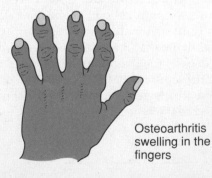

Osteoarthritis swelling in the fingers

of the changed appearance that we associate with the aging hand. As a rule, they cause relatively little pain or stiffness and don't need specific treatment other than exercise.

Numbness or tingling may indicate a problem with nerves or circulation. A call to the doctor will help you make a decision about what to do.

HOME TREATMENT

Listen to the pain message and avoid activities that cause or aggravate pain. Rest the finger joints so that they can heal, but use gentle stretching exercises to keep them limber and maintain motion. The key to managing finger problems is to use common sense.

With a bit of ingenuity, you can find a less stressful way to do almost any activity that puts stress on the joints. Because everyone's activities are a bit different, you will have to invent some of these new methods yourself. Here are a few hints to get you going:

- A big handle can be gripped with less strain than a small handle. Wrap pens, knives, and other similar objects with tape.

- Lift smaller loads. Make more trips. Plan ahead rather than blundering through an activity.

- Let others open a car door for you. Get power steering or a very light car.

- Find clothing that uses Velcro or large buttons instead of small buttons and snaps for fasteners.

- Use a gripper for opening tough jar lids or stop buying products that come in hard-to-open jars. When opening a tough lid, apply friction pressure on the top of the lid with your palm and twist with your whole hand, not with your grip.

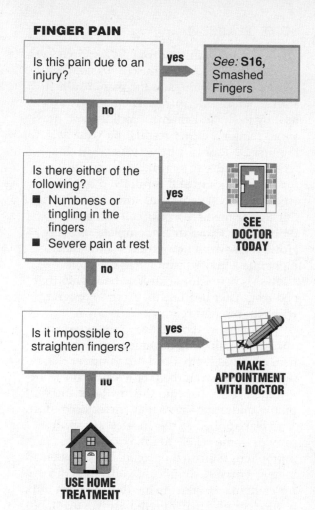

FINGER PAIN

Is this pain due to an injury? **yes** → *See:* **S16,** Smashed Fingers

no ↓

Is there either of the following?
- Numbness or tingling in the fingers
- Severe pain at rest

yes → **SEE DOCTOR TODAY**

no ↓

Is it impossible to straighten fingers? **yes** → **MAKE APPOINTMENT WITH DOCTOR**

no ↓

USE HOME TREATMENT

- Don't put heavy objects too high or too low. Organize your kitchen, workshop, study, and bedroom.

Don't use strong medicines that mask your pain because these may lead you to overdo an activity. Be sure to take any medication prescribed for inflammation just as instructed. If the problem persists after six weeks of home treatment, see the doctor.

WHAT TO EXPECT AT THE DOCTOR'S OFFICE

The doctor will examine your hands and the finger motions. Sometimes an X-ray is taken, but usually not more often than every two years. Anti-inflammatory medications such as aspirin, ibuprofen, and naproxen can help **(M4),** but doses should usually be low to moderate.

In rare cases, injecting corticosteroids into a particularly bad finger joint is helpful, but this is less effective with small joints such as fingers than with large ones. Surgery is also less effective with small joints and is often not appropriate. Operations such as replacement with plastic joints or removal of inflamed tissue usually succeed in making the hand look more normal and may decrease pain, but the hand often doesn't work much better than it did before the operation.

Stretch your joints gently twice a day to maintain motion. Putting your hands in warm water before stretching may help you get more motion.

1. Straighten one hand out against the table top.

2. Make a fist and then cock the wrist to increase the stretch.

3. Use one hand to move each finger of the other hand through its full range of motion. Don't force, but stretch just to the edge of discomfort. If the motion of a joint is normal, one repetition is enough. If the motion is limited, do up to ten repetitions.

73 Low Back Pain

Few problems can frustrate patient and doctor alike as much as low back pain. The pain is slow to resolve and often comes back. Frustration then becomes a part of the problem and may also require treatment.

Low back pain usually involves spasm of the large supportive muscles alongside the spine. Any injury to the back may produce such spasms. Pain — often severe — and stiffness result. The onset of pain may be immediate or may occur some hours after exertion or injury. Often the cause isn't clear.

Most muscular problems in the back are linked to some injury and must heal naturally. Give them time. Back pain that results from a severe blow or fall may require immediate attention. As a practical matter, if back pain is caused by an injury received at work, examination by a doctor is required by the workers' compensation laws.

Pain due to muscular strain is usually confined to the back. Occasionally it may extend into the buttocks or upper leg. Pain that extends down the leg to below the knee is called sciatica, and suggests pressure on the nerves as they leave the spinal cord. Sciatica often responds to home treatment, but the following symptoms mean that immediate help from a doctor may be required:

- loss of bladder or bowel control
- weakness in the leg

HOME TREATMENT

The low back pain syndrome is a vicious cycle in which injury causes muscle spasm, the spasm induces pain, and the pain results in additional muscle spasm. The injury must heal by itself. To heal most rapidly, you must avoid reinjury. Either rest flat on your back for the first 24 hours, or be very, very careful.

Severe muscle spasm pain usually lasts for 48 to 72 hours and is followed by days or weeks of less severe pain. Strenuous activity during the next six weeks can bring the problem back and delay complete recovery. However, several new studies show that moderate activity (as much as the pain allows) is better for acute low back pain than bed rest. After healing, an exercise program will help prevent reinjury.

The person should sleep, pillowless, in one of the following arrangements: on a very firm mattress, with a bed board under the mattress, on a waterbed, or even on the floor. A folded towel beneath the low back and a pillow under the knees may increase comfort.

Heat applied to the affected area will provide some relief. You may take acetaminophen, aspirin, ibuprofen, or naproxen as long as you feel significant pain. To avoid upset stomach, take the medication with milk or food, or else use buffered aspirin (M4). No drug will hasten healing; drugs only reduce symptoms and may actually encourage reinjury.

If there is no nerve damage, hospitalization and the doctor have little to offer. If significant pain persists beyond a week, call the doctor.

WHAT TO EXPECT AT THE DOCTOR'S OFFICE

Expect questions similar to those in the decision chart. The examination will center on

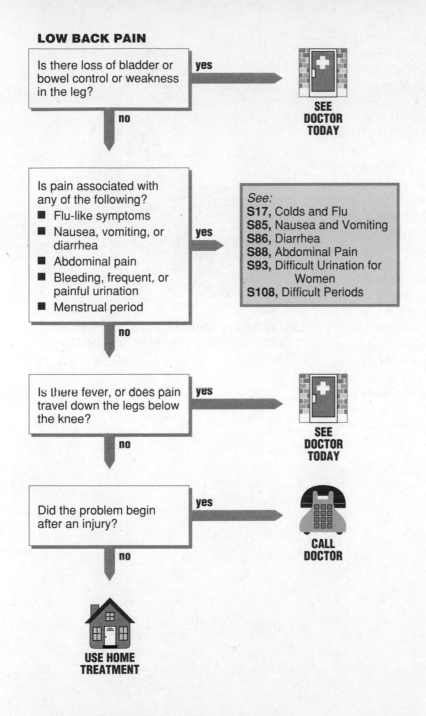

LOW BACK PAIN

Is there loss of bladder or bowel control or weakness in the leg? **yes** → **SEE DOCTOR TODAY**

no ↓

Is pain associated with any of the following?
- Flu-like symptoms
- Nausea, vomiting, or diarrhea
- Abdominal pain
- Bleeding, frequent, or painful urination
- Menstrual period

yes →

See:
S17, Colds and Flu
S85, Nausea and Vomiting
S86, Diarrhea
S88, Abdominal Pain
S93, Difficult Urination for Women
S108, Difficult Periods

no ↓

Is there fever, or does pain travel down the legs below the knee? **yes** → **SEE DOCTOR TODAY**

no ↓

Did the problem begin after an injury? **yes** → **CALL DOCTOR**

no ↓

USE HOME TREATMENT

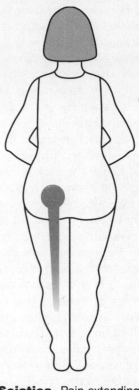

Sciatica. Pain extending from the lower back to below one knee indicates pressure on the sciatic nerve. See a doctor if you also have weakness in that leg or loss of bladder control.

the back, abdomen, arms, and legs, with special attention to testing the nerve function of the legs. If the injury is the result of a fall or a blow to the back, X-rays are indicated; otherwise, they usually aren't. X-rays reveal injury only to bones, not to muscles. The doctor's advice will usually be similar to that described above.

A muscle relaxant may be prescribed. If the history and physical examination indicate damage to the nerves leaving the spinal cord, a special X-ray, such as a myelogram, CT scan, or magnetic resonance imagery (MR or MRI) may be necessary. If there is pressure on nerves, hospitalization, traction, or surgery may be considered. Such treatments may be considered if pain is continuous over a long period, even if there is no pressure on any nerves. The chance that these treatments will help, however, is slim. For example, less than half of those who have surgery for chronic back pain have substantial relief. Chronic pain may respond best to increasing flexibility and strength of the muscles, as well as learning to control pain through mental relaxation and thought control techniques.

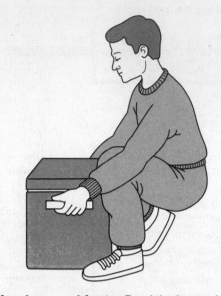

Lifting heavy objects. Bend the knees, but keep the back straight and erect, to avoid back strain.

SYMPTOM   S74

74 Hip Pain

The hip is a "ball-and-socket" joint. The largest bone in the body, the femur, is in the thigh. The femur narrows to a "neck" that angles into the pelvis and ends in a ball-shaped knob. This ball fits into a curved socket in the pelvic bones, providing a joint that can move in all directions. The joint is located under some big muscles so that it is protected from dislocation — that is, from coming out of its socket.

Two special problems arise because of this anatomical arrangement. The narrow neck of the femur can break rather easily, and this is usually what happens when an older person breaks a hip after a slight fall. Also, the ball portion of the femur gets its blood through the narrow neck. The small artery that supplies the head of the femur can get clogged, leading to death of the bone and a kind of arthritis called aseptic necrosis.

Among other causes of hip pain, the hip joint can get infected. The bursae (fluid-filled sacs) that lie over the joint can be inflamed (bursitis). Rheumatoid arthritis and osteo-arthritis can also injure the joint. Another arthritis condition, ankylosing spondylitis, can cause stiffness or loss of motion of the hip.

A flexion contracture is a common result of hip problems. This means that motion of the hip joint has been partly lost. The hip becomes partially fixed in a slightly bent position. When you are walking or standing, the pelvis tilts forward; and when you stand straight, the back has to curve a little more. This throws extra strain on the lower back.

For poorly understood reasons, pain in the hip is often felt down the leg, often at or just above the knee. This is called referred pain. Nonreferred hip pain may be felt in the groin or the upper outer thigh. Pain that starts in the low back is often felt in the hip region. Because the hip joint is so deeply located, it can often be difficult to identify the exact source of pain.

HOME TREATMENT

Listen for the pain message and try to avoid activities that aggravate your hip. You should avoid pain medication as much as possible. Rest the joint after painful activities.

Use a cane or crutches if necessary. The cane is usually best held in the hand opposite the painful hip because this allows greater relaxation in the large muscles around the sore hip joint. Move the cane and the affected side simultaneously.

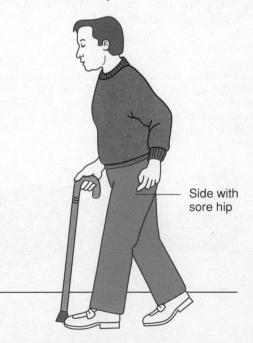

Side with sore hip

As the pain begins to resolve, exercise should be gradually introduced. First use gentle motion exercises to free the hip and prevent stiffness. Repeat these exercises gently two or three times a day:

- Stand with your good hip by a table and lean on the table with your hand. Let the leg with the bad hip swing side to side and front and back.

- Lie on your back with your leg hanging off the bed. Let the leg stretch backward toward the floor; bend your knees as little as possible (see diagram). Or you can get into this position by sitting on the edge of the bed and then easing down on your back while straightening your legs.

- See how far apart you can straddle your legs as you bend the upper body from side to side.

- With your legs together, try to turn your feet outward like a duck, so that the rotation ligaments get stretched.

Then introduce more active exercises to strengthen the muscles around the hips.

- Lie on your back and raise your legs one at a time. Keep straight and lift until you reach a 45° angle.

- Swim. This stretches muscles and builds good muscle tone.

- Bicycle or walk. When walking, start with short strides and gradually lengthen them as you loosen up. Gradually increase your efforts and distance, but not by more than 10% each day.

A good firm bed will help. The best sleeping position is on your back. Avoid pillows beneath the knees or under the lower back. Make sure you are taking anti-inflammatory medication as prescribed, especially if you have rheumatoid arthritis or ankylosing spondylitis.

If pain persists after six weeks of home treatment, see the doctor.

Hip exercise. With your shoulders, trunk, and one leg resting on the bed, allow the leg with the injured hip to dangle off the bed. Bend your knee as little as possible as you stretch the leg and hip backward, toward the floor.

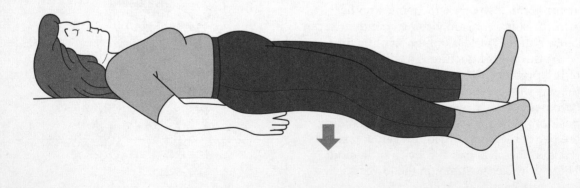

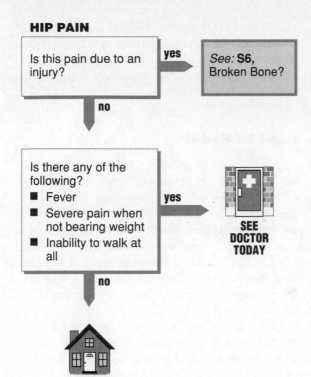

HIP PAIN

Is this pain due to an injury? → **yes** → *See:* **S6,** Broken Bone?

↓ **no**

Is there any of the following?
- Fever
- Severe pain when not bearing weight
- Inability to walk at all

→ **yes** → **SEE DOCTOR TODAY**

↓ **no**

USE HOME TREATMENT

WHAT TO EXPECT AT THE DOCTOR'S OFFICE

The doctor will examine the hip and take it through its range of motion. Your other leg joints and back will also be examined. X-rays may be necessary. Anti-inflammatory medication may be prescribed or the dosage increased. Injection is only rarely needed.

A surgical procedure may be recommended if the pain is intense and persistent, or if you are having real problems walking. Total hip replacement, while still major surgery, is a remarkable operation and has largely replaced many older techniques. This operation is almost always successful in stopping pain and may help mobility a great deal. An artificial hip should last at least 10 to 15 years with current techniques. You will be able to get up and around quite quickly after surgery, and complications are rather rare.

75 Knee Pain

The knee is a hinge. It is a large weight-bearing joint, but its motion is much more strictly limited than that of most other joints. It will straighten for stable support, and it will bend to more than a right angle, to approximately 120°. However, it won't move in any other direction. The limited motion of the knee gives it great strength, but it isn't engineered to take side stresses.

There are two cartilage compartments in the knee — one inner and one outer. If the cartilage wears unevenly, the leg can bow in or bow out. If you were born with crooked legs, there can be strain that causes the cartilage to wear more rapidly. If you are overweight, you are far more likely to have knee problems.

The knee must be stable, and it must be able to extend fully so that the leg is straight. If it lacks full extension, the muscles have to support the body at all times, and strain is continuous. If the knee wobbles from side to side, there is too much stress on the side ligaments, and the condition may gradually worsen.

When to See a Doctor

If the knee is unstable and wobbles, or if it cannot be straightened out, you need a doctor. This is also true if the knee is red or hot, which suggests the possibility of gout or an infection; the knee is the joint most frequently bothered by these serious problems.

Finally, if there is pain or swelling in the calf below the sore knee, you may have a blood clot. More likely, you have a Baker's cyst. These cysts start as fluid-filled sacs in an inflamed knee but enlarge through the tissues of the calf and may cause swelling quite a distance below the knee. You should see your doctor for this condition.

HOME TREATMENT

Listen to the pain message and try not to do anything that aggravates the pain. If you have arthritis, make sure you are taking your medication as directed. Otherwise, acetaminophen, aspirin, ibuprofen, or naproxen may be used to ease the pain (M4).

Using a cane can help; usually, the cane is best carried in the hand on the same side as the painful knee, but some prefer to carry it on the opposite side.

Do not use a pillow under the knee at night or at any other time. This can make the knee stiffen so that it cannot be straightened out.

Start exercising slowly, and work up to performing exercises several times daily, if possible.

1. From the beginning, pay close attention to flexing and straightening the leg. It may be more comfortable to have someone move the leg for you while you are sitting or lying down. Ask a friend to help. But work at getting it straight and keeping it straight.

2. Next, begin gentle exercises. Tense the muscles in your upper leg, front and back at the same time, so that you are exerting force but your leg isn't moving. Exert the force for two seconds, then rest two seconds. Do ten repetitions three times a day.

3. Begin gentle active exercises. A bicycle in low gear is a good place to start. Stationary

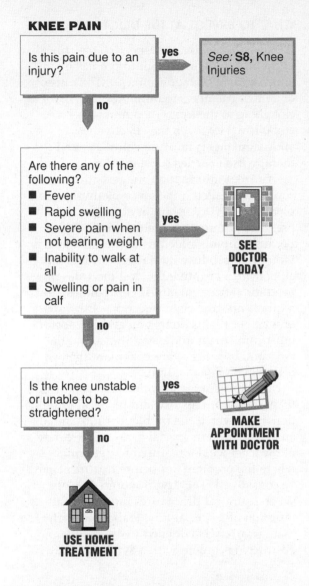

KNEE PAIN

Is this pain due to an injury? — **yes** → *See:* **S8**, Knee Injuries

no ↓

Are there any of the following?
- Fever
- Rapid swelling
- Severe pain when not bearing weight
- Inability to walk at all
- Swelling or pain in calf

yes → **SEE DOCTOR TODAY**

no ↓

Is the knee unstable or unable to be straightened?

yes → **MAKE APPOINTMENT WITH DOCTOR**

no ↓

USE HOME TREATMENT

Many people have wondered if exercise such as walking or running can cause knee problems. No. If the knee isn't injured, exercise and weight-bearing are good. They help nourish the cartilage, and they keep the side ligaments, the muscles, and the bones strong, which keeps the knee stable.

Avoid exercises or activities that simulate deep knee bends because they place too much stress on the knee. Knee problems can develop from the feet, so proper shoes can help.

See your doctor if pain remains after six weeks of home treatment.

WHAT TO EXPECT AT THE DOCTOR'S OFFICE

The knee and other joints will be examined and taken through their range of motion. An X-ray of the knee may be taken. Fluid may be drawn from the knee through a needle and tested if a Baker's cyst is suspected or for other diagnostic reasons. This procedure is easy, not too uncomfortable, and quite safe.

A number of operations are quite helpful for knee problems. Torn cartilage may be removed, or cartilage may be shaved through arthroscopic surgery. Increasingly, doctors are using the arthroscope to view the condition and often to help cure it. This is a minor procedure. For severe and persistent problems, total knee replacement may be recommended. This is an excellent operation and usually gives total pain relief. Next to hip replacement, knee replacement is the most successful total joint replacement surgery.

bicycles are fine. Be sure that the seat is relatively high. Your knee shouldn't bend to more than a right angle during the bicycle stroke.

4. Swimming and walking are probably the best overall exercises. Gradually increase your distances.

76 Leg Pain

Three types of problems account for most leg pain not associated with injuries:

- Inflammation and clots in veins — thrombophlebitis
- Narrowing of arteries — intermittent claudication
- "Overuse" problems associated with vigorous exercise, collectively referred to as "shin splints" **(S77)**

Thrombophlebitis is most likely to occur after a prolonged period of inactivity, such as a long car or plane ride. The pain is aching and usually not localized, but sometimes a firm and tender vein can be felt in the middle of the calf. Swelling doesn't always occur or may be so slight that it's hard to detect.

In older people or heavy smokers, the arteries in the leg may become narrowed so that not enough blood reaches the muscles during even such mild exercise as walking. The pain that this causes is called intermittent claudication, because the pain is brought on by exercise, but relief comes in a few minutes with rest.

Both thrombophlebitis and intermittent claudication will require the help of the doctor, but thrombophlebitis is more urgent. A decision on the method of treatment should be made as soon as possible.

Consult the physician by telephone for leg pain that doesn't fit the description of intermittent claudication, thrombophlebitis, or shin splints.

WHAT TO EXPECT AT THE DOCTOR'S OFFICE

If thrombophlebitis is suspected, the crucial question is whether or not to prescribe anticoagulants (blood thinners). The purpose of anticoagulants is to minimize the risk of a clot going to the lungs — pulmonary embolism. However, the effectiveness of anticoagulants is far from complete, and the therapy itself carries substantial risks.

Current information suggests that a simple test called impedance plethysmography (IPG) is very useful in detecting the presence of thrombophlebitis in the thigh. Because thrombophlebitis in the calf alone is thought to produce little risk of pulmonary embolism, a negative IPG test indicates no need for anticoagulants. IPG is painless and requires no surgery or injections. Regardless of whether IPG is done, you and the doctor must come to an understanding about the risks and benefits of anticoagulant therapy before making a decision.

Intermittent claudication can usually be diagnosed from history and physical examination. However, if the problem is substantial, an arteriogram (a special X-ray of the arteries of the legs) will be required to determine where the problem lies before treatment can be considered. Therapy, if required, is one of several surgical procedures ranging from insertion of a special tube (balloon catheter) so that the artery is widened to bypass the obstructed segment with a synthetic graft.

LEG PAIN

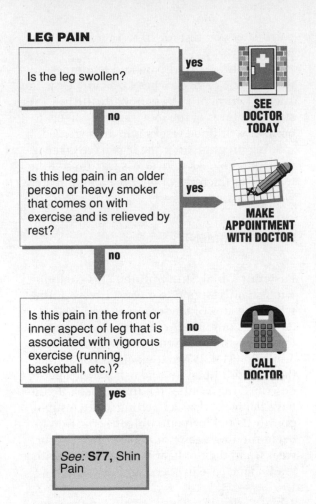

Is the leg swollen? — **yes** → **SEE DOCTOR TODAY**

no ↓

Is this leg pain in an older person or heavy smoker that comes on with exercise and is relieved by rest? — **yes** → **MAKE APPOINTMENT WITH DOCTOR**

no ↓

Is this pain in the front or inner aspect of leg that is associated with vigorous exercise (running, basketball, etc.)? — **no** → **CALL DOCTOR**

yes ↓

See: **S77,** Shin Pain

77 Shin Pain

Shin pain is often called "shin splints," a catch-all term that may indicate any one of four conditions associated with strenuous exercise, usually after a period of relative inactivity.

Posterior tibial shin splints are the "original" shin splints and account for about 75% of the problems affecting athletes in the front portion of their legs. Overstressing the posterior tibial muscle causes pain where the muscle attaches to the tibia, or shin bone, which is easily seen and felt in the front of your leg. Pain and tenderness are located in a three- to four-inch (8–10 cm) area on the inner edge of the tibia about midway between the knee and ankle. It is the muscle and the attachments to the bone that are painful; the front of the tibia itself, felt immediately beneath the skin, is not tender.

The front of the tibial bone is tender, however, in another form of shin splint, tibial periostitis. The pain and tenderness are similar to that in posterior tibial shin splints except that it is further toward the front of the leg and the bone itself is tender.

A third form of shin splint, anterior compartment syndrome, is located on the outer side of the front of the leg. You can readily feel the difference between the hard tibial bone and the muscles located in the anterior compartment. Pain arises when the muscles swell with blood during hard use. The compartment cannot increase in size so that the swelling squeezes the blood vessels and diminishes blood flow. The lack of adequate blood flow to the muscles causes the pain. After you rest for 10 to 15 minutes, the pain goes away.

Sharply localized pain and tenderness in the tibia one or two inches (3–5 cm) below the knee is typical of a stress fracture. Just as with stress fractures of the foot, these are likely to occur two or three weeks into an increased training program after the legs have taken a real pounding. As with stress fractures of the foot, stress fractures of the tibia aren't treated with casts, but with rest.

HOME TREATMENT

Posterior Tibial Shin Splints. This condition will usually respond to a week of rest during which the area of tenderness is iced twice a day for 20 minutes. Acetaminophen, aspirin, ibuprofen, or naproxen with every meal may also help **(M4)**. When the pain is gone, stretch the posterior tibial muscle using the exercises described for Achilles tendinitis **(S80)**. If you have flat feet, consider getting an arch support (orthotic) for your athletic shoe. Don't begin running again for another two to four weeks, and then only at half speed and with a gradual increase in speed and distance.

Tibial Periostitis. This is treated in the same way as posterior tibial shin splints, except that your gradual return to sports can begin after a week of rest; acetaminophen, aspirin, ibuprofen, or naproxen; and ice therapy. Athletic shoes with good shock absorption, especially in the heel, are very important.

Anterior Compartment Syndrome. This condition will almost always go away as the muscles gradually become accustomed to vigorous exercise. You can help by resting for ten minutes when pain occurs, and running slowly when you begin to run again.

SHIN PAIN

Is this pain in the front or inner aspect of the leg associated with vigorous exercises such as running or basketball?

no → *See:* **S76,** Leg Pain

yes ↓

USE HOME TREATMENT

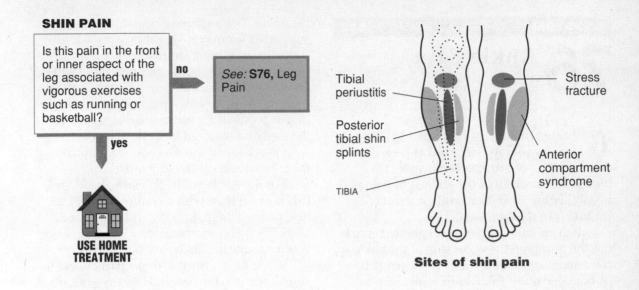

Tibial periustitis

Posterior tibial shin splints

TIBIA

Stress fracture

Anterior compartment syndrome

Sites of shin pain

Cooling the leg with ice for 20 minutes after each workout may also help. Complete rest is not necessary. Shoes and pain relievers are unimportant in the treatment of anterior compartment syndrome. If you're the one person in 1,000 with anterior compartment syndrome for whom the problem doesn't go away with home treatment, surgery can be considered.

Stress Fractures. These require rest from running, usually for a month, before gradually starting to recondition your legs. Complete healing requires between four and six weeks. Crutches can be used but usually aren't necessary.

Note again that only the anterior compartment syndrome has any treatment other than home treatment and that this treatment (surgery) is used only as a last resort. However, if you are unsure as to the nature of the problem or you have made no progress with home treatment after several weeks, consult the doctor.

WHAT TO EXPECT AT THE DOCTOR'S OFFICE

Home treatment will be prescribed for any of the four varieties of shin splints. In the very rare event that an anterior compartment syndrome doesn't go away over time, the pressure can be relieved by splitting the tough, fibrous tissue (fascia) that surrounds the muscles. This is a relatively simple surgical procedure and can be accomplished without requiring a stay in the hospital.

78 Ankle Pain

The ankle is a large weight-bearing joint that is unavoidably stressed at each step. Several kinds of arthritis can involve the bones and cartilage of the ankle, but pain and instability are more frequently a result of problems in the ligaments.

With an ankle sprain, the ligament attaching the bump on the outer side of the ankle to the outer surface of the foot is injured at one or both ends; the ankle itself is all right.

With arthritis, injured ligaments may let the joint slip and wobble. This results in further stress on the ligaments, pain, and instability. Walking on an unstable joint increases the damage, but with a stable joint, walking is usually all right.

If you look at your leg when you are lying down and again when you are standing, you can tell if the joint is stable. If it is unstable, the line of your leg won't be straight down to the foot when you stand. Perhaps the foot will be slipped a half-inch or an inch (1–3 cm) to the outside of where it should be. When you aren't bearing weight, it will move back in line toward a more normal position. The unstable joint may actually slip sideways if you try to move the foot with your hands. Instability is not just a swollen ankle **(S79)**; the ankle must be crooked to be unstable.

HOME TREATMENT

Listen to the pain message. It is telling you to rest your ankle a bit more, to provide support for an unstable ankle, to back off your exercise program, or to use an aid to take weight off the ankle. The unstable ankle should be supported for major weight-bearing activity.

Support is most simply obtained from high-lacing boots, but sometimes these will be too uncomfortable and you will need specially made boots or an ankle brace. Professional help is required for adequate fitting of such devices, and they can be quite expensive.

Crutches and even a cane can help you take the weight off the sore ankle.

For the stable ankle, an elastic bandage **(M21)** and a shoe with a comfortable, thick heel pad will help. Jogging shoes are good. Light hiking boots, resembling running shoes that go above the ankle, are often excellent.

If you have arthritis, make particularly sure that you have been taking any prescribed medication exactly as ordered. Sometimes a patient gets a little bored and lax with the pill-taking routine and a few days later experiences pain or swelling.

As soon as the pain begins to decrease, you can gently begin to exercise the joint again. Swimming is good because you don't have to bear weight. Start easily and slowly with your exercises.

1. Sit on a chair, let the leg hang, and wiggle the foot up and down and in and out.

2. Later, walk carefully with an ankle bandage for support. Stretch the ankle by putting the forefoot on a slightly raised surface, such as a step, and lowering the heel.

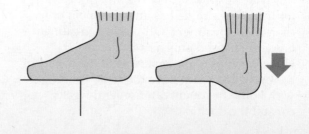

ANKLE PAIN

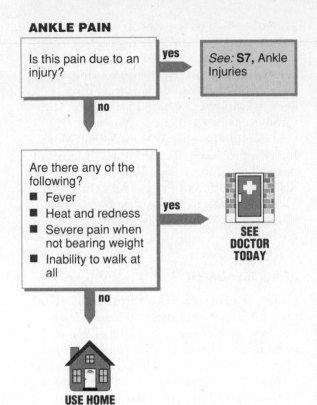

Is this pain due to an injury? — **yes** → *See:* **S7**, Ankle Injuries

no ↓

Are there any of the following?
■ Fever
■ Heat and redness
■ Severe pain when not bearing weight
■ Inability to walk at all

yes → **SEE DOCTOR TODAY**

no ↓

USE HOME TREATMENT

taking them. Special shoes or braces may be prescribed.

Surgery is occasionally necessary. Fusing some of the ankle bones together is generally the most useful procedure. A fixed, pain-free ankle is far preferable to an unstable and painful one. The artificial ankle joint isn't yet satisfactory for most people, but engineers are making rapid progress in this area.

3. As the ankle gains strength, you can walk on tiptoe and walk on your heels to stretch and strengthen the joint.

Do the exercises several times a day. The ankle shouldn't be a lot worse after exercising, if you aren't overdoing it. Keep at it, take your time, and be patient.

WHAT TO EXPECT AT THE DOCTOR'S OFFICE

The ankle and the area around it will be examined. X-rays may be necessary. The doctor may prescribe anti-inflammatory medications or increase the dosage if you are already

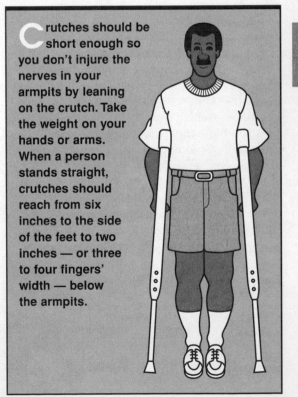

Crutches should be short enough so you don't injure the nerves in your armpits by leaning on the crutch. Take the weight on your hands or arms. When a person stands straight, crutches should reach from six inches to the side of the feet to two inches — or three to four fingers' width — below the armpits.

79 Ankle and Leg Swelling

Painless swelling of the ankles is a common problem, and the swelling usually affects both legs and may extend up the calves or even the thighs.

Usually the problem is fluid accumulation (edema). This is most pronounced in the lower legs because of the effects of gravity. If there is excess fluid and you press firmly with your thumb on the area that is swollen, it will squeeze the fluid out of that area and leave a deep impression. The depression will stay for a few moments.

Fortunately most swelling is due to local causes. Often, breakdowns in the veins over time have made it difficult for blood to be returned to the heart fast enough. This increases pressure in the smallest blood vessels (capillaries) and causes fluid to leak out into the tissues, which causes the leg swelling. This is what happens in "varicose veins," but the problem can happen with larger, deeper veins as well as with capillaries.

Serious Problems

If just one leg becomes swollen rapidly, thrombophlebitis (a blood clot in the vein) may be present, and a doctor is needed **(S76).**

Thrombophlebitis usually causes pain and redness also, but this isn't always true.

Accumulation of fluid in the body as a result of heart failure can also result in swollen ankles. With serious lung disease, such as emphysema, blood may "back up" through the heart, increase pressure in the veins, and thus cause ankle swelling. More rarely, a problem with the kidneys can result in swelling of the ankles. With serious liver disease, retention of fluid is very common. This fluid tends to accumulate primarily in the abdomen but is also frequently present in the legs.

HOME TREATMENT

If there is an associated medical problem, the most important treatment will come from your doctor. However, all kinds of ankle swelling can be helped by things you can do yourself. First, you need to exercise your legs. As you work the muscles, the fluid tends to work back into the veins and lymphatic channels, and the swelling tends to go down.

Ankle swelling is almost always a signal that your body has too much salt. A low-salt diet helps decrease the fluid retention and the ankle swelling.

Elevating your legs can help the fluid drain back into more proper parts of your circulatory system. Lie down and prop your legs up so they are higher than your heart as you rest. One or two pillows under the calves

Reducing swelling. Rest with your legs higher than your heart.

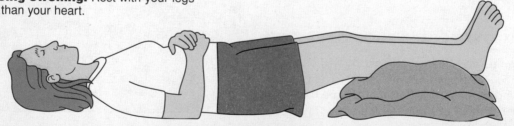

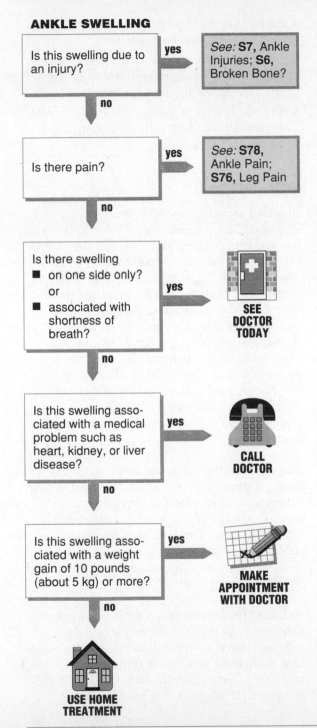

ANKLE SWELLING

Is this swelling due to an injury? — **yes** → *See:* **S7**, Ankle Injuries; **S6**, Broken Bone?

no ↓

Is there pain? — **yes** → *See:* **S78**, Ankle Pain; **S76**, Leg Pain

no ↓

Is there swelling
- on one side only? or
- associated with shortness of breath?

— **yes** → **SEE DOCTOR TODAY**

no ↓

Is this swelling associated with a medical problem such as heart, kidney, or liver disease? — **yes** → **CALL DOCTOR**

no ↓

Is this swelling associated with a weight gain of 10 pounds (about 5 kg) or more? — **yes** → **MAKE APPOINTMENT WITH DOCTOR**

no ↓

USE HOME TREATMENT

will help. Be sure not to place anything directly under the knees and don't wear any constricting clothing or garters on the upper legs.

Avoid sitting or standing without moving for long periods of time. If you must be in these positions, work the muscles in your calves by wiggling your feet and toes frequently. Support stockings, by applying constant external pressure, help reduce ankle swelling.

WHAT TO EXPECT AT THE DOCTOR'S OFFICE

The doctor will conduct a thorough examination including heart and lungs as well as the legs. Blood tests may be taken to check the function of your kidneys and your liver and to measure the proteins in your blood. The specific treatment will be directed at whatever underlying cause is found. Diuretics (pills that decrease fluids in the body by increasing urination) may be prescribed. These are effective but, of course, they have some side effects, such as causing loss of potassium from the body. If home treatment is successful, it is generally better than using drugs.

80 Heel Pain

The most frequent causes of heel pain are sometimes referred to as injuries, but they aren't due to a single event such as a fall or twist. Each of the following problems usually brings tenderness and some swelling.

Plantar fasciitis is a sprain of the tendon that is attached to the front of the heel bone and runs forward along the bottom of the foot. There are four main causes of plantar fasciitis:

- Feet that flatten and roll inwardly (pronate) excessively when walking or running
- Shoes with inadequate arch support
- Sudden turns that put great stress on the ligaments
- Running on hard surfaces or up hills

The retrocalcaneal bursa is a fluid-filled sac that surrounds the back of the heel. This may become inflamed (bursitis) due to pressure from shoes. For this reason, it is sometimes called a "pump bump." The inferior calcaneal bursa is located underneath the heel. Inflammation here is usually caused by landing hard or awkwardly on the heel.

The Achilles tendon is the large tendon that connects the calf muscles to the back of the heel. Achilles tendinitis occurs when the calf muscles repeatedly contract hard or suddenly. There are four factors that contribute to Achilles tendinitis:

- Shortening of and lack of flexibility in the calf muscle — Achilles tendon unit (the main cause)

- Shoes that don't provide good stability and shock absorption for the heel
- Sudden inward or outward turning of the heel when striking the ground (this is due to the shape of the foot, an inherited trait)
- Running on hard surfaces such as concrete or asphalt (running hills may contribute further to this factor)

HOME TREATMENT

Plantar Fasciitis. Give your feet as much rest as possible for a week or so. Pain relievers can be used for comfort **(M4).** Use that time to get proper-fitting shoes — that is, shoes with adequate arch supports and flexible soles. A one-quarter-inch (6 mm) heel pad is a good idea. Some people need to wear only well-padded shoes, such as running shoes. Lace the top two eyelets very firmly to take some tension off your ligaments. Try an orthotic device (obtained through a podiatrist or orthopedic surgeon), especially if there is excessive pronation of the foot. Be very patient. This problem can take a year or more to go away.

Bursitis. Resting for seven to ten days and taking a pain reliever with each meal will help relieve the initial problem **(M4).** For retrocalcaneal bursitis, getting a new shoe or stretching the old shoe so that there is no rubbing against the heel is recommended. Moleskin may be used to relieve pressure from the "pump bump."

Achilles Tendinitis. Stop exercising, apply ice twice daily to the tendon, and take a pain reliever with each meal for a week **(M4).** After that, stretching is the most important treatment. Remember to stretch and hold the stretched position. Do not bounce.

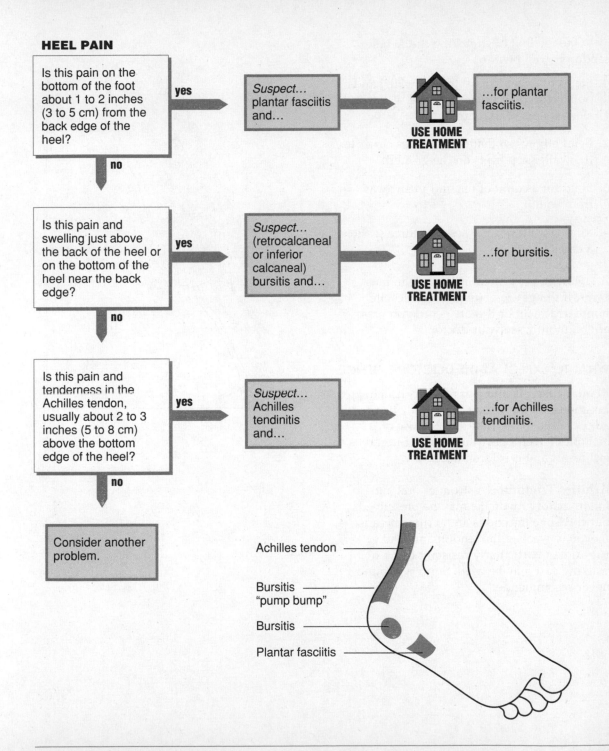

HEEL PAIN

Is this pain on the bottom of the foot about 1 to 2 inches (3 to 5 cm) from the back edge of the heel?

yes → *Suspect...* plantar fasciitis and... → **USE HOME TREATMENT** → ...for plantar fasciitis.

no ↓

Is this pain and swelling just above the back of the heel or on the bottom of the heel near the back edge?

yes → *Suspect...* (retrocalcaneal or inferior calcaneal) bursitis and... → **USE HOME TREATMENT** → ...for bursitis.

no ↓

Is this pain and tenderness in the Achilles tendon, usually about 2 to 3 inches (5 to 8 cm) above the bottom edge of the heel?

yes → *Suspect...* Achilles tendinitis and... → **USE HOME TREATMENT** → ...for Achilles tendinitis.

no ↓

Consider another problem.

Achilles tendon

Bursitis "pump bump"

Bursitis

Plantar fasciitis

One method of stretching the Achilles tendon is wall push-ups:

1. Stand two feet (0.7 m) from a wall, hands outstretched and placed on the wall (see shaded area of diagram).

2. Bend elbows so that body moves closer to the wall. Keep heels on the ground.

3. Hold for a count of ten and push away from wall.

4. Repeat ten times per session, three sessions a day.

Slow improvement is the rule in most cases. If things are getting worse despite home treatment or if there is little progress after a month, see your doctor.

WHAT TO EXPECT AT THE DOCTOR'S OFFICE

Plantar Fasciitis and Bursitis. Cortisone injections, no more than three, may be tried if adjustments to the shoe and the use of orthotics haven't been successful. Surgery is a last resort and is seldom necessary.

Achilles Tendinitis. A stronger oral anti-inflammatory medicine may be prescribed, but cortisone injections aren't done because they may weaken the tendon and lead to rupture. In particularly resistant cases, a walking cast may be tried. Surgery is almost never recommended.

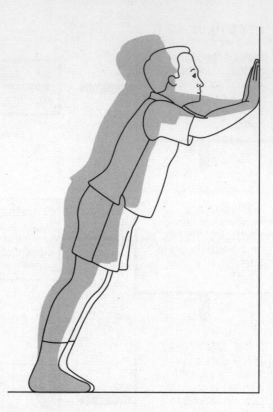

81 Foot Pain

There are a few foot problems that lead to unnecessary pain or an unnecessary visit to the doctor's office.

The nerves that supply sensation to the front portion of your foot and your toes run between the long bones of the foot, the metatarsals. (There is a metatarsal just behind each toe.) Tight-fitting shoes can squeeze the nerves between the bones, and this may cause swelling in a nerve, a Morton's neuroma. The swelling is very sensitive, and pressure can cause intense pain. If pressure is constant, some numbness between the toes may also occur. Morton's neuroma occurs most commonly between the third and fourth metatarsals (between the middle toe and the next toe toward the outside of the foot).

If your big toe points toward the other four toes on that foot, the end of the metatarsal behind the big toe may rub against the shoe. The skin thickens over the end of the metatarsal, and the metatarsal itself may develop a bony spur at that point. This is a bunion, and if it becomes inflamed and sore, it can make life miserable.

Corns and calluses are the results of friction, and friction is usually caused by ill-fitting shoes. Corns appear as lumps of thickened skin that may be hard with a clear core or soft and moist. They are usually found on the tops of toes. Calluses also appear as thickened skin but are less lumpy and are most often found across the ball of the foot.

Plantar warts are caused by a virus and are often found on the ball of the foot. They may be distinguished from calluses by small black dots within the wart, the interruption of normal skin lines, and the inward growth of the wart.

Unaccustomed, heavy use of the feet, as in beginning training for running or basketball, may produce enough stress to produce a crack — stress fracture — in the metatarsals. The fourth metatarsal is most vulnerable to this. A stress fracture usually occurs several weeks into an increased training session or other activity involving strenuous use of the feet. Pain usually comes on gradually.

HOME TREATMENT

Morton's Neuroma. Shoes with adequate room around the ball of the foot are necessary. Acetaminophen three times a day for two to three weeks may also help **(M4).**

Bunion. Place a small sponge or pad between the big and second toe so that the big toe becomes aligned with the other four toes. Moleskin or padding around the bunion may help relieve pressure. Shoes wide enough in the ball of the foot, so that pressure isn't applied, will help. Acetaminophen or other pain medication may be used as above **(M4).**

Corns and Calluses. The first step is to make sure your shoes fit properly. Sandals, if practical, and cushioning socks can be helpful. The "corn plasters" containing 40% salicylic acid available without prescription are effective. Be sure to follow their directions: cut the plaster so that it is smaller than the corn or callus, and be careful in removing the dead skin that the plaster produces. A doctor's visit is rarely needed.

Plantar Warts. Good shoes and corn plasters can be effective for plantar warts also, but the removal of dead skin may be more difficult and time-consuming. For this reason plantar warts end up in the doctor's office more often than corns and calluses. See the doctor if you are making no progress in decreasing the size of the problem. Meanwhile, wear slippers or bath shoes to decrease the likelihood of passing the virus on to someone else.

Metatarsal Stress Fracture. You are going to have to give your foot a rest. Using crutches for a week or so may be helpful in getting pressure off the foot if it is particularly painful. Remember that it may take from six weeks to three months for the fracture to heal completely so that you can return to full activity. A cast doesn't reduce the healing time and may create other problems, so most doctors avoid any kind of cast if at all possible.

WHAT TO EXPECT AT THE DOCTOR'S OFFICE

Morton's Neuroma. Cortisone injections, no more than three, may be tried if relief hasn't been obtained with oral medication and switching shoes. If these fail, the neuroma can be removed surgically. The operation usually leaves a region of skin on the foot permanently numb.

Bunion. If the bunion is particularly inflamed, a cortisone injection can provide temporary relief. If the big toe is so crooked that adjusting the shoes and using moleskin don't help, then surgery to realign the big toe may be needed.

Plantar Warts. The doctor may use cold (liquid nitrogen), heat (electrocoagulation), or surgery to remove a plantar wart. Unfortunately, plantar warts often recur.

Metatarsal Stress Fracture. The doctor has little to offer to relieve metatarsal stress

fractures. You can get crutches at the drug store. Casts are to be avoided if at all possible, and surgery is virtually never done. A walking cast for an incredibly painful foot is about the only thing the doctor can do that you can't.

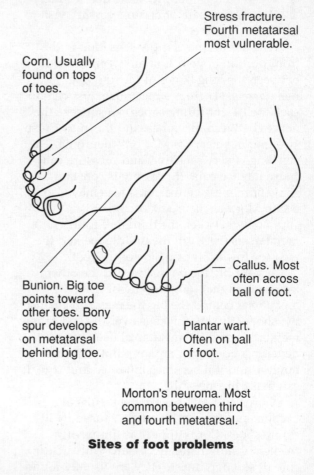

Stress fracture. Fourth metatarsal most vulnerable.

Corn. Usually found on tops of toes.

Callus. Most often across ball of foot.

Bunion. Big toe points toward other toes. Bony spur develops on metatarsal behind big toe.

Plantar wart. Often on ball of foot.

Morton's neuroma. Most common between third and fourth metatarsal.

Sites of foot problems

FOOT PAIN

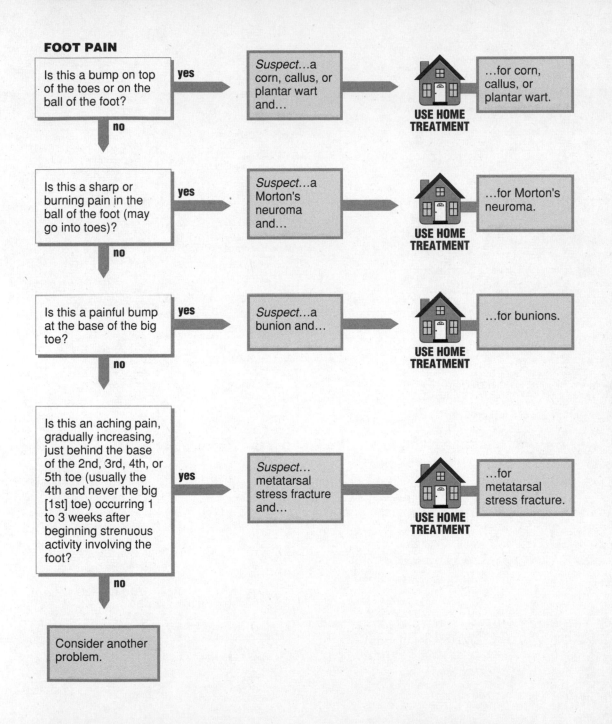

Is this a bump on top of the toes or on the ball of the foot? — **yes** → *Suspect*...a corn, callus, or plantar wart and... → **USE HOME TREATMENT** ...for corn, callus, or plantar wart.

no ↓

Is this a sharp or burning pain in the ball of the foot (may go into toes)? — **yes** → *Suspect*...a Morton's neuroma and... → **USE HOME TREATMENT** ...for Morton's neuroma.

no ↓

Is this a painful bump at the base of the big toe? — **yes** → *Suspect*...a bunion and... → **USE HOME TREATMENT** ...for bunions.

no ↓

Is this an aching pain, gradually increasing, just behind the base of the 2nd, 3rd, 4th, or 5th toe (usually the 4th and never the big [1st] toe) occurring 1 to 3 weeks after beginning strenuous activity involving the foot? — **yes** → *Suspect*... metatarsal stress fracture and... → **USE HOME TREATMENT** ...for metatarsal stress fracture.

no ↓

Consider another problem.

CHAPTER 7

Chest and Abdominal Symptoms

82 Chest Pain

Chest pain is a serious symptom meaning "heart attack" to most people. Serious chest discomfort should usually be evaluated by a doctor.

However, pain can also come from the:

- **Chest wall** — including muscles, ligaments, ribs, and rib cartilage
- **Lungs** and outside covering of the lungs — pleurisy
- **Outside covering of the heart** — pericarditis
- **Gullet**
- **Diaphragm**
- **Spine**
- **Skin**
- **Organs** in the upper part of the abdomen

Often it's difficult even for a doctor to determine the precise origin of pain. There are no absolute rules that determine which pains you may treat at home. The following guidelines usually work and are used by doctors, but there are exceptions.

Signs of Non-heart Pain

A shooting pain lasting a few seconds is common in healthy young people and means nothing. A sensation of a "catch" at the end of a deep breath is also trivial and doesn't need attention. Heart pain almost never occurs in previously healthy men under 30 years of age or women under 40 and is uncommon for the following ten years in each sex.

If you press a finger on the chest at the spot of discomfort and reproduce or aggravate the pain, it's probably chest wall pain. Heart and chest wall pain are rarely present at the same time.

The hyperventilation syndrome **(S101)** is a frequent cause of chest pain, particularly in young people. If you're dizzy or have tingling in your fingers, suspect this syndrome.

Pleurisy gets worse with a deep breath or cough. Heart pain doesn't. When the outside covering of the heart is inflamed (pericarditis), the pain may throb with each heartbeat. Ulcer pain burns with an empty stomach and gets better with food. Gallbladder pain often becomes more intense after a meal. Each of these four conditions, when suspected, should be evaluated by a doctor.

Signs of Heart Pain

Heart pain may be mild, but more often it is intense. Sometimes a feeling of pressure or squeezing on the chest is more prominent than the actual pain. Almost always the pain or discomfort will be just inside the breastbone. It may also be felt in the jaw or down the inner part of either arm. There may be nausea, sweating, dizziness, or shortness of breath. A person experiencing shortness of breath or irregular pulse along with the pain should see a doctor immediately.

Heart pains may occur with exertion and go away with rest. In this case they aren't an actual heart attack but are termed angina pectoris or "angina." Any new pains that might be angina should be brought to the attention of the doctor.

HOME TREATMENT

You should be able to deal effectively with pain arising from the chest wall. Pain

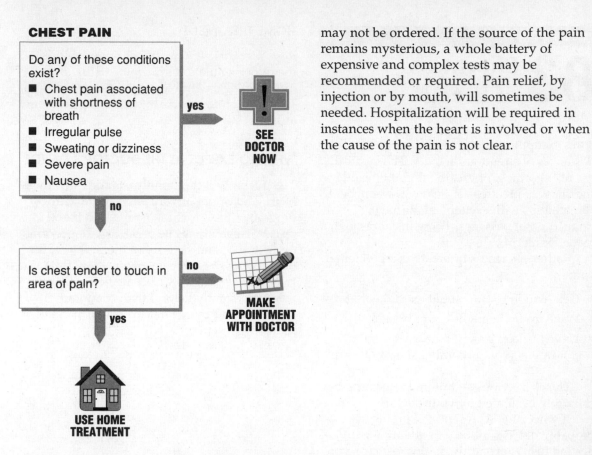

CHEST PAIN

Do any of these conditions exist?

- Chest pain associated with shortness of breath
- Irregular pulse
- Sweating or dizziness
- Severe pain
- Nausea

yes → SEE DOCTOR NOW

no ↓

Is chest tender to touch in area of pain?

no → MAKE APPOINTMENT WITH DOCTOR

yes ↓

USE HOME TREATMENT

may not be ordered. If the source of the pain remains mysterious, a whole battery of expensive and complex tests may be recommended or required. Pain relief, by injection or by mouth, will sometimes be needed. Hospitalization will be required in instances when the heart is involved or when the cause of the pain is not clear.

medicines (acetaminophen, aspirin, ibuprofen, or naproxen **[M4]**), topical treatments (Ben-Gay, Vicks Vaporub, etc.), and general measures such as heat and rest should help. If symptoms persist for more than five days, see a doctor.

WHAT TO EXPECT AT THE DOCTOR'S OFFICE

The doctor will thoroughly examine the chest wall, lungs, and heart and will frequently order an electrocardiogram (EKG) and blood tests. A chest X-ray is usually not helpful and

83 Shortness of Breath

This symptom is normal under circumstances of strenuous activity. The medical use of "shortness of breath" doesn't include shortness of breath after heavy exertion, being "breathless" with excitement, or having clogged nasal passages. These instances aren't cause for alarm.

Rather, shortness of breath is a problem if you:

- Get "winded" after slight exertion or at rest
- Wake up in the night out of breath
- Have to sleep propped up on several pillows to avoid becoming short of breath

This is a serious symptom that should be promptly evaluated by your doctor.

If wheezing is present, the problem is probably not as serious, but attention is needed just as promptly. In this instance, you may have asthma or early emphysema. See Wheezing **(S25).**

The hyperventilation syndrome **(S101)** is a common cause of shortness of breath in previously healthy young people and is almost always the problem if the fingers are tingling. In this syndrome the patient is actually overbreathing but has the sensation of shortness of breath.

A second emotional problem that may include the complaint of difficult breathing is mental depression **(S103).** Deep, sighing respirations are a frequent symptom in depressed individuals.

HOME TREATMENT

Rest, relax, use the treatment described for the hyperventilation syndrome **(S101)** if indicated. If the problem persists, see a doctor. There isn't much you can do for this problem at home.

WHAT TO EXPECT AT THE DOCTOR'S OFFICE

The doctor will thoroughly examine the lungs, heart, and upper airway passages. Electrocardiograms (EKGs), chest X-rays, and blood tests will sometimes be necessary. Depending on the cause and severity of the problem, the doctor may prescribe hospitalization, fluid pills, heart pills, or asthma medicine. Oxygen is less frequently helpful than commonly imagined and can be hazardous for patients with emphysema.

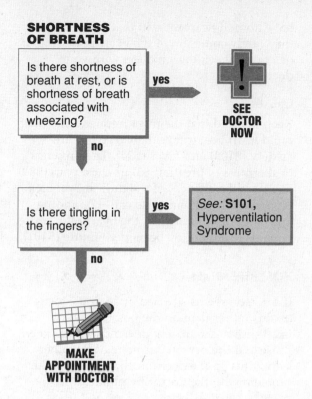

SHORTNESS OF BREATH

Is there shortness of breath at rest, or is shortness of breath associated with wheezing?

yes → **SEE DOCTOR NOW**

no ↓

Is there tingling in the fingers?

yes → *See:* **S101,** Hyperventilation Syndrome

no ↓

MAKE APPOINTMENT WITH DOCTOR

84 Palpitations

Everyone experiences palpitations. A pounding heart seems serious but is usually trivial. It can be brought on by strenuous exercise or intense emotion or can just happen. It is seldom associated with serious disease. Most people who complain of palpitations don't have heart disease but are overly concerned about the possibility of such disease and thus overly sensitive to normal heart actions. Often this anxiety stems from heart disease in parents, other relatives, or friends.

Understanding the Pulse

The pulse can be felt on the inside of the wrist, in the neck, or over the heart itself. On your next checkup, ask the nurse or doctor to check your method of taking pulses. Take your own pulse and those of your family, noting the variation with respiration. There is a normal variation in the pulse with respiration (faster when breathing in, slower when breathing out). Even though the pulse may speed up or slow down, the normal pulse has a regular rhythm.

Occasional extra heart beats, felt as "flip-flops" or thumps in the chest, occur in nearly everyone. The most common time to notice these extra beats is just before going to sleep. They are of no consequence unless they're frequent (more than five per minute) or if they occur in runs of three or more.

Rapid pulses may also mimic palpitations. In adults, a heart rate greater than 120 beats per minute (without exercise) is cause to check with your doctor. Young children may have normal heart rates in that range, but they rarely complain of the heart pounding. If one does, check the situation with your doctor.

Causes

Keep in mind that the most frequent causes of rapid heart beat (other than exercise) are anxiety **(S100)** and fever **(S94)**. The presence of shortness of breath **(S83)** or chest pain **(S82)** increases the chances of a significant problem. Hyperventilation may also cause pounding and chest discomfort, but the heart rate remains less than 120 beats per minute **(S101)**.

HOME TREATMENT

If a person seems stressed or anxious, focus on this rather than on the possibilities of heart disease. If anxiety doesn't seem a likely cause and the person has none of the other symptoms on the decision chart, discuss the problem with the doctor by phone. If it persists, see the doctor.

WHAT TO EXPECT AT THE DOCTOR'S OFFICE

Tell the doctor the exact rate of the pulse and whether or not the rhythm was regular. Usually the symptoms will disappear by the time you see the doctor, so the accuracy of your story becomes crucial. The doctor will examine your heart and lungs. An electrocardiogram (EKG) is unlikely to help if the problem is not present when the test is being done. A chest X-ray is seldom needed.

Don't expect reassurance from a doctor that your heart will be sound for the next month, year, or decade. Your doctor has no crystal ball, nor can he or she perform an annual tune-up or oil change. You, not the doctor, are in charge of preventive maintenance of your heart (see Chapter 1).

PALPITATIONS

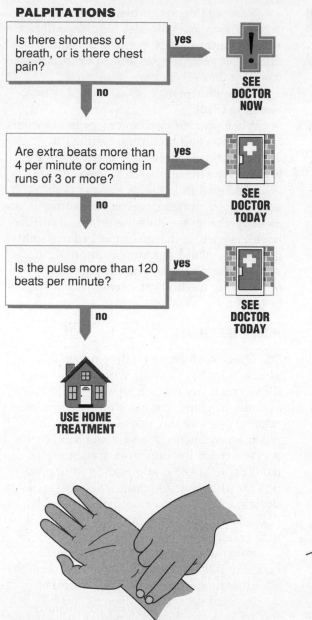

Is there shortness of breath, or is there chest pain? **yes** → **SEE DOCTOR NOW**

no ↓

Are extra beats more than 4 per minute or coming in runs of 3 or more? **yes** → **SEE DOCTOR TODAY**

no ↓

Is the pulse more than 120 beats per minute? **yes** → **SEE DOCTOR TODAY**

no ↓

USE HOME TREATMENT

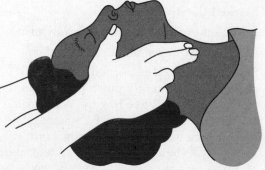

Wrist pulse. This drawing shows the technique for taking a pulse from the inside of the wrist. (*Caution:* Do not use your thumb, which has its own pulse.)

Neck pulse. This drawing shows the technique for taking a pulse from either side of the neck. (*Caution:* Do not take pulse from both sides of the neck at once.)

85 Nausea and Vomiting

Medications are the most common cause of nausea and vomiting in the elderly, whereas viral infections are the most common cause in children and young adults. When viruses are to blame, diarrhea is usually present as well.

Food poisoning is often blamed for stomach problems but is actually one of the less frequent causes of nausea and vomiting. In any event, nausea and vomiting caused by food poisoning are treated the same way as any other kind.

Dangers of Vomiting

Dehydration is the real threat with most vomiting. The speed with which dehydration develops depends on the size of the individual, the frequency of the vomiting, and the presence of diarrhea. Thus, infants with frequent vomiting and diarrhea are at the greatest risk. Signs of dehydration are:

- Marked thirst
- Infrequent urination or dark yellow urine
- Dry mouth or eyes that appear sunken
- Skin that has lost its normal elasticity. To determine this, gently pinch the skin on the stomach using all five fingers. When you release it, it should spring back immediately; compare with another person's skin if necessary. When the skin remains tented up and doesn't spring back normally, the person may be dehydrated.

Bleeding (bloody or black vomitus) or severe abdominal pain also requires a doctor's attention immediately. Some abdominal discomfort accompanies almost every case of vomiting, but severe pain is unusual.

Head injuries may be associated with vomiting (S10).

When pregnancy, diabetes, or medications cause nausea and vomiting, getting the doctor's advice by phone is usually sufficient to determine the approach you should take.

Headache and stiff neck along with vomiting are sometimes seen in meningitis, so an early visit to the doctor's office for further advice is wise. Lethargy or marked irritability in a young child has a similar implication.

Persistent nausea without vomiting is often due to medication, occasionally to ulcers or cancer.

HOME TREATMENT

The objective of home treatment is to take in as much fluid as possible without upsetting the stomach any further. Sip clear fluids such as water or ginger ale. Suck on ice chips if nothing else will stay down. Don't drink much at any one time, and avoid solid foods. As your condition improves, try soups, bouillon, Jell-O, and applesauce. Milk products may help but sometimes aggravate the situation. Work up to a normal diet slowly. Popsicles or iced fruit bars often work well with children.

If vomiting persists for more than 72 hours, or if the person isn't hydrated enough after that time, check with your doctor.

If a medication might be responsible, call the doctor to see if you should keep taking it.

If nausea persists for four weeks, call the doctor.

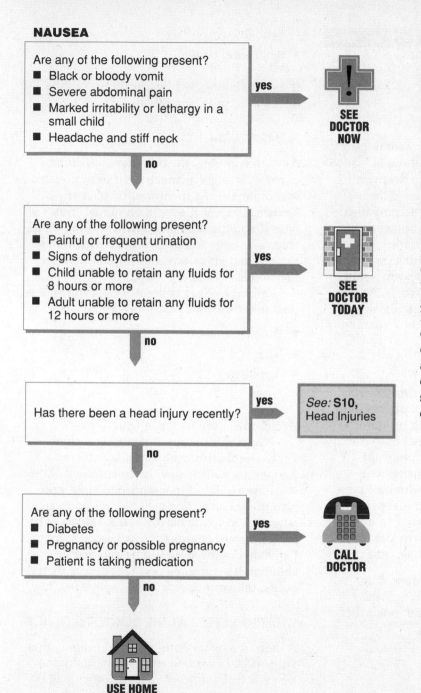

NAUSEA

Are any of the following present?
- Black or bloody vomit
- Severe abdominal pain
- Marked irritability or lethargy in a small child
- Headache and stiff neck

yes → **SEE DOCTOR NOW**

no

Are any of the following present?
- Painful or frequent urination
- Signs of dehydration
- Child unable to retain any fluids for 8 hours or more
- Adult unable to retain any fluids for 12 hours or more

yes → **SEE DOCTOR TODAY**

no

Has there been a head injury recently?

yes → *See:* **S10,** Head Injuries

no

Are any of the following present?
- Diabetes
- Pregnancy or possible pregnancy
- Patient is taking medication

yes → **CALL DOCTOR**

no

USE HOME TREATMENT

WHAT TO EXPECT AT THE DOCTOR'S OFFICE

The history and physical examination will focus on determining the degree of dehydration, as well as the possible causes. Blood tests and a urinalysis may be ordered but aren't always necessary. Ordinary X-rays of the abdomen are usually not very helpful, but special X-ray procedures may be necessary in some cases. If dehydration is severe, intravenous fluids may be given. This may require hospitalization, although it can often be done in the doctor's office. The use of antivomiting drugs is controversial, and they should be used only in severe cases.

86 Diarrhea

Many of the considerations with respect to diarrhea are the same as those in Nausea and Vomiting **(S85).** Viruses are the most common cause, and dehydration is the greatest risk. Diarrhea is often accompanied by nausea and vomiting. Vomiting and fever both increase the risk of dehydration. Bacteria or bacterial toxins (food poisoning) may also produce diarrhea, but antibiotics are rarely helpful and may make things worse. As with viral infections, the major danger in bacterial problems is dehydration, and the treatment is essentially the same.

Dangers of Diarrhea

Black or bloody diarrhea may signal significant bleeding from the stomach or intestines. However, medicines containing bismuth subsalicylate (Pepto-Bismol, etc.) or iron may also turn the stool black. Cramping and intermittent gaslike pains are usual with diarrhea, but severe, steady abdominal pain isn't. Bleeding or severe abdominal pain requires the immediate attention of a doctor.

Many medications may cause diarrhea. Frequent culprits include the following:

- Nonsteroidal anti-inflammatory drugs (NSAIDs), especially meclofenamate (Meclomen) — these are often prescribed for arthritis
- Antibiotics
- Gold compounds
- Blood pressure drugs
- Digitalis
- Anticancer drugs

If you are taking such medications, call the doctor who prescribed them.

HOME TREATMENT

As with vomiting, the objective in treating diarrhea is to get as much fluid in as possible without upsetting the intestinal tract any further. Sip clear fluids; plain old tap water is best. If nothing will stay down, sucking on ice chips is usually tolerated and provides some fluid. Avoid juices or sodas for children. Pedialyte is essential for infants.

Once the patient tolerates clear fluids, it is time to eat the foods that spell BRAT:

- Bananas
- Rice
- Applesauce
- Toast

Avoid milk and fats for several days.

Nonprescription preparations such as Pepto-Bismol (bismuth subsalicylate) or Kaopectate will change the consistency of the stool from a liquid to a semisolid state, and bismuth subsalicylate may reduce stool amount and frequency **(M13).** Adults may try narcotic preparations such as Parepectolin or Parelixir, but these should be avoided in children. If symptoms persist for more than 96 hours, call your doctor.

WHAT TO EXPECT AT THE DOCTOR'S OFFICE

A thorough history and physical examination with special attention to assessing dehydration will be completed. The abdomen will be examined. Frequently the stools will be

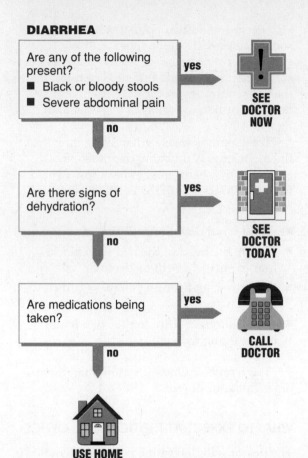

DIARRHEA

Are any of the following present?
- Black or bloody stools
- Severe abdominal pain

yes → **SEE DOCTOR NOW**

no ↓

Are there signs of dehydration?

yes → **SEE DOCTOR TODAY**

no ↓

Are medications being taken?

yes → **CALL DOCTOR**

no ↓

USE HOME TREATMENT

with vomiting, severe dehydration will require intravenous fluids. This may be taken care of in the doctor's office or may require hospitalization.

examined under the microscope, and occasionally a culture will be taken. A urine specimen may be examined to assist in assessing dehydration. An antibiotic may be prescribed. A narcotic-like preparation (such as Lomotil) may also be prescribed for adults to decrease the frequency of stools. Chronic diarrhea may require more extensive evaluation of the stools, blood tests, and often X-ray examinations of the intestinal tract. As

87 Heartburn

Heartburn is irritation of the stomach or the esophagus, the tube that leads from the mouth to the stomach. The stomach lining is usually protected from the effects of its own acid. Certain factors, however, such as smoking, caffeine, aspirin, and stress, cause this protection to be impaired. The esophagus is not protected against acid, and a backflow of acid from the stomach into the esophagus causes irritation.

Ulcers of the stomach or the upper bowel (duodenum) may also cause pain. Treatment for ulcers is the same as for uncomplicated heartburn, provided that pain isn't severe and there's no evidence of bleeding. Long-lasting stomach ulcers may demand antibiotic treatment (see Abdominal Pain, **S88**).

Vomiting black, "coffee ground" material or bright red blood means giving the doctor a call. Black stools, rather like tar, have the same significance; however, iron supplements and bismuth subsalicylate (Pepto-Bismol) will also cause black stools.

Heartburn pain ordinarily doesn't go through to the back, and such pain may signal involvement of the pancreas or a severe ulcer.

HOME TREATMENT

Avoid substances that aggravate the problem. The most common irritants are coffee, tea, alcohol, aspirin, ibuprofen, and naproxen. The contributing effect of smoking or stress must be considered in every sufferer.

Relief is often obtained by using nonabsorbable antacids (Maalox, Mylanta, Gelusil, etc.) every one to two hours **(M5).** Baking soda may provide quick relief but isn't suitable for repeated use. Nonfat milk may be substituted for antacid but adds calories. If the pain continues, you can try the new nonprescription formulas of Tagamet and Pepcid AC.

If the pain is worse when lying down, the esophagus is probably the problem. Measures that help prevent backflow of acid from the stomach into the esophagus should be employed:

- Avoid lying down or reclining after eating.
- Elevate the head of the bed with blocks four to six inches (10 to 15 cm).
- Don't wear tight-fitting clothes (girdles, tight jeans).
- Avoid eating or drinking for two hours before going to bed.

If the problem lasts for more than three days, call your doctor.

WHAT TO EXPECT AT THE DOCTOR'S OFFICE

The doctor will determine if the problem is due to stomach acid, a peptic acid syndrome. If so, treatment will be similar to that outlined above. Medications to reduce secretion of acid may be prescribed. X-rays of the esophagus and stomach (upper GI) may be done, after the patient has swallowed barium, to determine the presence of ulcers and to note if backflow of acid from the stomach into the esophagus, or hiatal hernia, is present. Because the treatment for any acid syndrome is essentially the same, an X-ray is usually not done on the first visit. Any indication of bleeding will require a more vigorous approach to therapy.

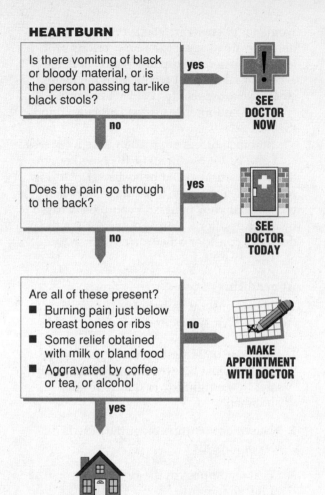

HEARTBURN

Is there vomiting of black or bloody material, or is the person passing tar-like black stools?

yes → **SEE DOCTOR NOW**

no ↓

Does the pain go through to the back?

yes → **SEE DOCTOR TODAY**

no ↓

Are all of these present?
- Burning pain just below breast bones or ribs
- Some relief obtained with milk or bland food
- Aggravated by coffee or tea, or alcohol

no → **MAKE APPOINTMENT WITH DOCTOR**

yes ↓

USE HOME TREATMENT

88 Abdominal Pain

Abdominal pain can be a sign of a serious condition. Fortunately, minor causes are much more frequent. Location of the pain can help in suggesting the cause.

- **Appendix pain** usually occurs in the right lower quarter of the abdomen
- **Diverticulitis** usually hurts in the left lower quarter of the abdomen
- **Kidney pain,** the back
- **Gallbladder,** the right upper quarter
- **Stomach,** the upper abdomen
- **Bladder** or female organs, the lower areas

Exceptions to these rules do occur.

Pain from hollow organs — such as the bowel or gallbladder — tends to be intermittent and resembles gas pains or colic. Pain from solid organs — kidneys, spleen, liver — tends to be more constant. Stomach ulcers tend to create burning pain in the upper abdomen which usually gets better after a meal or a dose of antacid. There are exceptions to these rules as well.

When to See a Doctor

If the pain is very severe or if bleeding from the bowel occurs, see a doctor. Similarly, if there has been a significant recent abdominal injury, see the doctor — a ruptured spleen or other major problem is possible.

Pain during pregnancy is potentially serious and must be evaluated. An "ectopic pregnancy" — in the fallopian tube rather than in the uterus — can occur before a woman is even aware she is pregnant. Pain in only one area suggests a more serious problem than generalized pain; again, there are exceptions. Pain that recurs with the menstrual cycle, especially premenstrually, is typical of endometriosis; see Difficult Periods **(S108).**

Stomach ulcers are made worse by excess acid and better by antacids. It's now known that a bacterium called helicobacter pylori is responsible for many, if not most, stomach ulcers. So if your pain isn't completely eased by antacids after a couple of weeks, see the doctor to consider other forms of therapy.

Appendicitis

The most constant signal of appendicitis is the *order* in which symptoms occur:

1. Pain — usually first around the belly button or just below the breast bone; only later in the right lower quarter of the abdomen

2. Nausea or vomiting or, at the very least, loss of appetite

3. Local tenderness in the right lower quarter of the abdomen

4. Fever ranging from 100°F to 102°F (38°C to 39°C)

The following signs make appendicitis unlikely:

- Fever precedes or is present at the time of initial pain
- There's *no* fever or a *high* fever, greater than 102°F (39°C), in the first 24 hours
- Vomiting accompanies or precedes the first bout of pain

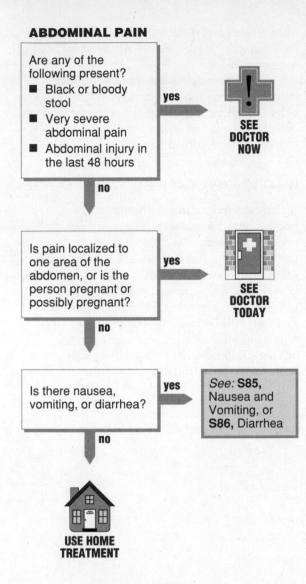

ABDOMINAL PAIN

Are any of the following present?
- Black or bloody stool
- Very severe abdominal pain
- Abdominal injury in the last 48 hours

yes → **SEE DOCTOR NOW**

no ↓

Is pain localized to one area of the abdomen, or is the person pregnant or possibly pregnant?

yes → **SEE DOCTOR TODAY**

no ↓

Is there nausea, vomiting, or diarrhea?

yes → *See:* **S85,** Nausea and Vomiting, or **S86,** Diarrhea

no ↓

USE HOME TREATMENT

HOME TREATMENT

Sip water or other clear fluids, but avoid solid foods. A bowel movement, passage of gas through the rectum, or a good belch may give relief — don't hold back. A warm bath helps some patients.

Antacid treatment for heartburn, indigestion, or suspected stomach ulcer should usually begin with 500 mg of calcium carbonate (Tums, etc.) every four hours **(M5).** You may also use liquid antacids and periodic drinks of nonfat milk. If antacids fail, try one of the two new nonprescription medications that help stop stomach acid secretion (Tagamet and Pepcid AC). And if these don't work either, a visit to the doctor is in order.

The key to home treatment is periodic reevaluation; any persistent pain should be treated at the emergency room or the doctor's office. Home treatment should be reserved for mild pains that resolve within 24 hours or are clearly identifiable as stomach flu, heartburn, or other minor problems.

WHAT TO EXPECT AT THE DOCTOR'S OFFICE

The doctor will give a thorough examination, particularly of the abdomen. Usually a white blood cell count and urinalysis, and often other laboratory tests, will be recommended. X-rays are generally not important for pain of short duration but are sometimes needed. Observation in the hospital may be required. If the initial evaluation is negative but pain persists, reevaluation is necessary.

Doctors have achieved impressive results treating stomach ulcers with antibacterial agents to kill the helicobacter pylori. If your doctor diagnoses a stomach ulcer, ask about such treatment.

89 Constipation

Many people are preoccupied with constipation. Concern about the shape of the stool, its consistency, its color, and the frequency of bowel movements is often reported to doctors. Such complaints are medically trivial. Only rarely (and then usually in older patients) does a change in bowel habits signal a serious problem.

Weight loss and thin, pencil-like stools suggest a tumor of the lower bowel.

Abdominal pain and a swollen abdomen suggest a possible bowel obstruction.

HOME TREATMENT

We like to encourage a healthy diet for the bowel, followed by a healthy lack of interest in the details of the stool-elimination process. The diet should contain fresh fruits and vegetables for their natural laxative action and adequate fiber residue. Fiber is present in brans, celery, and whole-grain breads and is absent from foods that have been overly processed. Fiber draws water into the stool and adds bulk; thus, it decreases the transit time from mouth to bowel movement and softens the stool.

Bowel movements may occur three times daily or once every three days and still be normal. The stools may change in color, texture, consistency, or bulk without need for concern. They may be regular or irregular. Don't worry about them unless there is a major deviation.

If you need to use laxatives, we prefer a bulk laxative such as Metamucil **(M12).** Milk of magnesia is satisfactory, but it and stronger traditional laxatives should not be used over a long period.

For an acute problem, an enema may help. Fleet's enemas are handy and disposable. If such remedies are needed more than occasionally, ask your doctor about the problem on your next routine visit.

WHAT TO EXPECT AT THE DOCTOR'S OFFICE

If you have had a major change in bowel habits, expect a rectal examination and, usually, inspection of the lower bowel through a long (sometimes cold) metal tube called a sigmoidoscope. An X-ray of the lower bowel (using a barium enema) is often needed. These procedures are generally safe and only mildly uncomfortable. If you have only a minor problem, you may receive advice similar to that under Home Treatment, without examination or procedures.

CONSTIPATION

Is constipation associated with the following?

- Very thin, pencil-like stools
- Abdominal pain and bloating
- Weight loss

yes →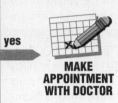

MAKE APPOINTMENT WITH DOCTOR

no ↓

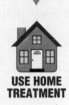

USE HOME TREATMENT

High-fiber diets not only prevent constipation but they also may prevent diverticulosis, hemorrhoids, intestinal polyps, even colon cancer. For more on fiber, see pages 11–12.

90 Rectal Problems

Seldom is a rectal problem major, but the discomfort it can cause may materially interfere with the quality of life. Unlike most other medical problems, rectal pain doesn't yield the dividend of a good topic for social conversation.

Hemorrhoids, or "piles," are the most common rectal problem. There is a network of veins around the anus, and they tend to enlarge with age, particularly in individuals who sit a great deal during the day. Straining to have a bowel movement and passing hard, compacted stools tend to irritate these veins, and they may become inflamed, tender, or clogged. The veins themselves are the "hemorrhoids." They may be outside the anal opening and visible, or they may be inside and invisible. Pain and inflammation usually disappear within a few days or a few weeks, but this interval can be extremely uncomfortable. After healing, a small flap, or "tag," of vein and scar tissue often remains.

Bleeding from the digestive tract should be taken seriously. We aren't talking here about the bright red, relatively light bleeding that originates from the hemorrhoids but about blood from higher in the digestive tract. This blood will be burgundy or black. Iron supplements or bismuth subsalicylate (Pepto-Bismol) may also turn the stool black. Blood from hemorrhoids may be on the outside of the stool but won't be mixed into the stool substance and frequently will be seen on the toilet paper after wiping. Such bleeding from hemorrhoids isn't medically significant unless it persists for several weeks.

Sometimes a child will suddenly awake in the early evening with rectal pain. This almost always means pinworms. Though these small worms are seldom seen, they're quite common. They live in the rectum, and the female emerges at night and secretes a sticky and irritating substance around the anus into which she lays her eggs. Occasionally the worms move into the vagina, causing pain and itching in that area. Although the Food and Drug Administration has approved the nonprescription sale of a drug effective against pinworms, the manufacturer refuses to sell it without a prescription. You'll have to call a doctor for a prescription even if you're sure the problem is pinworms.

If rectal pain persists more than a week, consult the doctor. In such cases, a crack in the wall of the rectum may have developed, or an infection or other problem may be present.

HOME TREATMENT

Soften the stool by including more fresh fruits and fiber (bran, celery, whole-grain bread) in the diet, or by using fiber bulk laxatives **(M12).** Keep the area clean. Use the shower as an alternative to rubbing with toilet paper.

After gently drying the painful area, apply zinc oxide paste or powder **(M16).** This will protect against further irritation. The various proprietary hemorrhoid preparations are less satisfactory. We prefer not to use compounds with a local anesthetic agent because these compounds may sensitize and irritate the area and may prolong healing. Such compounds have "-caine" in the brand name or in the list of ingredients.

Internal hemorrhoids sometimes may be helped by using a soothing suppository in addition to stool-softening measures. If relief isn't complete within a week, see the doctor.

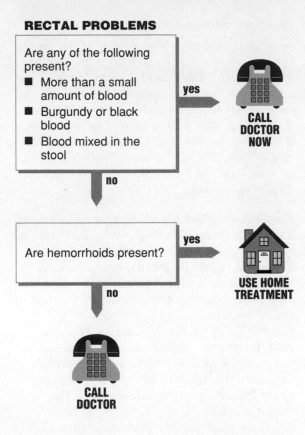

RECTAL PROBLEMS

Are any of the following present?
- More than a small amount of blood
- Burgundy or black blood
- Blood mixed in the stool

yes → CALL DOCTOR NOW

no ↓

Are hemorrhoids present?

yes → USE HOME TREATMENT

no ↓

CALL DOCTOR

Even if the problem resolves quickly, mention it to your doctor on your next visit.

WHAT TO EXPECT AT THE DOCTOR'S OFFICE

The doctor will examine the anus and rectum. If a clot has formed in a hemorrhoid, the vein may be lanced and the clot removed. Major hemorrhoid surgery is seldom required and should be reserved for the most persistent problems. Usually, advice such as that given in Home Treatment will be given.

91 Incontinence

Incontinence is the inability to hold feces or urine. We're all born incontinent, and as we grow older there's a tendency for this problem to return. Incontinence is a complicated issue because there are many causes and many treatments. It isn't a hopeless condition. The vast majority of people can be greatly helped.

Effects of Aging

In women, the uterus and pelvic floor sag with aging. This changes the angle of the urethra (the tube leading from the bladder) and disposes it to leak urine.

In men, harmless enlargement of the prostate gland tends to block passage of urine until finally the bladder must overflow.

With age, there are sometimes sudden contractions of the bladder muscles. This results in increased pressures at unexpected times. There can be decreased sensitivity to the presence of a full bladder, and once the condition is realized, it can be difficult to get to the toilet in time.

Causes of Incontinence

Drugs such as diuretics ("water pills") can cause major surges in urine flow. Other drugs, such as tranquilizers, sedatives, anticholinergics, pain pills, and antidepressants, can block the normal voiding mechanisms; this results in retention of urine and then incontinence.

Stones in the bladder can predispose a person to infection. Infections of the urinary tract can cause an urgency for which there is no time to react.

Fecal Incontinence

Fecal incontinence is usually due to the presence of hard or impacted stool in the rectum. This results in diarrhea and incontinence around the impacted stool. Problems with fecal incontinence should be reported to your doctor. This isn't a complaint to be shy about. If you let it persist, it will begin to affect every part of your life and even your self-image.

HOME TREATMENT

For fecal incontinence, it's important that your diet contain adequate fiber, water, and bulk. A soft stool passed twice a week is normal, but you should consider a hard, impacted stool (even if passed in small amounts twice daily) a problem. Fiber — as in whole grains, bran, celery, fresh fruits, and vegetables — is helpful. Preparations (Metamucil, Fiberall, etc.) can be used to add bulk (M12). Because the presence of impacted feces in the rectum can make you feel bad all over, it is important to get this taken care of immediately. The doctor will help.

Performance of the bladder can often be improved by exercising the muscles that control the urinary outlet. Practice stopping urination in midstream and then starting again. This exercise is often difficult, especially for women, but it will build stronger sphincter muscles. Deliberately contracting the muscles around your anus and urinary tract for a second or two, then relaxing, then repeating, will build strength in these muscles and help tighten the pelvic floor. Many doctors recommend that these exercises be done up to 100 times daily.

Double voiding techniques can be helpful. Here, you empty the bladder as much as you can, wait a minute or so and then empty it again. It is surprising how much additional

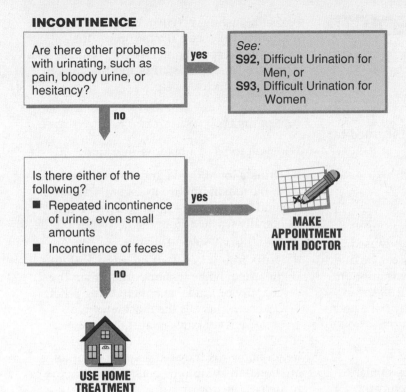

INCONTINENCE

Are there other problems with urinating, such as pain, bloody urine, or hesitancy?

yes → *See:*
S92, Difficult Urination for Men, or
S93, Difficult Urination for Women

no ↓

Is there either of the following?
- Repeated incontinence of urine, even small amounts
- Incontinence of feces

yes → **MAKE APPOINTMENT WITH DOCTOR**

no ↓

USE HOME TREATMENT

---

urine will sometimes be present. "Bladder drill" consists of urinating at fixed intervals, perhaps every four hours, during the day, whether the sensation of urgency is present or not; this can help. If you have trouble getting to the toilet on time, consider keeping a urine receptacle close at hand.

Always suspect that drugs that you're taking might be aggravating the problem; be sure to bring this possibility to the attention of your doctor.

WHAT TO EXPECT AT THE DOCTOR'S OFFICE

The doctor will perform a complete examination, with emphasis on the abdomen, rectum, and the urinary opening. Urinalysis will usually be performed. If there are abnormalities, cystoscopy (inspection of the inside of the bladder) may be performed.

The gynecologist and the urologist are the specialists most familiar with these problems. If simple treatments don't work, a variety of specialized tests may pinpoint the problem.

In women, the doctor will sometimes prescribe a local estrogen cream, which can be surprisingly effective. Uterine or pelvic suspension operations are sometimes needed.

Men may choose prostatectomy, drugs, or simple "watchful waiting." Internal or external tubes (catheters) are sometimes used.

---

92 Difficult Urination for Men

Infections of the bladder may be signaled by:

- Pain or burning upon urination
- Frequent, urgent urination
- Blood in the urine

These symptoms aren't always caused by infection due to bacteria. They can be due to a viral infection or excessive consumption of caffeine-containing beverages (coffee, tea, and some soft drinks), or they may have no known cause and may be blamed on "nerves."

Infection of the prostate gland — *prostatitis* — may cause symptoms similar to those of a bladder infection. Difficulty in starting urination, dribbling, or decreased force of the urinary stream — symptoms of *prostatism* — may also be present. However, prostatism is much more likely to be due to benign prostatic hypertrophy (BPH) than prostatitis. Some degree of BPH is universal in elderly men. Prostatic cancer may also cause prostatism.

Vomiting, back pain, or teeth-chattering, body-shaking chills aren't typical of bladder or prostate infections and suggest kidney infection. This requires a more vigorous treatment and follow-up. A history of kidney disease (infections, inflammations, and kidney stones) also alters the treatment.

Most, if not all, bacterial bladder infections will respond to home treatment. Nevertheless, using antibiotics has become standard medical practice. Given this and the difficulty of distinguishing between bladder infection and prostatitis, see a doctor unless the symptoms respond quickly and completely to home treatment. Prostatitis and prostatism require the doctor's help.

HOME TREATMENT

For symptoms of a bladder infection:

- Drink a lot of fluids. Increase fluid intake to the maximum (up to several gallons of fluid in the first 24 hours). Bacteria are literally washed from the body during the resulting copious urination.
- Drink fruit juices. Putting more acid into the urine, while less important than the quantity of fluids, may help bring relief. Cranberry juice is the most effective because it contains a natural antibiotic.

Begin home treatment as soon as symptoms are noted. If symptoms persist for 24 hours or recur, see the doctor.

WHAT TO EXPECT AT THE DOCTOR'S OFFICE

A urinalysis and culture should be performed. The back and abdomen are usually examined. With symptoms of prostatitis or prostatism, a rectal examination (so that the prostate can be felt) should be expected. With pre-existing kidney disease or symptoms of kidney infection, a more detailed history and physical as well as extra laboratory studies may be needed.

If bacterial infection is determined, the doctor will prescribe an antibiotic. A surgical procedure — there are several — may be chosen to relieve prostatism, but drugs or simple "watchful waiting" may be best for you.

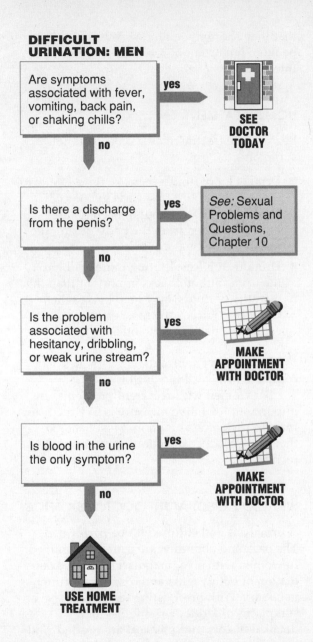

DIFFICULT URINATION: MEN

Are symptoms associated with fever, vomiting, back pain, or shaking chills?

yes → **SEE DOCTOR TODAY**

no ↓

Is there a discharge from the penis?

yes → *See:* Sexual Problems and Questions, Chapter 10

no ↓

Is the problem associated with hesitancy, dribbling, or weak urine stream?

yes → **MAKE APPOINTMENT WITH DOCTOR**

no ↓

Is blood in the urine the only symptom?

yes → **MAKE APPOINTMENT WITH DOCTOR**

no ↓

USE HOME TREATMENT

93 Difficult Urination for Women

The best-known symptoms of bladder infection are:

- Pain or burning on urination
- Frequent, urgent urination
- Blood in the urine

These symptoms aren't always caused by infection due to bacteria. They can be due to a viral infection, excessive use of caffeine-containing beverages (coffee, tea, and cola drinks), bladder spasm, or they can have no known cause (i.e., "nerves").

Bladder infection is far more common in women than it is in men. The female urethra, the tube leading from the bladder to the outside of the body, is only about one-half inch (1 cm) long — a short distance for bacteria to travel to reach the bladder. Sometimes bladder infection is related to sexual activity; hence, "honeymoon cystitis" has become a well-known medical syndrome.

Bladder infections are common during pregnancy. Treatment may be more difficult and must take the pregnancy into account.

Vomiting, back pain, or teeth-chattering, body-shaking chills aren't typical of bladder infections but suggest kidney infection. This requires more vigorous treatment and follow-up. A history of kidney disease (infections, inflammations, and kidney stones) also alters the treatment.

Most, if not all, bacterial bladder infections will respond to home treatment alone. Nevertheless, using antibiotics has become standard medical practice, and it is possible that they shorten the illness. Antibiotics may be more important in recurrent bladder infections.

HOME TREATMENT

Begin home treatment as soon as you note symptoms.

- Drink a lot of fluids. Increase fluid intake to the maximum (up to several gallons of fluid in the first 24 hours). Bacteria are literally washed from the body during the resulting copious urination.
- Drink fruit juices. Putting more acid into the urine, although less important than the quantity of fluids, may help bring relief. Cranberry juice is the most effective, as it contains a natural antibiotic.

If relief isn't substantial in 24 hours and complete in 48, call the doctor.

For women with recurrent problems, an important preventive measure is to wipe from front to back after urination. Most bacteria that cause bladder infections come from the rectum.

WHAT TO EXPECT AT THE DOCTOR'S OFFICE

A urinalysis and culture will be performed. The back and abdomen are usually examined. In women with a vaginal discharge, an examination of both vagina and discharge is often necessary. With pre-existing kidney disease or symptoms of kidney infection, a more detailed history and physical are needed, and extra laboratory studies may be necessary. If tests prove there is a urinary tract infection, the doctor will prescribe an antibiotic.

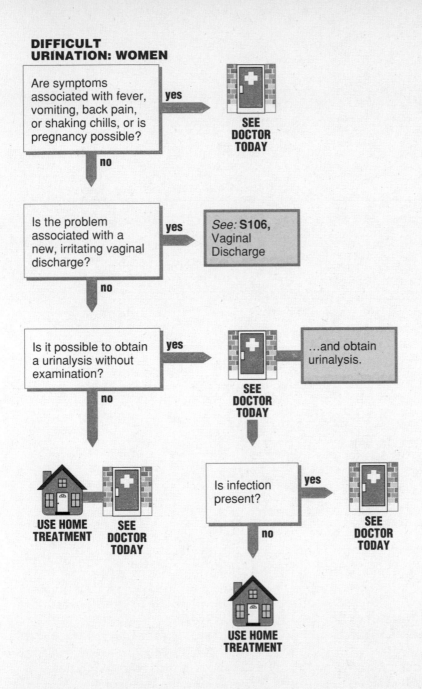

DIFFICULT URINATION: WOMEN

Are symptoms associated with fever, vomiting, back pain, or shaking chills, or is pregnancy possible?

yes → SEE DOCTOR TODAY

no ↓

Is the problem associated with a new, irritating vaginal discharge?

yes → *See:* **S106,** Vaginal Discharge

no ↓

Is it possible to obtain a urinalysis without examination?

yes → SEE DOCTOR TODAY ...and obtain urinalysis.

no ↓

USE HOME TREATMENT   SEE DOCTOR TODAY

Is infection present?

yes → SEE DOCTOR TODAY

no ↓

USE HOME TREATMENT

CHAPTER 8

Generalized Problems

94 Fever

Many people, including doctors, speak of fever and illness as if they were one and the same. Surprisingly, an elevated temperature is not necessarily a sign of illness. Normal body temperature varies from individual to individual. If we measured the body temperatures of a large number of healthy people while they were resting, we would find a difference of 1.5°F (about 1°C) between the lowest and highest temperatures. We are all individuals, and there is nothing absolute about a 98.6°F (37°C) temperature.

Normal body temperature varies greatly during the day. Temperature is generally lowest in the morning upon awakening. Food, excess clothing, excitement, and anxiety can all elevate body temperature. Vigorous exercise can raise body temperature to as much as 103°F (39.5°C). Other mechanisms also influence body temperature. Hormones, for example, account for a monthly variation of body temperature in ovulating women. Normal temperature is 1 to 1.5°F (1°C) higher in the second half of the menstrual cycle. In general, children have higher body temperatures than adults and seem to have greater daily variation because of their greater levels of excitement and activity.

Having said all this, we know you would like a rule to follow. Take the patient's temperature by mouth **(M3)** and:

- If the patient's temperature is 99 to 100°F (38°C), start thinking about the possibility of fever.
- If it is 100°F (38°C) or above, it's a fever.

Causes of Fever

The most common causes for persistent fevers are viral and bacterial infections, such as colds, sore throats, earaches, diarrhea, urinary infections, roseola, chicken pox, mumps, measles, and occasionally pneumonia, appendicitis, and meningitis.

The height of the temperature isn't a reliable measurement of how serious the underlying infection is. A viral infection can result in a temperature below normal, normal, or as high as 105°F (40.5°C).

Febrile Seizures (Fever Fits)

The danger of an extremely high temperature is the possibility that the fever will cause a seizure, also termed a convulsion, fit, or "falling-out spell." During a seizure, the brain, which normally transmits electrical impulses at a fairly regular rhythm, begins misfiring. This causes involuntary muscular responses. The first sign may be a stiffening of the entire body. Children may have rhythmic beating of

Starve a fever? This folk remedy probably originated from people who noticed the relationship between food and temperature elevation. However, there are many reasons why people should eat during a fever. Calories are burned faster by a person whose body temperature is high, so the person needs to take in more calories. More important, there is an increased demand for fluid. Liquids should never be withheld from a feverish person. If a person won't eat because of the discomfort caused by fever, it is still essential that he or she drink fluids.

a single hand or foot, or any combination of the hands and feet. The eyes may roll back and the head may jerk. Urine and feces may pass involuntarily.

All of us are capable of "seizing" if our body temperature becomes too high. Febrile seizures are relatively common in normal, healthy children; about 3 to 5% will experience a febrile seizure. Nevertheless, these seizures must be given due consideration.

Febrile seizures occur most often in children between the ages of six months and four years. Illnesses that cause rapid elevations to high temperatures, such as roseola, have been frequently associated with febrile seizure. Rarely, a seizure is the first sign of a serious underlying problem such as meningitis.

Most seizures last only one to five minutes. There is very little evidence that such a short seizure is of any long-term consequence. On the other hand, prolonged seizures of more than 30 minutes are often a sign of a more serious underlying problem. Fewer than half of all children who have a short febrile seizure will ever experience a second, and fewer than half who experience a second will ever have a third.

Although a "seizing" child is a terrifying sight to a parent, the dangers to the child during a seizure are small. The following commonsense rules should be followed during a seizure:

- Protect your child's head from hitting anything hard. Place the child on a bed.

- Do not force an object into the child's mouth to prevent biting of the tongue. Considerable damage can be done by this. Surprisingly, cut tongues are uncommon, and they usually heal quickly.

- Make sure the child's breathing passage is open. Forcing a stick into your child's

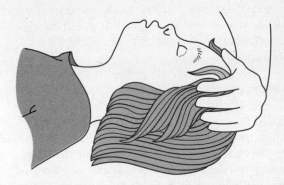

Open airway. If a child is having a febrile seizure, pull the head back slightly. Do not force anything into the mouth.

mouth doesn't ensure an open airway. To facilitate breathing, (1) clear the nose and mouth of vomit or other material, and (2) pull the head backward slightly to hyperextend the neck. Artificial respiration is almost never necessary. If it is, hyperextend the neck and breathe ten times each minute through the child's nose while keeping the mouth covered (or through the child's mouth while keeping the nose pinched closed with your fingers). Only blow air in; the child will blow the air out naturally. These techniques are best learned in demonstrations.

- Begin fever reduction (discussed below) and seek medical attention immediately. Do *not* give medicine by mouth to a seizing or unconscious patient. Fortunately, once the seizure has stopped, the child is usually temporarily resistant to a second seizure. However, because there are exceptions to this rule, prompt medical attention is important.

After a seizure has subsided, some children may be very groggy and have no memory of what happened. Others may show signs of extreme weakness and even paralysis of an arm or leg. This paralysis is almost always temporary but must be carefully evaluated.

The doctor will do a careful study to determine the cause of a febrile seizure. For the first febrile seizure, this will usually include a spinal tap (lumbar puncture) and fluid analysis to make certain that the seizure wasn't caused by meningitis. After the fever ends, the doctor will stress the importance of controlling the fever for the next few days and will often place the child on medications to prevent further seizures.

Chills

A chill is another symptom of a fever. The feeling of being hot or cold is maintained by a complex system of nerve receptors in our skin and in a part of our brain known as the hypothalamus. This system is sensitive to the difference between body temperature and the temperature outside the body. We sense cold both when the temperature of what surrounds our bodies is lowered and when our body temperature is raised.

The body responds to a chill in a similar manner as it would to a drop in the outside temperature. All of the normal systems that increase heat production, such as shivering, become active.

Because eating is a means of increasing heat production, hunger may be experienced. The body tries to conserve heat by causing constriction of the blood vessels near the skin. Children will sometimes curl up in a ball to conserve heat. Goose bumps are intended to raise the hairs on our body to form a layer of insulation. Don't bundle up the person in blankets if he or she shivers or becomes chilled; this will only cause the fever to go

higher. Use home treatment as described below.

HOME TREATMENT

There are two ways to reduce a fever: sponging and medication. If fever remains above 103°F (39.5°C) after an hour or so of home treatment, call the doctor.

Sponging

Evaporation has a cooling effect on the skin and hence on the body temperature. Evaporation can be enhanced by sponging the skin with water. Although alcohol evaporates more rapidly, it is somewhat uncomfortable and the vapors can be dangerous. Generally, sponging with tepid water (water that is comfortable to the touch) will be sufficient. Heat is also lost when a person is sponged while sitting in a tub of water about 70°F (21°C). Although cold water will work somewhat faster, the discomfort makes this less desirable. A child will tolerate cold bathing and sponging for a much shorter period. During the bath, wet the patient's hair as well. After drying, keep the patient in a cool room, wearing little or no clothing.

Medication

Remember that fever is the body's natural way of responding to a variety of conditions. A fever may signify that the patient's immune system is responding well to an infection. Nonetheless, fevers are uncomfortable. Controlling a fever that is high enough to interfere with eating, drinking, sleeping, or other important activities will make the person feel better. In short, if he or she is *suffering* from the fever, treat it. If the fever is

Heat exhaustion is a problem caused by being in a warm (and often humid) climate, usually without drinking enough water or other fluids. A person with heat exhaustion may complain of weakness, headache, or dizziness but can respond to questions and feels hot and thirsty. There may be some nausea or even vomiting, but this isn't severe. The person's skin is sweaty. Body temperature may be elevated slightly, but it isn't above 101°F (38.5°C). In other words, the person is ill from the heat and lack of fluid, but the body is still trying to lower its temperature by sweating, and the person is aware of the need to cool off. Heat exhaustion can be treated successfully by moving into a cool environment and drinking a lot of water.

If a person with heat exhaustion doesn't do this, the condition can become **heat stroke.** This is an emergency that requires *immediate medical care,* including rapid cooling of the body by ice baths, ice packs on wet sheets, or any other means possible. Heat stroke occurs when the body loses its battle with heat exhaustion. Sweating stops and body temperature rises rapidly. The victim no longer complains of heat or thirst and may be confused and delirious; seizures and loss of consciousness may follow. By definition, anyone with a rectal temperature above 105°F (40.5°C) has heat stroke and must be treated immediately; damage to the brain and other organs becomes almost certain if the temperature doesn't fall. When heat stroke occurs, cool the person's body immediately and get medical help. Treatment can be very effective. For example, one patient brought to an emergency room with a temperature of 116°F (46.5°C) survived and had no aftereffects!

mild and the patient shows no effects, it may be unnecessary to treat.

The temperature of a conscious, alert person can be controlled with several over-the-counter medications. We recommend acetaminophen. Aspirin, ibuprofen, and naproxen are also effective and usually safe when used correctly. For more about all these medications and the correct dosages for different ages, see **M4.**

Here are some important cautions:

- Never give medication by mouth to a person who is seizing or unconscious. A child who has just had a febrile seizure and must be treated can be given an aspirin suppository instead.

- Children and teenagers who take aspirin when they have chicken pox or the flu stand a higher chance of later developing Reye's syndrome, a rare but serious problem of the brain and liver. Because it's hard to recognize chicken pox and flu in their early stages, we recommend that parents give children and teenagers acetaminophen.

- Never give medication prescribed for one person to another, especially to a child. Some fever medications come in different strengths, available with and without a prescription; don't mix them up.

WHAT TO EXPECT AT THE DOCTOR'S OFFICE

Treatment depends on how long you have had a fever and how sick you appear. To determine whether an infection is present, the doctor will examine the skin, eyes, ears, nose, throat, neck, chest, and belly. If no other symptoms are present and the exam doesn't reveal an infection, watchful waiting may be advised. If the fever has been prolonged or the patient appears ill, tests of the blood and urine may be done. A chest X-ray or spinal tap may be needed. Specific infections will be treated appropriately; fever will be treated as discussed in Home Treatment.

FEVER

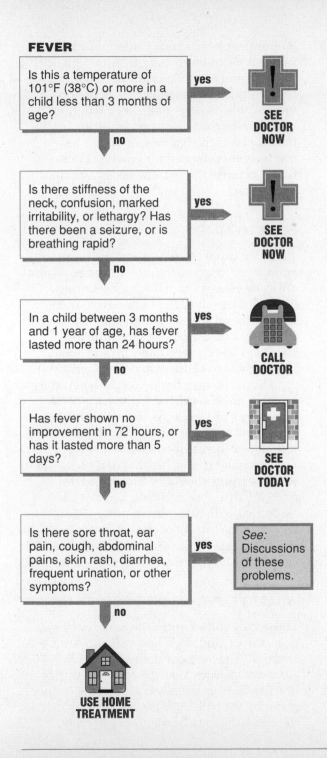

Is this a temperature of 101°F (38°C) or more in a child less than 3 months of age?

yes → SEE DOCTOR NOW

no

Is there stiffness of the neck, confusion, marked irritability, or lethargy? Has there been a seizure, or is breathing rapid?

yes → SEE DOCTOR NOW

no

In a child between 3 months and 1 year of age, has fever lasted more than 24 hours?

yes → CALL DOCTOR

no

Has fever shown no improvement in 72 hours, or has it lasted more than 5 days?

yes → SEE DOCTOR TODAY

no

Is there sore throat, ear pain, cough, abdominal pains, skin rash, diarrhea, frequent urination, or other symptoms?

yes → *See:* Discussions of these problems.

no

USE HOME TREATMENT

95 Headache

Headache is the most frequent single complaint of modern times. Most commonly, the causes are tension and muscle spasms in the neck, scalp, and jaw. Headache without any other associated symptoms is almost always caused by tension. Fever and a neck so stiff that the chin can't be touched to the chest suggest the possibility of meningitis (inflammation of the membranes covering the brain and spinal cord) rather than an ordinary tension headache. But even with these symptoms, meningitis is rare. Flu is much more likely. Muscle aches and pains are seldom seen in meningitis.

Migraines

Most so-called migraine headaches are really tension headaches. True migraine headaches are often associated with nausea or vomiting and are preceded by seeing flashes of light or "stars." They are caused by the tightening and then relaxing of blood vessels in the head. True migraine headaches occur on only one side of the head during any particular attack.

Signs of Trouble?

Increased internal pressure due to head injury (S10) can cause headache and may also cause vomiting and difficulties with vision.

Although headaches aren't a reliable indicator of high blood pressure, if they are worse in the morning, check the blood pressure.

Headache patients frequently worry about brain tumors. In the absence of paralysis or personality change, the possibility that an intermittent headache is caused by a brain tumor is exceedingly remote. Although constant and slowly increasing headaches are frequently noted in patients with brain tumors, it is usually some other symptom that leads the doctor to begin an investigation for tumor. Headache patients shouldn't be routinely investigated for possible brain tumor because the tests are costly and/or hazardous.

HOME TREATMENT

All of the usual over-the-counter drugs (acetaminophen, aspirin, ibuprofen, and naproxen) are quite effective in relieving headache. Aspirin, ibuprofen, and naproxen may be taken with milk or food to prevent stomach irritation. Because of a serious problem known as Reye's syndrome, aspirin should not be given to children and teenagers (M4).

Headache may frequently be relieved by massage or heat applied to the back of the upper neck or by simply resting with eyes closed and the head supported. Relaxation techniques such as meditation may work also.

Persistent headaches that don't respond to such measures should be brought to the attention of a doctor. Headaches that are associated with difficulty in using the arms or legs or with slurring of speech, as well as those that rapidly increase in frequency and severity, also require a visit to the doctor.

WHAT TO EXPECT AT THE DOCTOR'S OFFICE

The doctor will examine the head, eyes, ears, nose, throat, and neck, and will also test nerve function. The temperature will be taken. Abnormalities are rarely found. The diagnosis of a headache is usually based on the history given by the patient. If the doctor feels that the headache may be migraine, an ergot

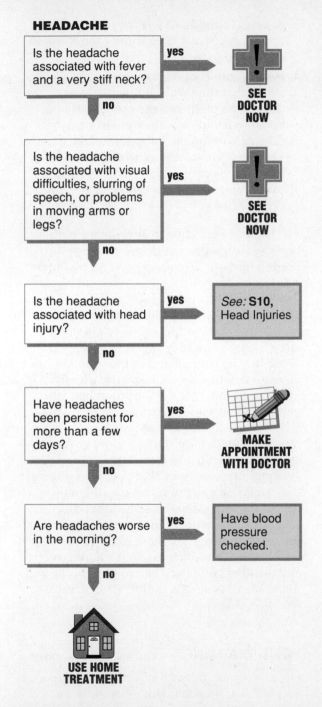

HEADACHE

Is the headache associated with fever and a very stiff neck? — **yes** → **SEE DOCTOR NOW**

no ↓

Is the headache associated with visual difficulties, slurring of speech, or problems in moving arms or legs? — **yes** → **SEE DOCTOR NOW**

no ↓

Is the headache associated with head injury? — **yes** → *See:* **S10,** Head Injuries

no ↓

Have headaches been persistent for more than a few days? — **yes** → **MAKE APPOINTMENT WITH DOCTOR**

no ↓

Are headaches worse in the morning? — **yes** → Have blood pressure checked.

no ↓

USE HOME TREATMENT

preparation (Cafergot, etc.) may be prescribed. Other uncommon types of headaches, such as cluster headaches, may also be treated with this medicine. However, most headaches are caused by tension, and the basic approach will be that outlined under Home Treatment.

96 Insomnia

Insomnia isn't a disease, but it is a continuing problem for some 15 to 20 million Americans and causes occasional problems for almost everyone else. It is a frequent cause of doctor visits, many of which could be avoided.

For most people, occasional insomnia is a response to excitement. Both good and bad events in your life can keep you awake and thinking at night. Other people develop poor sleeping schedules; sleeping late or napping during the day makes sleep at night more difficult.

Diseases are unlikely to cause insomnia, but some can affect sleep. A disease that causes pain (such as arthritis) or shortness of breath (such as heart and lung diseases) may make sleep difficult. Depression and similar problems often interfere with sleep. Clearly, in these cases treating the disease is the best way to restore sound sleep.

Sleep Apnea

People with sleep apnea actually stop breathing many times during sleep. There are two types of sleep apnea, *obstructive* and *central*. Both types cause people to feel tired during the day, but otherwise they differ in significant ways:

- Obstructive sleep apnea is sneaky in that most individuals who have it are unaware that they are having difficult sleeping at night. On the other hand, their sleeping partners are keenly aware of the loud, repeated snoring that is a hallmark of this disease. Individuals with obstructive sleep apnea are usually tired during the day and often take naps.

- People with central sleep apnea are usually aware that they wake up many times during the night and may feel short of breath when they wake up. They may complain of fatigue but seldom take naps. They may snore but not with the loud, repeated snoring characteristic of obstructive sleep apnea. Most central sleep apnea occurs in men.

There are effective treatments for both types of sleep apnea. A doctor's help is needed for both firm diagnosis and treatment.

Medications

Nonprescription sleep aids seem to depend mostly on what doctors call the "placebo effect": they work only if you think they're going to. The antihistamines they contain can increase daytime drowsiness and actually make you think that the sleep problem is getting worse. Older drugs available by prescription are more likely to really knock you out, but they don't produce a natural, restful sleep. As a result, you feel more fatigued than ever and may conclude that you need more of the drug. The more of it you use, the more disturbed your sleep. This vicious cycle is called drug-dependent insomnia. Newer prescription drugs are more likely to promote restful sleep, but doctors will try to remove any cause of poor sleep before prescribing them. Many drugs, including alcohol, interfere with sleep.

HOME TREATMENT

Here are some suggestions for developing a successful approach to your insomnia:

INSOMNIA

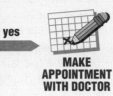

Has faithfully applied home treatment been unsuccessful for 3 weeks or more?

yes → **MAKE APPOINTMENT WITH DOCTOR**

no ↓

USE HOME TREATMENT

- Avoid drinking alcohol in the evening; this leads to disturbed sleep at best.

- Avoid caffeine for at least two hours before bedtime.

- Establish a regular bedtime, but don't go to bed if you feel wide awake.

- Use the bedroom for bedroom activities only. If the bedroom is used for activities such as paying bills, studying, and so on, entering the bedroom can be a signal to become active rather than to go to sleep.

- Break your chain of thought before retiring. Relax by reading, watching television, taking a bath, or listening to soothing music — something that helps to keep your mind from working overtime on life's more serious activities.

- A bedtime snack seems to help many people, as does the traditional glass of warm milk. However, don't eat a big meal before going to bed because this seems to cause problems with sleep.

- Exercise regularly, but not in the last two hours before going to bed.

- Give up smoking. Smokers have more trouble getting to sleep than nonsmokers.

- Once you get into bed, use creative imagery and relaxation techniques to keep your mind off unrestful thoughts. Counting sheep is the oldest kind of creative imagery. Another image technique is to concentrate on a pleasant scene that relaxes you, such as walking along a beach and hearing the sounds of the ocean.

- Finally, many researchers believe that the most effective natural sleep inducer is — you guessed it — sex.

It may take several weeks or more to establish a new, natural sleeping routine. If you are unable to make progress after giving these methods an honest try, a visit to the doctor may be necessary.

WHAT TO EXPECT AT THE DOCTOR'S OFFICE

The doctor will focus on your sleeping schedule, reasons that could be causing stress and anxiety, and other factors related to sleep such as the use of drugs. The physical examination is less important than the history and may be brief. In some instances, the doctor may want to obtain further studies such as an electroencephalogram (EEG) during sleep. On rare occasions it may be necessary to refer you to a center for the study of sleep disturbances where complex studies of your sleep pattern may be conducted.

97 Weakness and Fatigue

Weakness and fatigue are often considered to be similar, but in medicine they have distinct and separate meanings.

Weakness refers to lack of *strength*. Weakness is usually the more serious condition and is particularly important when it is confined to one area of the body. Such weakness in one area is often due to a problem in the muscular or nervous system, such as a stroke.

Fatigue is lack of *energy*. It is tiredness or lethargy. Fatigue is typically associated with a viral infection or with feelings of anxiety, depression, or tension. It's caused by a large variety of illnesses.

Hypoglycemia means "low blood sugar," and many patients fear that this problem is the cause of their tiredness. A few individuals do in fact feel shaky several hours after a meal because their blood sugar level drops at that point. However, they do *not* feel fatigued. Low blood sugar throughout the day can cause fatigue, but this is a rare condition.

Chronic fatigue is common; about one in every four adults seen in doctors' offices say it is one of their problems. But chronic fatigue syndrome (CFS) is unusual; perhaps only one in a thousand of the adults who complain of chronic fatigue meet the criteria for this diagnosis.

CFS created a stir in the 1980s because some doctors believed it to be a new disease, probably due to an acute infection (perhaps Epstein-Barr virus, or even yeast). However, a link to infection has never been demonstrated, and there is little evidence that treating for infections is useful. As a result, other doctors believe that CFS is actually a collection of diseases that have been with us for a long time under such names as neurasthenia and even "the vapors." To try to resolve this issue, groups of experts have created a standard list of criteria for diagnosing chronic fatigue immune-deficiency syndrome (CFIDS, pronounced "see-fids"). This list excludes almost all people with chronic fatigue. But the problem still may be one such as fibromyalgia **(S67)** or depression **(S103).**

HOME TREATMENT

There is time and need for careful reflection on the causes of fatigue. The most common situation was once termed "the tired housewife syndrome." Many young and middle-aged women come to the doctor's office complaining of fatigue and requesting tests for anemia or thyroid problems. Many adult women are mildly iron deficient, and thyroid problems may cause fatigue, but it is very unusual for one of these conditions to be the cause of fatigue. In most cases, fatigue is more closely related to boredom, unhappiness, some disappointment, or just plain hard work. The patient should consider these possibilities before consulting the doctor.

Vitamins are rarely helpful, but in moderation they don't hurt.

WHAT TO EXPECT AT THE DOCTOR'S OFFICE

If the problem is weakness of only part of the body, the doctor will concentrate the examination on the nerve and muscle functions. A typical stroke will be identified by such an examination, whereas more uncommon ailments may require further testing and special procedures.

If the problem is fatigue, the medical history is the most important part of the en-

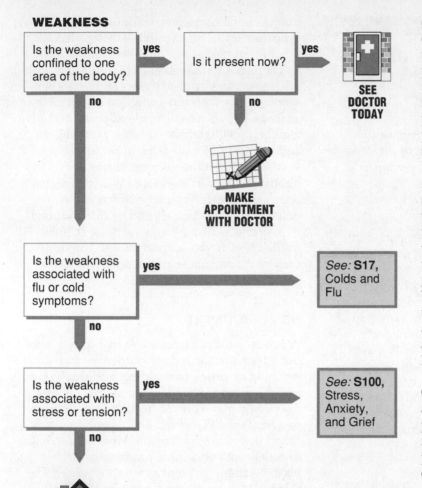

WEAKNESS

Is the weakness confined to one area of the body? — **yes** → Is it present now? — **yes** → **SEE DOCTOR TODAY**

no ↓

Is it present now? — **no** → **MAKE APPOINTMENT WITH DOCTOR**

Is the weakness associated with flu or cold symptoms? — **yes** → *See:* **S17**, Colds and Flu

no ↓

Is the weakness associated with stress or tension? — **yes** → *See:* **S100**, Stress, Anxiety, and Grief

no ↓

USE HOME TREATMENT

counter. Physical examination of heart, lungs, and the thyroid gland can be expected. The doctor may test for anemia and thyroid dysfunction, as well as other problems. Inquiry into the patient's lifestyle and feelings is important.

There are no direct cures for the most common fatigue syndromes. Pep pills don't work, and the downswing when the pills wear off usually makes the problem worse. Tranquilizers generally intensify fatigue. Vacations, job changes, undertaking new activities, and making marital adjustments are far more helpful.

Up to 80% of people with CFS have depression or anxiety as a part of the problem, and many doctors feel that treating those problems is the best way to deal with CFS.

98 Dizziness and Fainting

Three different problems are frequently introduced by the complaint of dizziness or fainting: loss of consciousness, vertigo, and lightheadedness.

Unconsciousness

True unconsciousness includes a period in which the victim has no control over the body and of which there is no recollection. Therefore, if consciousness is lost while standing, the victim will fall and may sustain injury in doing so. The common symptom of "blackout," in which the person finds it difficult to see and needs to sit or lie down but can still hear, isn't true loss of consciousness. Such blackouts may be related to changes in posture or to emotional experiences. True loss of consciousness needs to be investigated promptly by a doctor.

Vertigo

Vertigo is caused by a problem in the balance mechanism of the inner ear. Because this balance mechanism also helps control eye movements, there is loss of balance and the room seems to be spinning around. Walls and floors may seem to lurch in crazy motions. Most vertigo has no definite cause and is thought to be due to a viral infection of the inner ear. A doctor should be seen.

Feeling Lightheaded

"Lightheadedness" is by far the most common of these problems. It is that woozy feeling that is such a common part of flu or cold syndromes. If such a feeling is associated with other flu or cold symptoms, see section S17.

Lightheadedness that isn't associated with other symptoms is usually not serious either. Many people with this condition are tense or anxious. Others have low blood pressure and regularly feel lightheaded when standing up suddenly. This is called "postural hypotension" and doesn't require treatment. If lightheadedness is associated with the use of drugs, the doctor should be contacted to determine if the drug should be discontinued.

Alcohol is also a frequent cause of lightheadedness. If you suspect excess drinking may be the real cause of the problem, see section S104.

HOME TREATMENT

A person most often feels a momentary blackout after he or she moves suddenly from reclining or sitting to standing upright. Blood stops flowing to the brain for an instant, and the person may notice a fleeting loss of vision or a lightheaded feeling. This phenomenon is called postural hypotension. Most people will experience it at one time or another, but it becomes more frequent as we grow older. The therapy is to avoid sudden changes in posture. Unless postural hypotension suddenly becomes worse, you don't need to visit the doctor. You may report the feeling on your next routine visit.

A persistent lightheaded feeling without any other symptoms doesn't indicate a brain tumor or other hidden disease. This type of lightheadedness often disappears when the person resolves anxiety. Not infrequently, it's a problem the person must learn to live with.

If the problem persists for more than three weeks, call the doctor.

DIZZINESS

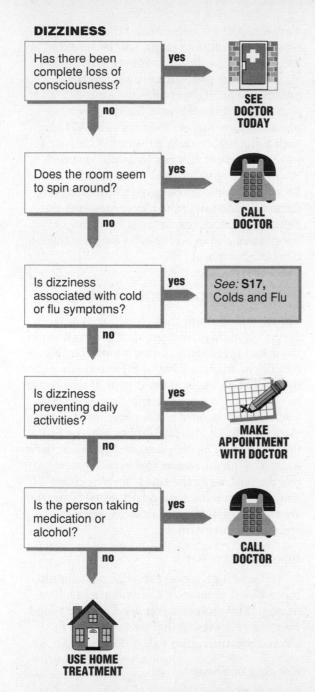

Has there been complete loss of consciousness?

yes → SEE DOCTOR TODAY

no ↓

Does the room seem to spin around?

yes → CALL DOCTOR

no ↓

Is dizziness associated with cold or flu symptoms?

yes → See: **S17,** Colds and Flu

no ↓

Is dizziness preventing daily activities?

yes → MAKE APPOINTMENT WITH DOCTOR

no ↓

Is the person taking medication or alcohol?

yes → CALL DOCTOR

no ↓

USE HOME TREATMENT

WHAT TO EXPECT AT THE DOCTOR'S OFFICE

The doctor will obtain a history with emphasis on making the distinctions outlined above. If loss of consciousness is the problem, the heart and lungs will be examined and nerve function will be tested. Special testing for irregular heartbeat or sudden drop in blood pressure may be necessary. If vertigo is the problem, the head, ears, eyes, and throat will be examined, along with neurological testing. Sometimes further tests of hearing or balance may be required. A search for predisposing factors, such as anxiety, will be made. Often a period of "watchful waiting" will be advised.

99 High Blood Pressure

High blood pressure, or hypertension, is among the most common and most treatable chronic health problems. It has been estimated that 30 to 40 million Americans have high blood pressure — more than one out of every ten.

Many of those who have high blood pressure don't know it. This is a uniquely silent disease. There are no symptoms until it's too late: the catastrophe of a heart attack or stroke is all too often the first indication of a problem. Don't wait for headaches or nosebleeds to give you fair warning; these aren't reliable indicators of high blood pressure. (Even if you have these symptoms, it's quite unlikely that they're due to high blood pressure.)

HAVE YOUR BLOOD PRESSURE CHECKED

Because high blood pressure is silent and can be treated effectively, early detection (screening) is important. Once a year, have your blood pressure checked. This is a reliable, cheap, and painless test. Often the doctor's office isn't the best place to have this done because just being in the doctor's office can raise the blood pressure. Blood pressure checks are available without charge through corporations, public health departments, and voluntary health agencies; an extra visit to the doctor's office is almost never necessary. The blood pressure machines available in many stores are reasonably accurate.

Don't be panicked by just one reading. Because your blood pressure varies, you'll need to have several readings if the first one is

elevated. At least one-third of the people whose first reading is high will be found to have normal readings on subsequent checks.

The blood pressure reading has two numbers. The higher one is the systolic pressure, and the lower is the diastolic pressure. Blood pressure is considered to be high if the higher number (systolic) exceeds 140 or the lower number (diastolic) exceeds 90. Traditionally, "normal" is said to be 120/80, but this has been overemphasized. Generally, the lower the blood pressure, the better. Low readings are usually found in youngsters and in adults who are in excellent physical condition.

IF YOU HAVE HIGH BLOOD PRESSURE

The most important thing to realize is that you must manage this problem yourself. After the initial investigation, you should be able to handle the management of this problem with relatively few visits to the doctor. It will be up to you to control your weight, your exercise, your salt intake, and to take your medicines. We think that it also should be up to you to take your own blood pressure. No matter how much the doctor would like to take care of this for you, he or she can't. Your doctor should be no more than a trusted advisor. You are in control, and good doctors will emphasize this point.

Blood Pressure Kit

If you have high blood pressure, you should buy a blood pressure kit. If you are going to manage this problem, you need regular blood pressure readings so that you can report changes or difficulties to the doctor.

Keeping in Shape

Make exercise, weight control, and diet a part of your program. Aerobic exercise conditions

Don't buy a **blood pressure cuff** unless you actually have high blood pressure or you plan to perform many blood pressure readings as a public service or for some other reason. While taking blood pressure isn't difficult or mysterious, you do need some practice, and doing it once or even several times a year isn't enough.

the cardiovascular system so that blood pressure is reduced. Too high a weight means too high a blood pressure, and reducing your weight (see pages 16–18) is a reliable method for reducing blood pressure. Decreasing the salt, fat, and cholesterol in your diet and increasing the potassium and calcium help to lower blood pressure and decrease the risk of heart disease.

It is true that you can have high blood pressure even though you are slim and exercise regularly. But it is also true that being overweight and out of shape increases the risk of high blood pressure. Recent studies have confirmed that people with high blood pressure can lower their blood pressure by losing weight and exercising regularly. Many can control their blood pressure entirely without the use of drugs. Most others can reduce the amount of medication they require. That means less expense and fewer risks and side effects.

Managing Any Drugs

If you do take drugs for hypertension, understand how to manage them. Each drug has its own side effects and warning signs of which you should be aware. Chart the use of your drugs along with your blood pressure

readings. This is essential. It is the only way that you and your doctor can make rational decisions about your program.

Drug treatment of high blood pressure is effective but is expensive and has risks and side effects. Getting off drugs is very desirable and is only surpassed by never needing the drugs in the first place. In both cases, exercise, weight control, and relaxing can be the keys for most hypertensive people.

Stick With It

Managing high blood pressure is a lifelong undertaking. You can't stop your program because you feel good or wait for signs or symptoms to tell you what you need to do. This is a silent disease. If you take care of your blood pressure, the odds are overwhelmingly against it causing you a major problem. If you ignore high blood pressure or hope that someone else will take care of it, you are needlessly endangering your life and well-being.

100 Stress, Anxiety, and Grief

Stress is a normal part of our lives. It isn't necessarily good or bad. It isn't a disease. But reactions to stress can vary enormously, and some of these reactions are undesirable.

Anxiety

The most frequent undesirable reaction is anxiety. The degree of anxiety is much more a function of the individual than the degree of stress. A person who reacts with excessive anxiety to everyday stress has a personal rather than a medical problem. The person who doesn't recognize anxiety as the problem will have difficulty solving the problem.

Some common symptoms of anxiety are insomnia and an inability to concentrate. These symptoms can lead to a vicious cycle that aggravates the situation. But the symptoms are effects, not causes. The person who focuses on the insomnia or on the lack of concentration as the problem is far from a solution.

Most communities have several resources that can help with anxiety. Members of the clergy, social workers, friends, neighbors, and family may all play a beneficial role. The doctor is an additional resource but isn't necessarily the first or the best place to seek help for these problems.

Grief

Grief is an appropriate reaction to certain situations, such as death of a loved one or loss of a job. In such cases, time is the healer, although significant help may be gained from family, friends, and community resources.

Working through grief is an important part of getting over a loss. If the grief persists for several months, seek outside help.

The limitations of drugs, such as tranquilizers or alcohol, when a person is grieving must be understood. While they may provide short-term symptomatic relief, they are brain depressants that don't enhance mental processes or solve problems. They are a crutch. In this instance, the long-term use of a crutch ensures that the person using it will become a cripple. The underlying problem must be confronted.

HOME TREATMENT

An honest attempt to identify the cause of the anxiety is a requisite first step in resolving the problem. When physical symptoms are due to job pressures, marital woes, wayward children, or domineering parents, the situation must be accurately identified, admitted, and confronted. When anxiety or depression is a reaction to something, the cause is often obvious; simply talking about it with friends or counselors will help.

In other instances, identifying the source of the anxiety will be difficult, painful, time-consuming, and may eventually require the help of a professional counselor or psychiatrist.

Unfortunately, no scientific studies have been able to show which particular type of therapy produces the best results. So your choice should depend on what makes you feel you are making progress.

In addition, sometimes the symptoms of anxiety are associated with too much caffeine. Try cutting down on your caffeine intake and see if you feel more relaxed. Remember that caffeine is found in coffee, soft drinks, tea, a variety of cold and headache remedies, and even chocolate. Caffeine is also the active

STRESS

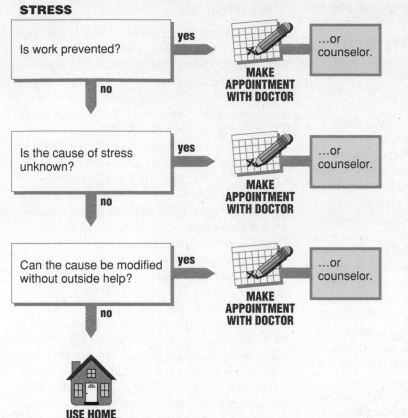

Is work prevented? — **yes** → MAKE APPOINTMENT WITH DOCTOR …or counselor.

no ↓

Is the cause of stress unknown? — **yes** → MAKE APPOINTMENT WITH DOCTOR …or counselor.

no ↓

Can the cause be modified without outside help? — **yes** → MAKE APPOINTMENT WITH DOCTOR …or counselor.

no ↓

USE HOME TREATMENT

ingredient in nonprescription stimulants (NoDoz, Vivarin, etc.).

Exercise can be helpful, as can relaxation techniques (see Lump in the Throat, **S102**).

WHAT TO EXPECT AT THE DOCTOR'S OFFICE

The family doctor will attempt to identify the problem and determine if the help of a psychiatrist or psychiatric social worker is required. Personal questions may be asked, and frank, honest answers must be given. Try to report the underlying problems and avoid emphasis on the effects, such as insomnia, muscle aches, headache, or inability to concentrate.

101 Hyperventilation Syndrome

Anxiety, especially unrecognized anxiety, can lead to physical symptoms. The hyperventilation syndrome is such a problem. In this syndrome, a nervous or anxious person becomes concerned about his or her breathing and feels unable to get enough air into the lungs. This is often associated with chest pain or tightness.

The sensation of being out of breath leads to overbreathing and a lowering of the carbon dioxide level in the blood. The lower level of carbon dioxide brings on symptoms of numbness and tingling of the hands, and dizziness. The numbness and tingling may extend to the feet and may also be noted around the mouth. Occasionally muscle spasms may occur in the hands.

This syndrome is almost always a disease of young adults. While it is more common in women, it is also frequently seen in men. Usually this syndrome afflicts people who recognize themselves as being nervous and tense. It often happens when such people have additional stress, use alcohol, or are in situations where it is advantageous to have a sudden, dramatic illness. A classic example is the occurrence of the hyperventilation syndrome during separation or divorce proceedings, so that the event becomes a call for help to the estranged spouse.

However, hyperventilation is also a natural response to severe pain. When in doubt, take a person who is hyperventilating to the doctor's office rather than discount a potentially serious problem.

HOME TREATMENT

The symptoms of hyperventilation syndrome are due to carbon dioxide loss from overbreathing. If the person breathes into a paper bag, so that the carbon dioxide is taken back into the lungs rather than being lost into the atmosphere, the symptoms will be alleviated. This usually requires five to fifteen minutes with a small paper bag held loosely over both the nose and the mouth. This isn't always as easy as it sounds because a major feature of the hyperventilation syndrome is panic and a feeling of impending suffocation. Approaching such a person with a paper bag for the mouth and nose may prove difficult, so be sure to reassure the person first.

Repeated attacks may occur. Once the person has honestly recognized that the problem is anxiety rather than a disease, the attacks will stop because the panic component won't come into play; convincing the person is the main obstacle. Having the person voluntarily hyperventilate (50 deep breaths while lying on a couch) to demonstrate that this reproduces the symptoms of the previous episode is frequently helpful. People are usually afraid that they are having a heart attack or are on the verge of a nervous breakdown. Neither is true, and when the fear has dissipated, hyperventilation usually ceases.

WHAT TO EXPECT AT THE DOCTOR'S OFFICE

The doctor will obtain a history and direct attention primarily to the examination of the heart and lungs. In the young person with a typical syndrome, with a normal physical examination and no abdominal pain, the diagnosis of hyperventilation is easily made. Electrocardiograms (EKGs) and chest X-rays are seldom needed. These procedures may

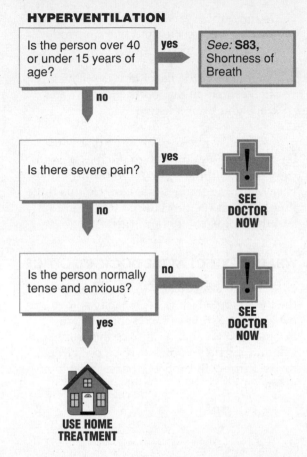

HYPERVENTILATION

Is the person over 40 or under 15 years of age?

yes → *See:* **S83,** Shortness of Breath

no ↓

Is there severe pain?

yes → **SEE DOCTOR NOW**

no ↓

Is the person normally tense and anxious?

no → **SEE DOCTOR NOW**

yes ↓

USE HOME TREATMENT

occasionally be necessary in less clear-cut cases.

If hyperventilation syndrome is diagnosed, the doctor will usually provide a paper bag and the instructions given above. A tranquilizer may be administered; we prefer merely to reassure the patient. It is seldom possible to deal effectively with the cause of the anxiety during the hyperventilation episode. The patient shouldn't assume that the underlying problem is solved simply because the hyperventilation has been controlled.

102 Lump in the Throat

The feeling of a "lump in the throat" is the best known of all anxiety symptoms. There may even be some difficulty swallowing, although eating is possible if an effort is made. The sensation is intermittent and is made worse by tension.

The difficulty in swallowing is worst when the person concentrates on swallowing and on the sensations within the throat. As an experiment, try to swallow rapidly several times without any food or liquid, and concentrate on the resulting sensation. You will then understand this symptom.

Several serious diseases can cause difficulty swallowing. In these cases, the symptom begins slowly, is noticed first with solid foods and then with liquids, results in loss of weight, and is more likely to be found in those over 40. "Lump in the throat," like the hyperventilation syndrome, is likely to be found in young adults, most frequently women.

HOME TREATMENT

The central problem isn't the symptom but, rather, the underlying cause of the anxiety state (see Stress, Anxiety, and Grief, **S100**). Recognition that the symptom is minor is crucial to its disappearance.

Relaxation techniques may be helpful. One such technique is called progressive relaxation:

1. Imagine that your toes weigh a thousand pounds and you couldn't move them if you wanted to. Let them go completely limp.

2. Do the same with each part of your body, relaxing the muscles and working your way up to the top of your head.

3. Don't neglect the facial muscles. Tension often centers in the forehead or jaw and keeps you from relaxing.

An alternative is to imagine that your breath is coming in through the toes of your right foot, all the way up to your lungs, and back out through the same foot. Do this three times. Repeat the procedure for the left foot and then for each of your arms.

WHAT TO EXPECT AT THE DOCTOR'S OFFICE

After taking a medical history and examining the throat and chest, a doctor may sometimes believe that X-rays of the esophagus are necessary. If an abnormality of the esophagus is found, further studies may be performed. Reassurance will probably be the treatment given.

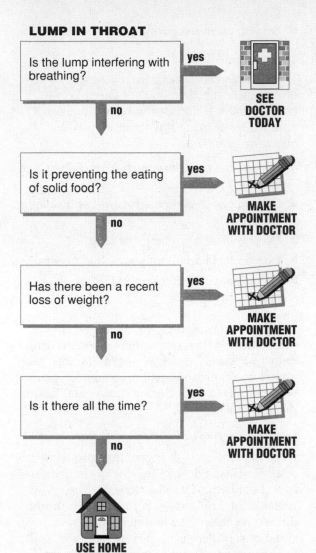

LUMP IN THROAT

Is the lump interfering with breathing?

yes → **SEE DOCTOR TODAY**

no ↓

Is it preventing the eating of solid food?

yes → **MAKE APPOINTMENT WITH DOCTOR**

no ↓

Has there been a recent loss of weight?

yes → **MAKE APPOINTMENT WITH DOCTOR**

no ↓

Is it there all the time?

yes → **MAKE APPOINTMENT WITH DOCTOR**

no ↓

USE HOME TREATMENT

103 Depression

The blues and the blahs — everybody gets them sometimes. No problem is more common. It can range from a feeling of no energy all the way to such an overwhelming sense of unhappiness and defeat that ending it all looks like the only way out.

Depression may appear to be simple fatigue or a general feeling of ill health: you just don't feel good, and you may not know the reason why. The future may seem to hold no promise. There is a sense of loss: a feeling of defeat or of having lost something — or someone — important. In medical terms, most depression is "reactive," meaning that it is a reaction to an unhappy event. It is natural to have some depression after a loss, such as the death of a friend or relative, or after a significant disappointment at home or work. If, however, the depression is so great as to disrupt your work or family life for a substantial period, put a time limit on it by making an appointment with your doctor.

Here are some questions that doctors think are important to determining whether you are depressed and to what degree. Let's start with depression itself:

- Are you sad or blue for most of the day, for more days than not?
- Do you often cry even though you aren't sure of the reason?
- Do you think that unhappiness is the rule in your life?
- Do you no longer get pleasure from things you used to like to do?

- Do you often have feelings of hopelessness?

If the answer to any two of these questions is yes, then you are very likely to be depressed. If depression seems likely, ask yourself these questions about its possible effects on your life:

- Do you have a poor appetite, or do you overeat?
- Do you not sleep enough, or do you sleep too much?
- Do you have low energy or fatigue?
- Do you feel bad about yourself in general?
- Do you have trouble concentrating or making decisions?

If you answered yes to any of the above questions and these symptoms are interfering with your family, work, or social life, then the depression is creating real problems for you. Seek help from your doctor or a mental health professional.

Suicidal Feelings

If the depression is so severe that you have considered suicide, call the doctor immediately and get help. If you have no doctor or you prefer to find help elsewhere, many communities have telephone hotlines for such situations. If there is no service near you, call the nearest emergency room or health care facility. They will arrange help for you.

HOME TREATMENT

Activity, both mental and physical, has long been recognized as the natural antidote for depression. Regular exercise is as effective for mild depression as the drugs usually prescribed by doctors. Make a plan for activity

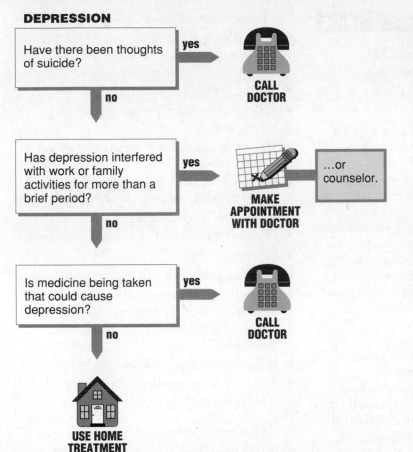

DEPRESSION

Have there been thoughts of suicide? **yes** → **CALL DOCTOR**

no ↓

Has depression interfered with work or family activities for more than a brief period? **yes** → **MAKE APPOINTMENT WITH DOCTOR** ...or counselor.

no ↓

Is medicine being taken that could cause depression? **yes** → **CALL DOCTOR**

no ↓

USE HOME TREATMENT

and there may be some suggestions the listener can make to ease the burden.

WHAT TO EXPECT AT THE DOCTOR'S OFFICE

The doctor will explore the issues and events associated with depression. Listening and responding are the most important things. The doctor will often make some suggestions about activities and exercise. If the patient is taking drugs that could cause depression, the doctor will change them. Antidepressant drugs may be prescribed, but usually only after other ways of helping have been tried or, at least, been given careful consideration. Hospitalization is best if the patient might commit suicide.

that includes regular exercise. Stay involved with others and let them support you.

Drugs may cause depression. Tranquilizers, high blood pressure medicines, corticosteroids (prednisone, etc.), codeine, and indomethacin are often culprits. If you suspect you are suffering depression, call your doctor about your prescription medicines. Decrease your use of alcohol and other nonprescription drugs.

Make a point of telling someone about your problems. Getting them out is a relief,

104 Alcoholism

Addiction to alcohol isn't hopeless, but a person with a drinking problem seldom changes this harmful behavior alone. Although recovery must come from within, the decisive nudge often comes from without. The drinker needs input, feedback, and support from a relative, friend, or coworker. If, like most people, you know someone who drinks too much, you can provide that help.

If in reading this section you recognize yourself as a person who drinks too much, be your own best friend and get help now.

Warning Signs

Following are some of the signs of problem drinking, when a person may not be medically addicted to alcohol but drinking is causing harm and the person needs treatment. Exhibiting many of the behaviors on this list may indicate an even deeper need for treatment:

- Drinking to get drunk

- Trying to solve or avoid problems by drinking

- Becoming loud, angry, or violent after drinking

- Drinking at inappropriate times, such as in the morning, before driving, or before going to work

- Drinking that causes problems, harm, or concern to others

- Developing an ulcer or gastritis

These are the signs of alcoholism:

- Spending time thinking about drinking, or planning where and when to get the next drink

- Hiding bottles for quick pick-me-ups

- Receiving citations for driving while intoxicated

- Having an automobile accident after any alcohol intake

- Starting to drink without planning to, and losing track of the amount of alcohol consumed

- Denying the amount of alcohol consumed

- Drinking alone

- Needing a drink before stressful situations

- Having no memory of what occurred while drinking, although the alcoholic may have appeared normal to others at the time — "blackouts"

- Incurring malnutrition and neglect

- Suffering from withdrawal symptoms, including delirium tremens (DTs)

A pregnant woman who drinks heavily is at risk of harming the fetus in her womb, a condition called fetal alcohol syndrome.

In addition to these signs, consult the decision chart for this section. It is derived from a questionnaire created to help physicians decide if their patients have drinking problems.

Barriers to Helping

There are many reasons why people hesitate to suggest that someone has a drinking problem. You might feel that you are butting into a painful and private area. Remember that you wouldn't be concerned in the first place unless the problem has already affected you. It is best to think of the alcohol abuser as someone with a problem that harms your ability to enjoy each other's company. That means you are responsible for helping the alcoholic own up to problem behavior toward you.

Don't wait for a person to hit rock bottom. Alcoholism is a progressive disease, and early intervention can halt the person's decline. It can also save you and the person from the grief that usually accompanies problem drinking.

It is easy but harmful to let yourself be drawn into the "alcoholic's game." The alcoholic creates a crisis by drinking (passes out at a party, smashes up the car, loses a job); you condemn the alcoholic; this person then seeks and obtains your forgiveness — until the cycle begins again. The drinker needs this periodic forgiveness and sympathy to sustain this destructive cycle. As long as you play this game, the alcoholic's behavior is reinforced.

Alcoholism can be a frightening subject. It helps to know as much as possible. Seek information from self-help groups, counselors, and your doctor. Then put that information to use when you talk to your friend.

What to Say

Pick a good time: not when the person is drunk but not long after a crisis, so that the experience is fresh. Tell the person what you have observed and how it causes problems. Describe your feelings and ask how the person feels about the situation. Suggest a way out.

Try not to sound as if you are charging the person with a crime. Don't try to punish, bribe, or emotionally blackmail the person, but remain calm, detached, and factual. Use your leverage, but use it fairly. For instance, if you are a drinker's supervisor, give fair

warning before threatening him or her with loss of a job. Make sure you leave the responsibility for the negative behavior and for changing it with the drinker; set limits on what you will tolerate, and be sure the drinker understands these limits.

The person may deny having a problem. Indeed, denial is one of the alcoholic's biggest fallbacks. Stating your concern and pointing out examples of trouble may be all you can do this time. Let the person know that you are learning about alcoholism. If the problem recurs, talk to the drinker again. People with drinking problems need to help themselves, but it is unlikely they can do so without a push from friends like you.

HOME TREATMENT

Alcoholism isn't a problem that is easily solved at home, but a doctor can't cure it either. The focus of any treatment must be on the drinker changing his or her behavior. There are many worthwhile methods, some involving physicians or professional counselors and some not. Certain techniques insist on abstinence, and others aim to reduce drinking to within acceptable limits.

The route to recovery pioneered by Alcoholics Anonymous (AA) has been as successful as any and more so than most. AA is based in local communities. It uses a self-help format to encourage the problem drinker to face up to his or her alcoholism and come to grips with the consequences. Almost all clinic- and hospital-based alcohol treatment programs refer their patients to AA once they have gotten off to a good start. Successful recovery requires a long-term commitment, and AA provides such sustained support.

Allied with AA are Al-Anon (for people affected by a family member's alcoholism) and Alateen (for teens with family members or friends who are alcoholics). Other groups follow some, but not all, of the AA precepts. There is a group for just about every approach. The most important ingredient in every program is commitment on the part of the drinker.

Where to Find Help

Start by looking in your phone book's white pages under "alcohol abuse"; there are many information hotlines that operate around the clock. Alcoholics Anonymous and its related groups are community-based, meaning that there is almost certainly a branch in your area. For more information you can contact these central offices:

- Alcoholics Anonymous (AA)
  General Service Office
  P.O. Box 459 Grand Central Station
  New York, NY 10163
  (212) 870-3400

- Al-Anon and Alateen
  Family Group Headquarters
  P.O. Box 862 Midtown Station
  New York, NY 10018-0862
  (212) 302-7240

- National Council on Alcoholism and Drug
    Dependence
  12 West 21st Street, 7th Floor
  New York, NY 10010
  (800) 622-2255

- National Clearinghouse for Alcohol and
    Drug Information
  P.O. Box 2345
  Rockville, MD 20847-2345
  (800) 729-6686

WHAT TO EXPECT AT THE DOCTOR'S OFFICE

Tell your doctor if you are recovering from alcoholism or suspect you have a drinking problem. A history of drinking can affect many aspects of your medical care, from the possible causes of certain illnesses to how strongly you might react to anesthetics or pain relievers.

If you ask your doctor for help for an alcoholic friend, the doctor will probably suggest counseling for your friend. Don't expect the doctor to suggest a clinic to "dry out." Many clinics do a fine job of starting people on the road to recovery, but an alcoholic's success rides on the ability to control drinking in the everyday world. Since the cost of outpatient treatment is less than one-tenth the cost of inpatient care, hospitals best serve:

- Patients whose bodies are so poisoned with alcohol that they require acute detoxification

- Patients who may go into severe withdrawal, requiring medical care

- The rare patient who suffers from profound psychological problems beyond alcoholism

ALCOHOLISM

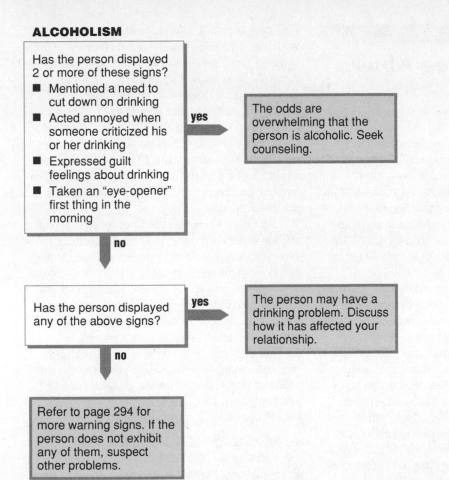

Has the person displayed 2 or more of these signs?
- Mentioned a need to cut down on drinking
- Acted annoyed when someone criticized his or her drinking
- Expressed guilt feelings about drinking
- Taken an "eye-opener" first thing in the morning

yes → The odds are overwhelming that the person is alcoholic. Seek counseling.

no ↓

Has the person displayed any of the above signs?

yes → The person may have a drinking problem. Discuss how it has affected your relationship.

no ↓

Refer to page 294 for more warning signs. If the person does not exhibit any of them, suspect other problems.

105 Drug Abuse

From 5 to 13% of adults in this country abuse or depend on some kind of psychoactive substance other than alcohol. This problem extends beyond illegal drugs, such as cocaine and some narcotics, to abuse of prescription drugs. People addicted to drugs need someone to push them into getting help. You, as a loved one or colleague, can start that process and improve both your lives.

Overdoses and withdrawal symptoms are just two of the dangers of drug dependency. Abusers need the substance so much that they will harm themselves or others to have it, causing many more medical and nonmedical problems. The craving for a drug may lead people to steal, share needles, engage in risky sex, neglect their health, and take other risks. Addictions also make abusers more emotionally volatile, and thus more prone to violence. At least one-half of all spouse abuse cases and one-third of all child abuse cases are related to substance abuse. More than one-third of all suicides are drug-related.

Teenagers who drink alcohol and smoke tobacco are a cause for concern. These substances are addictive and harmful, it is illegal for teenagers to buy them in most states, and they are "gateway" substances that often lead to drug abuse. About one-quarter of all youngsters between 12 and 17 used an illicit drug in the last year.

HOME TREATMENT

It isn't your role to diagnose or treat a drug problem. Let the professionals do that. Your first task is to acknowledge the situation, which is difficult. The decision chart lists some of the signs of substance abuse. Unfortunately, they aren't all as easy to spot as the chronic runny nose of a cocaine abuser.

If you suspect that a person is abusing drugs, find out more about the problem for your own sake. Talk to counselors, self-help groups, and your doctor. Phone hotlines are available locally and nationwide. Groups like Nar-Anon can provide support during this troubled period.

You may then be able to confront the drug abuser with your worry. There is nothing wrong in saying: "I'm concerned about your behavior. You seem troubled. Why not speak to someone about it?" See Alcoholism (S104) for more advice on bringing up the subject. If the person agrees to seek help, share your knowledge about counseling services.

Many substance abusers resist such advice, however. Again, it isn't your role to force them to stop their behavior, only to protect yourself from its consequences. Don't assist the drug abuser to continue abusing by:

- Covering up his or her behavior from others
- Hiding the full impact of the behavior from him or her
- Taking over the abuser's responsibilities in the home or at work
- Rationalizing the drug as a benefit for the abuser
- Cooperating in buying, selling, or using the drug

WHAT TO EXPECT AT THE DOCTOR'S OFFICE

For the drug abuser who refuses your entreaty to get help, a doctor or other professional advisor might recommend a method

DRUG ABUSE

Does the person exhibit any of these signs?

- Unhealthy lifestyle — neglect of appearance
- Secretive behavior
- Frequently being absent or late
- Mood swings
- Weight loss
- Money problems
- Anxiety and nervousness
- Impulsive behavior
- Troubled relationships
- Denial that problem exists

yes →

MAKE APPOINTMENT WITH DOCTOR

...or counselor.

no →

Consider other problems.

Anabolic steroids are drugs that target the muscles instead of the brain, encouraging muscle cell growth. They have positive medical uses, but taking them without a prescription can lead to dependency. Anabolic steroids have become very popular among young men and teenage boys, both those involved in athletics and those who want larger muscles to improve their appearance. Ironically, steroid abusers risk acne, stunted growth, impaired fertility, and psychological problems.

called intervention. After meeting several times with an advisor, family members and friends confront the user. Led by the advisor, they express their concerns, citing specific examples. If the abuser agrees to get help, he or she immediately enters a treatment program. If the abuser still refuses help, it is critical that family members receive counseling so that they don't inadvertently enable the abuser to continue his or her behavior.

After diagnosing substance abuse, most doctors will refer the patient to a treatment program run by specialists. There is no cure for substance dependence; the craving can persist for life. But, it can be controlled. Treatment programs are geared to the long haul. Successful rehabilitation or recovery can be expected for 50 to 70% of all substance abusers.

Sometimes a short stay in a hospital is necessary to prevent a patient from dying of an overdose or withdrawal, to hold a dangerously unstable person, or to treat complications of drug abuse, such as infections. The average stay for drug abuse problems is 12 days. The hospital should guide the patient to continuing treatment after discharge.

Where to Find Help

Narcotics Anonymous (NA) and Cocaine Anonymous (CA) are self-help groups

organized on the principles of Alcoholics
Anonymous. Nar-Anon serves people affected
by a family member's drug abuse. These
organizations are listed in most phone
directories, and you can contact these central
offices:

- Narcotics Anonymous (NA)
  World Service Office
  19737 Nordhoff Place
  Chatsworth, CA 91311
  (818) 773-9999

- Nar-Anon
  Family Group Headquarters
  P.O. Box 2562
  Palos Verdes Peninsula, CA 90274
  (310) 547-5800

For immediate help, look in your phone
book's white pages under "drug abuse."
There are many information hotlines, including these two national numbers:

- National Institute of Drug Abuse Hotline
  (800) 662-HELP

- Cocaine Hotline 24-hour information and
    referral
  (800) COCAINE

CHAPTER 9

Women's Health

How to Do a Breast Self-examination

Most lumps in the breast are not cancerous. Most women will have a lump in a breast at some time during their life. Many women's breasts are naturally lumpy (so-called benign fibrocystic disease). Obviously, every lump or possible lump cannot and should not be subjected to surgery.

Cancer of the breast does occur, however, and is best treated early. Regular self-examination of your breasts gives you the best chance of avoiding serious consequences. Self-examination should be done monthly, just after the menstrual period.

The technique is as follows:

1. Examine your breasts in the mirror, first with your arms at your sides (A1) and then with both arms over your head (A2). The breasts should look the same. Watch for any change in shape or size, or for dimpling of the skin. Occasionally a lump that is difficult to feel will be quite obvious just by looking.

2. Next, while lying flat, examine the left breast using the inner finger tips of the right hand and pressing the breast tissue against the chest wall. Don't pinch the tissue between the fingers; all breast tissue feels a bit lumpy when you do this. The left hand should be behind your head while you examine the inner half of the left breast (B1) and down at your side when you examine the outer half (B2). Don't neglect the part of the breast underneath the nipples or that which extends outward from the breast toward the underarm (B3). A small pillow under the left shoulder may help.

3. Repeat this process on the opposite side.

Any lump detected should be brought to the attention of your doctor. Regular self-examination will tell you how long it has been present and whether it has changed in size. This information is very helpful in deciding what to do about the lump; even the doctor often has difficulty with this decision. Self-examination is an absolute necessity for a woman with naturally lumpy breasts. She is the only one who can really know whether a lump is new, old, or has changed size. For all women, regular self-examination offers the best hope that surgery will be performed when, and only when, it is necessary. Many doctors recommend repeating a self-examination in the shower, where smooth, slightly soapy skin can make lumps easier to detect.

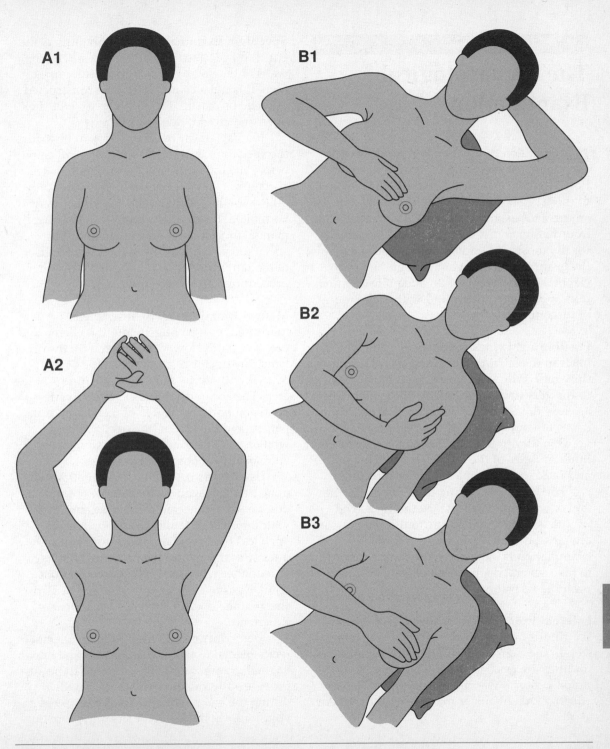

The Gynecological Examination

Examination of the female reproductive organs, usually called a "pelvic examination," may be expected for complaints related to these organs, along with the annual Pap smear. This examination yields a great deal of information and is often absolutely essential for diagnosis. By understanding the phases of the examination and your role in them, you can make it possible for an adequate examination to be done quickly and with a minimum of discomfort.

Positioning. Lying on your back, put your heels in the stirrups (the nurse may assist in this step). With your knees bent, move down to the very end of the examination table. Get as close to the edge as you can. Now let your knees fall out to the sides as far as they will go. Don't try to hold the knees closed with the inner muscles of the thigh. This will tire you and make the examination more difficult.

The key word during the examination is "relax"; you may hear it several times. The vagina is a muscular organ, and if the muscles are tense, a difficult and uncomfortable examination is inevitable. You may be asked to take several deep breaths in an effort to promote relaxation.

External Examination. Inspection of the labia, the clitoris, and vaginal opening is the first step in the examination. The most common findings are cysts in the labia, rashes, and so-called venereal warts. These problems have effective treatments or may need no treatment at all.

Speculum Examination. The speculum is the "duck-billed" instrument used to spread the walls of the vagina so that the inside may be seen. It is not a clamp. It may be constructed of metal or plastic. The plastic ones will click open and closed; don't be alarmed.

If a Pap smear or other test is to be made, the speculum examination usually will come before the finger (manual) examination. The speculum will be lubricated with water only; otherwise the results of the Pap smear may be spoiled. If these tests aren't needed, the manual examination may come first. The speculum also opens the vagina so that insertion of an intrauterine device (IUD) or other procedures can be accomplished.

Manual Examination. By inserting two lubricated, gloved fingers into the vagina and pressing on the lower abdomen with the other hand, the doctor can feel the shape of the ovaries and uterus as well as any lumps in the area. The accuracy of this examination depends on both the degree of relaxation of the patient and the skill of the doctor. Obese women can't be examined as easily; this is another reason not to be overweight.

Usually the best pelvic examinations are done by those who do them most often. You don't need a gynecologist, but be sure that your internist or family practitioner does "pelvics" on a regular basis before you request a yearly gynecological exam. A nurse practitioner who does pelvic examinations regularly is usually an expert also. The Pap smear alone doesn't require a great deal of experience.

Many doctors will also perform a rectal or recto-vaginal (one finger in rectum and one in vagina) examination. These examinations can provide additional information. Usually during the examination there is a drape over your knees and the doctor sits on a stool out of your line of sight. Ask the doctor to explain what is going on.

THE PAP SMEAR

You should be familiar with the basics of this test, in which a scraping of the cervix and a sample of the vaginal secretions are obtained with the aid of a speculum. This provides cells for study under the microscope. A trained technician (a cytologist) can then classify the cells according to their microscopic characteristics. There are five classes:

- Classes I and II are negative for tumor cells.
- Classes III and IV are suspicious but not definite for tumors; your doctor will ask you to return for another Pap test or a biopsy of the cervix. This doesn't mean that cancer is definite.
- Class V is a definite indication of tumors.

Your doctor will explain the approach to confirming the diagnosis and starting treatment.

A single Pap smear detects up to 90% of the most common cancers of the womb and 70 to 80% of the second most common. Both of these common types of cancer grow slowly. Current evidence indicates that it may take ten years or more for a single focus of cancer of the cervix to spread. Thus, there is an excellent chance that regular Pap smears will detect the cancer before it spreads.

Cancer of the cervix is more frequent with moderate-to-heavy sexual activity, especially, and perhaps only, if you have multiple partners. Regular Pap testing probably should begin when regular sexual activity begins or at age 21, whichever is earlier. Testing is done annually for the first three years. If these first Pap smears are normal, then tests are done every three years. Some experts suggest that the tests can be discontinued at age 65 if all previous tests have been normal. While this recommendation probably carries little risk, we think that a Pap smear every three years is a small burden and prefer to continue the tests. There is almost no evidence that the use of birth control pills requires more frequent Pap smears.

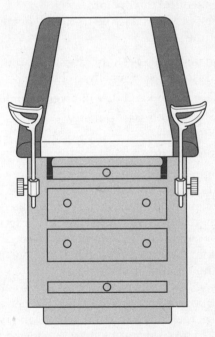

Examination table with stirrups

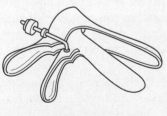

Speculum

106 Vaginal Discharge

Abnormal discharge from the vagina is common but shouldn't be confused with the normal vaginal secretions, which are thin, clear, and painless. Some of the many possible causes require the doctor.

The problem may be treated at home — for a time — if:

- The discharge is slight, doesn't hurt or itch, and isn't cheesy, smelly, or bloody
- There is no possibility of a venereal disease
- The patient is past puberty

Signs of Trouble

Abdominal pain suggests the possibility of serious disease, ranging from gonorrhea to an ectopic pregnancy in the fallopian tube. Bloody discharge between periods, if recurrent or significant in amount, suggests much the same. Discharge in a girl before puberty is rare and should be evaluated.

If sexual contact in the past few weeks might possibly have resulted in a venereal disease, the doctor must be seen. Don't be afraid to take this problem to the doctor. Be frank in naming your sexual contacts, for their own benefit. Information will be kept confidential, and the doctor will not embarrass you; doctors are commonly confronted with this situation.

Monilia is a yeast that may infect the walls of the vagina and cause a white, cheesy discharge. Trichomonas is a common microorganism that can cause a white, frothy discharge and intense itch. A mixture of bacteria may be responsible for a discharge, so-called nonspecific vaginitis. These infections aren't serious and don't spread to the rest of the body, but they are bothersome. They will sometimes but not always go away by themselves. If discharge persists beyond a few weeks, make an appointment with the doctor.

In older women, lack of hormones can cause dryness of the vagina. Prescription creams are sometimes needed if symptoms are bothersome. Foreign bodies, particularly forgotten tampons, are a surprisingly frequent cause of vaginitis and discharge.

HOME TREATMENT

Hygiene and patience are the home remedies. If you have a discharge, douche daily and following intercourse with a Betadine solution (two tablespoons to a quart of water, or 30 ml to a liter) or baking soda (one teaspoon to a quart, or 5 ml to a liter).

If you are taking an antibiotic such as tetracycline for some other condition, call your doctor for advice on changing medication.

If the discharge persists despite treatment for more than two weeks or becomes worse, see the doctor. Do not douche for 24 hours prior to seeing the doctor.

Medications active against yeast (Monistat, etc.) are now available without prescription.

WHAT TO EXPECT AT THE DOCTOR'S OFFICE

You should anticipate a pelvic examination (see The Gynecological Examination, pages 304–305). If a venereal disease is suspected, a culture of the mouth of the womb, the cervix, is mandatory. If not, examination of the discharge under the microscope or a culture of the discharge is sometimes, but not always, needed. Suppositories or creams are the usual

VAGINAL DISCHARGE

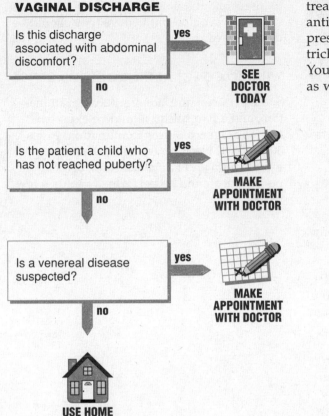

Is this discharge associated with abdominal discomfort?

yes → **SEE DOCTOR TODAY**

no ↓

Is the patient a child who has not reached puberty?

yes → **MAKE APPOINTMENT WITH DOCTOR**

no ↓

Is a venereal disease suspected?

yes → **MAKE APPOINTMENT WITH DOCTOR**

no ↓

USE HOME TREATMENT

treatment. If venereal disease is at all likely, antibiotics, normally penicillin, will be prescribed. Oral medication for fungus or trichomonas may be used in severe cases. Your sexual partner(s) may require treatment as well.

107 Bleeding Between Periods

Most often the interval between two menstrual periods is free of bleeding or spotting. Many women experience such bleeding, however, even though no serious condition is present. Women with an intrauterine birth control device (IUD) are particularly likely to have occasional spotting. If the bleeding is slight and occasional, it may be ignored.

Serious conditions such as cancer and abnormal pregnancy may be first suggested by bleeding between periods. However, many less serious problems, such as fibroids (benign tumors in the uterus), may have the same sign. If bleeding is severe or occurs three months in a row, a doctor must be seen. Often a serious problem can be detected best when the bleeding isn't active. The gynecologist or the family doctor is a better resource than the emergency room.

Any bleeding after the menopause should be evaluated by a doctor.

HOME TREATMENT

Relax and use pads or tampons. Avoid taking aspirin, ibuprofen, or naproxen if possible; it may prolong the bleeding. If in doubt about the effect of any medication, call your doctor.

The relationship between tampons and toxic shock syndrome is a subject of medical controversy, but many doctors believe that leaving tampons in place too long increases the risk of this problem. Change tampons regularly, at least twice daily. Be sure that tampons are removed: it is surprisingly easy to forget about them. We don't think tampons should be avoided but believe they should be used with care.

WHAT TO EXPECT AT THE DOCTOR'S OFFICE

Some personal questions, a pelvic examination, and a Pap smear should be expected (see The Gynecological Examination, pages 304–305). If bleeding is active, the pelvic examination and Pap smear may be postponed but should be performed within a few weeks.

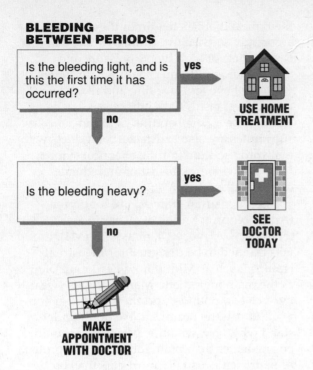

**BLEEDING
BETWEEN PERIODS**

Is the bleeding light, and is this the first time it has occurred?

yes → **USE HOME TREATMENT**

no ↓

Is the bleeding heavy?

yes → **SEE DOCTOR TODAY**

no ↓

MAKE APPOINTMENT WITH DOCTOR

108 Difficult Periods

Adverse mood changes and fluid retention are very common in the days just prior to a menstrual period. Such problems are vexing and can be difficult to treat but are a result of normal hormonal variations during the menstrual cycle.

The menstrual cycle varies from woman to woman. Periods may be regular, irregular, light, heavy, painful, pain-free, long, or short, and yet still be normal. The rhythm of a menstrual cycle is medically less significant than bleeding, pain, or discharge between periods. Only when problems are severe or recur for several months is medical attention required. The doctor can find such problems as endometriosis — the presence of the sort of tissue that lines the uterus in other parts of the body, where it can cause problems. Emergency treatment is seldom needed.

HOME TREATMENT

We believe that diuretics (pills that help the body get rid of fluids through increased urination) and hormones are rarely needed. As we have said in other sections of this book, we prefer the simple and natural to the complex and artificial. We have all too frequently seen hormone treatment lead to mood changes that are worse than premenstrual tension, and diuretics lead to potassium loss, gouty arthritis, and psychological drug dependency.

Salt tends to hold fluid in the tissues. The most natural way to start fluids moving is to cut down on salt intake. In the United States,

the typical diet has ten times the required amount of salt. Many authorities feel that this is one cause of high blood pressure and arteriosclerosis. If you can eliminate some salt, you may have less swelling and fluid retention. If food tastes flat without salt, try using lemon juice as a substitute. Commercial salt substitutes are also satisfactory. Products with the word "sodium" or the chemical symbol "Na" anywhere in the list of ingredients contain salt.

For menstrual cramps, use ibuprofen (Advil, Nuprin, Midol, etc.), naproxen (Naprosyn, Aleve, etc.), or aspirin **(M4)**. Products claimed to be designed for menstrual cramps (such as Midol) now have ibuprofen as the main ingredient. Many patients swear by such compounds, and they are fine if you want to pay the premium. We don't understand why, on a scientific basis, they should be any better than plain ibuprofen. Ibuprofen or naproxen is usually most effective, but sometimes aspirin or acetaminophen may be preferred.

WHAT TO EXPECT AT THE DOCTOR'S OFFICE

The doctor will give you some advice. Frequently a prescription for diuretics or hormones will be given. For menstrual cramps, ibuprofen (Motrin, etc.) or another prostaglandin-inhibiting drug is often prescribed. Note that ibuprofen is also available in lower doses (Advil, Nuprin, Midol, etc.) without prescription **(M4).**

Pelvic examination is often unrewarding and sometimes may not be performed. However, if endometriosis is suspected, the pelvic exam should be done during the premenstrual phase of the menstrual cycle.

In cases of heavy bleeding, dilatation and curettage, or "D and C," may be required. The removal of the uterus (hysterectomy)

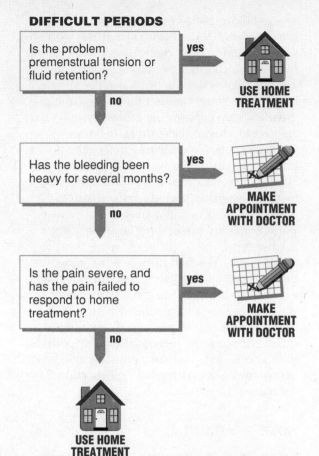

DIFFICULT PERIODS

Is the problem premenstrual tension or fluid retention?

yes → **USE HOME TREATMENT**

no ↓

Has the bleeding been heavy for several months?

yes → **MAKE APPOINTMENT WITH DOCTOR**

no ↓

Is the pain severe, and has the pain failed to respond to home treatment?

yes → **MAKE APPOINTMENT WITH DOCTOR**

no ↓

USE HOME TREATMENT

shouldn't be performed for this complaint alone. If a tumor is found, surgery will sometimes be required; but the common fibroid tumor will often stop growing by itself, and surgery may not be needed. Such tumors often grow slowly and stop growing at menopause, so an operation can be avoided by waiting. If the Pap smear is positive, however, surgery is often appropriate.

109 Missed Periods

Although pregnancy is often the first thought when a period is missed, there are many reasons for being late. Obesity, excessive dieting, strenuous exercise, and stress may cause missed or irregular periods. Diseases such as hyperthyroidism that upset the hormonal balance of the body may also be the cause of missed periods, but this is only infrequently the case. It is normal for periods to be irregular before they stop completely with menopause.

Pregnancy Tests

Testing for pregnancy has become faster, easier, and more sensitive in the last decade. Home test kits that provide a reasonable degree of accuracy are now available and may show a positive result as early as two weeks after the missed period. The most sophisticated laboratory test available through your doctor's office may turn positive within a few days after the period should have started. In both instances, a negative result is less reliable when the test is used soon after the period is missed. Thus, it is common to repeat the test after a negative result if periods don't resume.

Because a positive result is less likely to be misleading than a negative one, the rule is to believe a positive test, but not to trust a negative test until it has been repeated at least once.

Other Causes

Two opposites, obesity and starvation, often lead to irregular periods. If either of these conditions is severe and persistent, it can cause the complete cessation of periods. At the other end of the health spectrum, women who are undergoing rigorous athletic training often have irregular periods. The missed periods themselves do not harm the athlete, but there is some concern that the hormonal imbalance that causes the missed periods may also lead to loss of calcium from bones. Currently it isn't possible to determine if this poses any real risk to women athletes.

Emotional as well as physical stress may result in irregular periods. Indeed, anxiety over possible pregnancy may cause a missed period, thereby increasing the anxiety even further.

If you've reached the age when menopause is possible or likely, then this inevitable event must move to the top of your list of possible causes for the missed period. You may have already experienced some of the other symptoms of menopause. Your periods may also be irregular for a considerable time before they cease altogether. (See section S110 for more information.)

HOME TREATMENT

In this instance, home treatment consists of giving yourself some time to consider the various causes of missed periods. You can do something about obesity (see Chapter 1). If you are dieting to the point of starvation, you may have a condition known as anorexia nervosa, and you should consult a doctor or a psychotherapist. If you are following a course of strenuous physical exercise, be alert for further information concerning the possible harmful effects of hormonal imbalance associated with missed periods. Finally, knowing that emotional stress may lead to missed periods will help you focus on the cause of the stress rather than on a potential symptom.

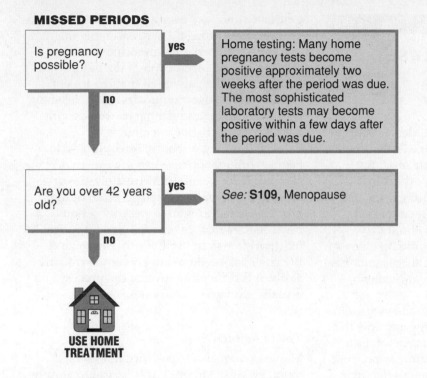

MISSED PERIODS

Is pregnancy possible? — **yes** → Home testing: Many home pregnancy tests become positive approximately two weeks after the period was due. The most sophisticated laboratory tests may become positive within a few days after the period was due.

no ↓

Are you over 42 years old? — **yes** → *See:* **S109,** Menopause

no ↓

USE HOME TREATMENT

If you feel that there is no satisfactory explanation for the missed period or are unable to develop a plan for dealing with the cause on your own, a phone call to your doctor should provide the advice you need.

WHAT TO EXPECT AT THE DOCTOR'S OFFICE

Because diseases are relatively infrequent causes of missed periods, most doctors won't rush into a series of tests in an effort to detect these diseases. The doctor will consider the common causes of missed periods discussed above; this is best done with a careful history and physical examination. If pregnancy is the only real possibility, the doctor may refer you by phone to the laboratory for a pregnancy test so that you can avoid an unnecessary office visit.

110 Menopause

The anthropologist Margaret Mead once said, "The most creative force in the world is the menopausal woman with zest." But many premenopausal women expect that menopause will be a time of difficulties and unhappiness. Understanding menopausal changes and what you can do about the problems that may come up is the best way to minimize the negative side of the menopause. You may even find that, on balance, menopause is a positive experience.

Menopause occurs because the ovaries' production of estrogen and progesterone, the female hormones, is greatly decreased quite suddenly. The ovaries do continue to produce low levels of androgens, hormones that help maintain muscle strength and sexual drive. The decrease in estrogen is responsible for the menopausal changes of most concern.

Changes in the Body

Menstrual periods usually become lighter and irregular before they stop altogether. The end of menstrual periods also means the end of fertility and with it the need for any form of contraception. These menopausal events are the ones most often considered to be positive.

Hot flashes — sudden feelings of intense heat usually lasting for two or three minutes — are most likely to occur in the evening but may happen at any time of the day. They may be aggravated by caffeine or alcohol, and some doctors believe they are lessened by exercise. For most women, hot flashes gradually decrease over a period of about two years and eventually disappear altogether.

Estrogen hormones are responsible for stimulating the production of the natural lubricants in the vagina, so that the loss of estrogen can cause vaginal dryness. This may lead to irritation and itching as well as soreness during and after intercourse.

The thinning of bones, osteoporosis, that begins with menopause usually causes no symptoms for years. Unfortunately, the first symptom is usually a fracture, often of the hip. These fractures are especially serious because they may cause prolonged physical inactivity, a risk in itself. Furthermore, once the bone has become thin enough to fracture easily, it is difficult to reverse the process and actually strengthen the bones.

The Emotional Side

Many women also experience unexpected mood swings. Although it is logical to assume that these changes are also related to the decrease in hormone production, the link is less clear than with other menopausal changes. More important, there seems to be an important difference between the mood changes that are actually experienced by women during menopause and those anticipated by premenopausal women. Many people, including men, expect that menopause will be characterized by unhappy and angry moods that come without warning and can't be avoided or improved.

In fact, the medical literature suggests that the mood changes aren't necessarily unpleasant, just unexpected. For example, a feeling of wakefulness in the middle of the night may be unusual for an individual but not uncomfortable; however, it might cause some worry if it isn't understood as a normal

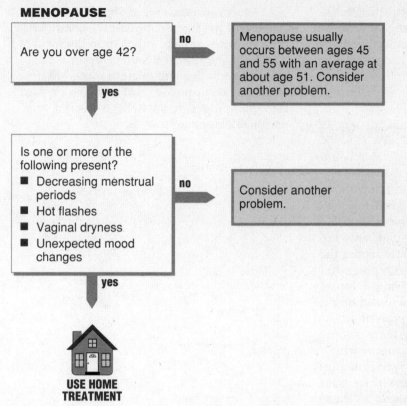

MENOPAUSE

Are you over age 42?

→ no → Menopause usually occurs between ages 45 and 55 with an average at about age 51. Consider another problem.

↓ yes

Is one or more of the following present?
- Decreasing menstrual periods
- Hot flashes
- Vaginal dryness
- Unexpected mood changes

→ no → Consider another problem.

↓ yes

USE HOME TREATMENT

part of the menopause. Most experts now believe that the menopause itself isn't a cause of depression.

Aging and wrinkling of the skin can't be blamed on menopause. Exposure to the sun and smoking are the most significant negative influences on the health of your skin.

HOME TREATMENT

Keeping cool is the rule for hot flashes. Keep the home or office cool, dress lightly, drink plenty of water. Go easy on alcohol and caffeine, and maintain a regular exercise program. You don't have a fever, so there's no need for medicines such as acetaminophen or aspirin.

Lubricants such as water-based gels (Lubifax, K-Y, etc.), unscented creams (Albolene, etc.), or a host of over-the-counter preparations (Lubrin, etc.) provide relief from vaginal dryness for many women. Many women also find that regular sexual activity actually decreases the problem of soreness with intercourse.

Regular exercise and adequate calcium in the diet are important in preventing osteoporosis. A regular aerobic exercise program (30 minutes a day, 4 days a week) is the foundation of a good program, but all types of activity — walking, climbing stairs rather than riding the elevator, and the like — will help maintain strong bones. Some studies have shown that the usual loss of calcium over these years can be almost entirely blocked by weight-bearing exercise. Swimming probably doesn't help.

Current recommendations are for post-menopausal women to obtain 1,200 to 1,500 mg of calcium per day. This is the equivalent of a quart (1 l) of skim milk. A calcium supplement may be needed if the required amount can't be obtained through dairy products.

Finally, understanding and acceptance of the unexpected mood changes is the best approach to these events.

Hot flashes, vaginal dryness, and osteo-porosis can be treated with estrogen. Such treatment requires a doctor's prescription and some careful consideration by you before you request or accept such a prescription.

WHAT TO EXPECT AT THE DOCTOR'S OFFICE

The doctor will interview and examine you to confirm that the symptoms are associated with menopause. The major question will then be whether to use estrogen replacement therapy. Current research suggests that pills consisting of estrogen alone may increase the risk of uterine cancer very slightly so that the estrogen should be combined with progestin, a chemical like progesterone. Such combina-tions appear to eliminate the increased uterine cancer risk and might even be protection against breast cancer. However, there is some indication that this combination approach might increase the risk of high blood pressure, heart disease, and stroke, and that there is an interaction with smoking that increases these risks dramatically. A careful discussion of these risks with your doctor is required before you embark on estrogen replacement; most doctors believe the risks are minimal. Many doctors recommend estrogen skin patches, which have a low dose and appear to have very few side effects; some of these may not have enough estrogen to strengthen the bones. Remember that estrogen replacement therapy won't make you young again or prevent aging.

Vaginal dryness can be treated with vaginal creams or suppositories that contain estrogen. This is effective, and because only a very little of the estrogen is absorbed, it may be a safer way of using estrogen for this problem than the taking of pills.

Osteoporosis is a more difficult question because of the silent nature of the condition until it causes a major problem in the form of a fracture. Almost all doctors emphasize exercise and adequate calcium intake. Many recommend supplements of estrogen or estrogen/progestin. We believe this is a reasonable approach.

CHAPTER 10

Sexual Problems and Questions

SEXUALLY TRANSMITTED DISEASES

If you think you might have a sexually transmitted disease (STD), you need the help of the doctor. The only noteworthy exception to this rule is when you are sure that you have genital herpes and you have chosen to manage the problem without the use of acyclovir **(S111).** Other than this, home treatment consists of prevention only. Consult Table 8 for further information.

TABLE 8 *Sexually Transmitted Diseases*

Disease	Type of Infection	Symptoms	Diagnosis
Chlamydia	Bacterial	When present, symptoms similar to those of gonorrhea	Microscopic examination of vaginal discharge; culture
Genital warts	Virus	Small, fleshy growths, called "condylomas," in the genital or anal area; soft, reddish internal growths; firmer, darker external growths	Physical examination
Pubic lice	Parasite	Itching that is worse at night; lice visible in pubic hair; eggs, called "nits," attached to pubic hair	Physical examination
AIDS (acquired immunodeficiency syndrome)	Virus	Unusual susceptibility to illness; development of rare, opportunistic diseases; persistent fatigue; fever; night sweats; unexplained weight loss; swollen glands; persistent diarrhea; dry cough	Blood test to check for antibodies to the AIDS virus; medical history
Gonorrhea	Bacterial	Males — discharge from penis, burning upon urination. Females — usually none; sometimes vaginal discharge and abdominal discomfort	Microscopic examination of vaginal discharge or culture from a suspected infection
Syphilis	Bacterial	Initially a sore called a "chancre," usually located in the genital or anal area, or mouth; later a rash, slight fever, and swollen joints	Examination of fluid from a chancre; blood test
Genital herpes	Virus	Painful sores, or blisters, in the genital area; sometimes fever, enlarged lymph glands, and flulike illness; sores heal, but tend to recur	Physical examination; Pap smear; laboratory tests

TABLE 8 *Sexually Transmitted Diseases*

Disease	Treatment	Special Concerns
Chlamydia	Can be cured with antibiotics	Chlamydia that is not cured can lead to pelvic inflammatory disease, infertility in women, and complications in pregnancy
Genital warts	Large condylomas may be removed surgically or burned off with caustic preparation	Genital warts can recur following treatment
Pubic lice	Medication is given to kill lice	None
AIDS (acquired immunodeficiency syndrome)	Several drugs now available can help fight the virus and slow the progression; there is no cure and no vaccine	AIDS is a fatal illness. AIDS-related complex, a less serious set of symptoms, will generally develop into AIDS over time.
Gonorrhea	Can be cured with antibiotics	If left untreated, gonorrhea can develop into a severe pelvic inflammation — a serious condition in women — or cause infertility, arthritis, or other problems
Syphilis	Penicillin or other antibiotics are given	If syphilis is not treated, it can cause severe problems many years later, including blindness, brain damage, and heart disease, as well as birth defects in the children of infected mothers
Genital herpes	Medications can ease symptoms, but there is no cure	Genital herpes is most contagious during an outbreak. Avoid sexual contact at these times. Genital herpes can cause complications during pregnancy and may be passed on to an infant during vaginal birth, so a cesarean delivery may be advised.

111 Genital Herpes Infections

Herpes infections of the genitalia (herpes progenitalis) are well on their way to occupying a major place in medicine. An estimated 20 million Americans have a recurrent problem with herpes.

There are two types of herpes simplex virus. Infections of the genitalia are usually caused by type 2 but may be due to type 1, especially in children. Herpes type 1 is responsible for the all-too-frequent fever blisters and cold sores of the lips and mouth (see Mouth Sores, S35). Whereas type 1 infections are usually spread by kissing and other similar contact, herpes type 2 infections are almost always spread by sexual contact. The virus takes up a permanent home in about one-third of the people it infects and causes recurrent outbreaks of painful, red blisters. These recurrences may be triggered by other illnesses, trauma, or emotional distress. The blisters usually last from five to ten days.

Not Infecting Others

Herpes is most contagious during and just before the period when the blisters are present. Many people with recurrent herpes can tell a day or two before an outbreak actually occurs. They develop an itchy or tingling feeling called a prodrome. The key to preventing transmission of herpes is to avoid sexual contact when the prodrome or blisters are present. Condoms probably give some protection against transmitting the disease but may be painful when sores are present, and they aren't complete protection.

Medication

There is no drug that cures herpes, but acyclovir (Zovirax) ointment may make an initial attack go away in 10 to 12 days rather than 14 to 16 days with no treatment. Recurrent attacks seem resistant to the ointment.

Oral acyclovir also speeds healing of initial attacks but is somewhat less effective with a recurrence. It will decrease the number and severity of recurrences if taken continuously, but attacks return when the drug is stopped, sometimes worse than before. Oral acyclovir is associated with side effects including nausea, vomiting, diarrhea, dizziness, joint pain, rash, and fever.

Dangers of Herpes

The painful, reddened, grouped blisters of herpes are seldom mistaken for the painless shallow ulceration (chancre) that is the initial sign of syphilis. However, if you are unsure, a call or a visit to your doctor may be necessary.

Herpes infections are associated with cancer of the cervix, but it isn't known if herpes causes this cancer. If you have recurrent herpes infections, this is another reason for a Pap smear. (Pap smears should be part of your health care routine anyway.)

HOME TREATMENT

The painful truth is that the treatment of herpes primarily consists of "grin and bear it." Various salves such as calamine lotion, alcohol, and ether have been tried; they may provide some relief in individual cases but none have been remarkably successful. A hot bath for five to ten minutes can inactivate the virus and seems to speed healing. We think that preventing the spread of herpes as indicated above should be a major concern.

Some people believe that reducing stress and anxiety may be helpful. This is one of the

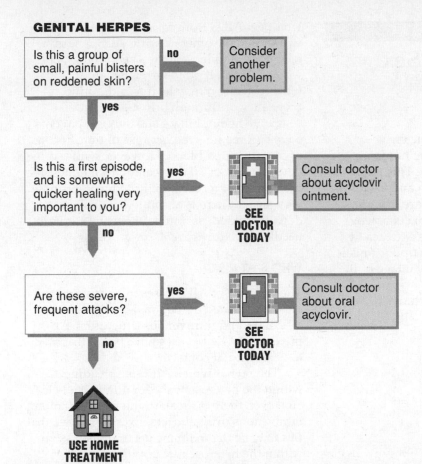

GENITAL HERPES

Is this a group of small, painful blisters on reddened skin? — **no** → Consider another problem.

↓ **yes**

Is this a first episode, and is somewhat quicker healing very important to you? — **yes** → **SEE DOCTOR TODAY** → Consult doctor about acyclovir ointment.

↓ **no**

Are these severe, frequent attacks? — **yes** → **SEE DOCTOR TODAY** → Consult doctor about oral acyclovir.

↓ **no**

USE HOME TREATMENT

approaches advocated by HELP, a program of the American Social Health Association that provides personal support:

- HELP
  American Social Health Association
  P.O. Box 100
  Palo Alto, California 94302

If the problem lasts for more than two weeks or you are unsure of the diagnosis, a call or visit to the doctor is called for.

WHAT TO EXPECT AT THE DOCTOR'S OFFICE

The history will focus on recurrences, possible exposure to herpes and other venereal diseases, and how the blisters developed. On occasion a microscopic examination of material scraped from the bottom of a blister will be made, but this is usually not necessary. If herpes is diagnosed, treatment for a first attack may include acyclovir ointment. If there are recurrent attacks, the problem is probably severe enough to warrant the risks associated with oral acyclovir.

AIDS and Safer Sex

AIDS (acquired immunodeficiency syndrome) is caused by the human immunodeficiency virus (HIV). This virus suppresses the immune system and leaves the body susceptible to normally rare disorders, including the type of pneumonia characterized as pneumocystis, Kaposi's sarcoma (a form of skin cancer), and other opportunistic diseases (diseases that take advantage of the body's low immune defenses).

The symptoms of AIDS include:

- Persistent fatigue
- Unexplained fever
- Drenching night sweats
- Unexplained weight loss
- Swollen glands
- Persistent diarrhea
- Dry cough

However, it can take many years before any of these symptoms appear.

MODES OF TRANSMISSION

HIV is transmitted through sexual intercourse — oral, vaginal, or anal — when semen or vaginal fluids are exchanged. The virus finds an entry into the bloodstream, usually through a tear in the mucous membrane.

A second mode of transmission is through sharing needles or syringes with an infected person.

HIV has not been shown to be spread from saliva, sweat, tears, urine, or feces. You won't get AIDS from casual contact, such as working with someone with AIDS. A kiss, a telephone, a toilet seat, or a swimming pool won't spread HIV. However, babies of infected women may be infected during pregnancy or through breast-feeding.

Some hemophiliacs and surgical patients have become infected because of transfusions of contaminated blood. However, with the development of HIV screening techniques, the probability of receiving infected blood is now very small. There is absolutely no risk in donating blood, assuming the usual sterile needle procedures are used.

WHO'S AT RISK?

The majority of AIDS cases in North America are concentrated among male homosexuals, bisexuals, and intravenous drug users. Approximately 4% of cases have been attributed to heterosexual contact.

The rate at which AIDS is spreading within the heterosexual community isn't clear. However, there is an alarming increase among intravenous drug abusers. Experts believe that this may be the main means of transmission within the heterosexual population in the future. It is important to stress that though AIDS has been predominant in certain groups (that is, gay men and intravenous drug abusers), it's not who you are, it's what you do, that increases your risk of infection. Casual sex, whether homosexual or heterosexual, is the biggest threat for most people. Having sex with many different people can be very dangerous, even when condoms are used. Therefore, reducing risky behavior is the first step to preventing and controlling the spread of AIDS.

Especially risky behaviors are the following:

- Having sex with multiple partners

- Sharing drug needles and syringes
- Anal sex with or without a condom
- Vaginal or oral sex with someone who shoots drugs or engages in anal sex
- Sex with a stranger (pick-up or prostitute) or with someone who is known to have multiple sex partners
- Vaginal sex without a condom when there is any chance the other person is infected with HIV

AIDS TESTING

Here are some ground rules for AIDS testing.

WHO: Men or women who have had sex with many partners or with prostitutes, who use intravenous drugs, who have gonorrhea or syphilis, who have had sex with anyone who has engaged in these behaviors, or who have received a blood transfusion or blood products between 1978 and 1985.

WHEN: Every three to six months for as long as the behavior creating the risk continues.

WHY: To detect infection with HIV. If you test positive, there are treatments that can reduce the risks of complications in some patients.

Current tests for AIDS, made with a sample of blood, are not able to identify HIV. Rather, they look for antibodies manufactured by the body in response to the infection. The standard screening test is the enzyme-linked immunosorbent assay, or ELISA. When an ELISA is positive, the finding is always confirmed with the more accurate, more expensive test known as the Western Blot.

Although these tests accurately diagnose HIV infection in high-risk groups, their performance is erratic in populations that aren't at high risk. A study conducted by the Congressional Office of Technology Assessment found that when HIV-antibody tests are performed under ideal conditions, fully one-third of the positive results in a low-risk group — such as blood donors from downstate Illinois — could be expected to be falsely positive. Worse, if the test conditions resembled those that actually prevail in U.S. laboratories, almost nine out of ten positive tests in this low-risk group would be false positives.

AIDS testing is further complicated by a number of other issues. Testing needs to be accompanied by counseling with respect to prevention of AIDS as well as interpretation of results. Keeping results confidential may require special strategies, but notification of sexual partners is essential when results are positive.

PREVENTING AIDS

Currently a number of researchers are testing AIDS vaccines. However, a vaccine for mass inoculation isn't on the immediate horizon. Some experts believe that it may be extremely difficult to provide an effective vaccine because HIV is a retrovirus. This means that it periodically changes its genetic code, thus requiring a different vaccine for each new strain.

Therefore, the primary means of prevention are:

- Celibacy — not having sex
- Maintaining a monogamous relationship with an uninfected person
- Practicing safer sex in relationships where risk of infection is possible
- Not sharing needles and/or syringes, or better yet not shooting drugs

The risk of AIDS is somewhat decreased by using a latex condom; wear the condom for a time before and after oral, anal, and vaginal intercourse, as well as during. Safety is increased by using a water-based lubricant such as K-Y jelly, Gynol II, Today, or Corn Husker's Lotion. Don't use petroleum jelly, cold cream, or baby oil as a lubricant. These products weaken the latex and can cause it to break.

A recent study has shown that the use of a spermicide containing nonoxynol-9 in conjunction with a condom may provide further protection from HIV infection if the condom breaks.

TREATMENT

Currently being tested are more than 70 drugs that are designed to slow or stop the AIDS virus or to help bolster the body's immune response. To date, zidovudine (AZT) is the most widely used drug and has shown some positive results in extending the longevity of AIDS sufferers and preventing HIV-infected pregnant women from passing the virus to their infants. Two newer drugs that have substantial promise are ddI and ddC. However, there is no cure. Drugs like Septra and inhaled pentamidine can reduce the frequency of some AIDS infections.

For the foreseeable future, the best way to prevent AIDS is to avoid risky behavior and practice safer sex when in doubt of your partner's status. Individuals who engage in risky behavior should consider having a blood test to detect the presence of HIV antibodies. Confidential HIV testing is offered through county health departments, hospitals, blood banks, sexually transmitted disease clinics, and your personal doctor.

PREVENTION OF OTHER SEXUALLY TRANSMITTED DISEASES (STDS)

The rules for AIDS prevention also decrease the risk of developing other STDs. Again, the effectiveness of condoms as a barrier to infection is not complete but can be substantial if properly used.

Preventing Unwanted Pregnancy

Every woman must decide to abstain from sex, have babies, or use a contraceptive technique. Ideally, the male partner participates in this decision, but through a well-known quirk of nature he doesn't participate in the most direct consequences. This chapter is concerned with the medical considerations involved in making decisions about contraception and childbearing. These decisions have a major effect on your health, both directly and indirectly, whether you are male or female. Childbearing and every form of contraception have definite risks.

Few women will pursue one course of action for all their childbearing years. Not having sex is most effective but will be a reasonable choice for only a few people. For most it is neither a practical nor healthy suggestion. The majority of women employ some form of contraception except for specific times when they are attempting to get pregnant or aren't engaging in sexual intercourse. Choosing a method of contraception is one of the most intensely personal decisions you will make, and the rest of us should respect your right to make up your own mind. Ideally, your choice depends on you and your partner.

FORMS OF CONTRACEPTION

Here are brief descriptions of the most popular forms of contraception:

Surgeries. If you are sure that you don't want any more children, the safest methods for ensuring this are surgeries. Women can have their fallopian tubes tied (tubal ligation), preventing sperm from reaching their eggs. Men can have a vasectomy operation, which keeps sperm out of their semen. Neither surgery interferes with sexual performance or pleasure.

Birth-control hormones. Birth control pills ("the pill"), Depo-Provera, and Norplant are the most common medications taken by women to prevent pregnancy.

Birth control pills use hormones to prevent pregnancy and must be taken on a daily basis. When used correctly they are very effective in preventing pregnancy. However, the pill may cause blood clots, which have been fatal on occasion. It may also contribute to high blood pressure. There are less dangerous but annoying side effects such as weight gain, nausea, fluid retention, migraine headaches, vaginal bleeding, and vaginal yeast infections.

Birth control pills can also be used as emergency contraception on "the morning after." Up to 72 hours after intercourse a woman who is worried that she may have been impregnated can take two doses of birth control pills 12 hours apart. This will reduce her chance of becoming pregnant by at least 75%. Depending on which pill is used, each dose is two or four times the usual daily dose of birth control pills. Therefore, it is helpful to ask advice from a doctor or clinic before trying this method. Since the dosages of hormone are so much higher, side effects are more common: nausea occurs for 50 to 70% of women using this method and vomiting occurs for about 20%.

Depo-Provera is a long-lasting injection of hormones that provides contraception for about three months. Norplant provides five years of contraceptive hormones from six slender, flexible capsules surgically placed under the woman's skin — in the fleshy part of the upper arm, for instance. The capsules are designed to be removed if the woman desires, but there have been reports of problems in doing this. These options have side effects similar to birth control pills since they also depend on hormones for their effect.

Intrauterine device (IUD). This device is inserted into the uterus by a doctor and remains there until removed or expelled. If the IUD is expelled, it may not be noticed. In such cases, some pregnancies have resulted. The IUD may also cause bleeding and cramps. In rare instances, it is associated with serious infections of the uterus, although the type of IUD most frequently associated with these uterine infections — the Dalkon Shield — has been removed from the market.

Diaphragm, cervical cap, sponge. A diaphragm is a rubber membrane that fits over the opening to the uterus in the vagina. It

must be inserted before intercourse and kept in place for at least six hours afterwards. There are no side effects or complications from diaphragms. They are best used with a spermicidal foam or jelly. Cervical caps and contraceptive sponges are more sturdy variations of the diaphragm and always contain spermicide. Caps and sponges are more effective for women who have never given birth than for those who have. However, the sponge is no longer being made for the U.S. market.

Foams, jellies, and suppositories. These ointments contain chemicals that kill or immobilize the man's sperm. In the past they have been used by themselves but now are almost always used in conjunction with a diaphragm. Side effects are unusual and consist of some irritation to the walls of the vagina. Their effect lasts only about 60 minutes, and many people find these preparations inconvenient and just plain messy.

Contraceptive devices. A: Norplant; B: intrauterine device, or IUD (this figure shows a Lippes Loop; other types are available); C: female condom; D: male condom; E: diaphragm; F: cervical cap; G: contraceptive sponge.

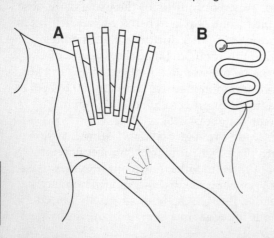
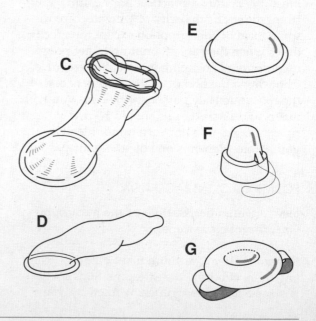

Condoms. Male condoms are enjoying a resurgence of popularity. If used correctly, latex condoms are 90% effective in preventing pregnancy. They have no side effects, and they are inexpensive and widely available. However, the male must remember to use a condom properly, and some designs decrease the male's physical sensitivity. Female condoms have been used less but appear to have similar advantages and disadvantages. Condoms are the only form of birth control to give substantial protection against sexually transmitted diseases, including AIDS. They work best when used with a spermicide.

Periodic abstinence. In this technique the couple avoids intercourse during the time when they expect the woman to ovulate. Such techniques are often taught as "natural family planning," and are preferred by many couples with a religious or moral dislike for other forms of birth control. The "rhythm method" requires the woman to have fairly regular periods and to carefully take daily temperatures in order to predict the time of ovulation. Under the best of circumstances, it is only moderately effective. More recently developed techniques based on frequent measurement of the acidity of the cervical mucus are a slight improvement. All such methods require highly motivated people to make them work.

Finally, we will mention two actions that reduce the chance of pregnancy somewhat, but in the long run aren't reliable enough to prevent it. In withdrawal (coitus interruptus) the male removes his penis from the vagina just before ejaculation. Because there are sperm present in the secretions of the penis *before* ejaculation occurs and because withdrawal at just the right time is a tricky business at best, this method rather frequently fails. Douching after intercourse also de-

TABLE 9

Effectiveness of Contraceptive Methods

Percentage of women who become pregnant during the first year of using each contraceptive method (the lower the number, the more effective the method)

Method	Typical Use	Perfect Use
No contraception	85%	85%
Spermicides only	21	6
Periodic abstinence	20	4*
Withdrawal	19	4
Cervical cap women who have never given birth	18	9
women who have given birth	36	26
Sponge women who have never given birth	18	9
women who have given birth	36	20
Diaphragm	18	6
Female condom	21	5
Male condom	12	3
Pill	3	0.3*
IUD	1*	0.6*
Female sterilization	0.4	0.4
Depo-Provera	0.3	0.3
Male sterilization	0.2	0.1
Norplant (6 capsules)	0.1	0.1

* This number is an average of the percentages produced by different methods within this category.

creases the number of sperm in the vagina, but it too is far from reliable.

Relative Risks

Table 10 presents information on the risks women face in using different forms of birth control or no birth control at all (thus increasing the chance that they become pregnant). The risks in Table 10 were calculated by measuring both the number of women who died during childbirth after trying contraception and the number who died from fatal complications of their contraceptive method. The higher the number, the greater the risk. (Note, however, that even the most hazardous action — smoking and taking birth control pills — resulted in death less than 1% of the time; the more frequent complication of poor birth control choice is having an unwanted child.)

Note the results:

- The risk to women who smoke and take birth control pills is substantially higher than the risk to nonsmokers — yet another good reason to stop smoking.

- Unprotected intercourse is one of the most hazardous choices women can make because of the death rates associated with pregnancy or childbirth.

- The least hazardous birth control techniques for women, aside from sterilization, require that abortion be available.

As far as your health is concerned, you might consider "mechanical" forms of contraception (IUD, condom, diaphragm with foam) and assure yourself of access to facilities for abortion. We present this information not to promote any particular method, but to ensure that you can make an informed decision. To risk your health without knowing it is the only bad choice.

TABLE 10

Safety of Contraceptive Methods

Number of women out of 100,000 aged 15 to 44 who died as a result of the side effects of each contraceptive method or of becoming pregnant while using that contraceptive method (the lower the number, the safer the method)

Pill (for smokers)	977
No birth control	462
Pill (for nonsmokers)	251
Periodic abstinence	68
Diaphragm and spermicide	53
IUD	45
Abortion	41
Condom	23
Condom and abortion	1

Please note: If a birth control method in table 9 does not appear in Table 10, it does not mean that the method is free from safety risks. It simply means that not enough research data exist to provide useful risk statistics.

DECIDING TO GIVE BIRTH

You may decide to become pregnant for the best of reasons — your own reasons. One of the most popular reasons to have sex without birth control is that you wish to raise a family, a desire that can easily outweigh the health risks. Many women have ethical or religious objections to abortion — or to other forms of contraception, for that matter. A pregnant woman who won't be able to care for her baby but can't accept an abortion has the option of allowing the newborn to be adopted.

Another common reason not to use contraception is simply not wanting to bother with it. Remember that deciding to have sex without birth control is, over the long run, the same as deciding to become pregnant.

In any case, a woman who chooses to give birth to a child deserves good medical care. This lowers the health risks of pregnancy and childbirth and provides for a healthier, happier baby. We and Dr. Robert Pantell discuss pregnancy and birth in detail in *Taking Care of Your Child.*

Questions About Sex

We all feel some insecurity about sex. Every person has anxieties and fears; everyone thinks that friends and colleagues are free from such problems. There are no experts in what sex means for you individually. No personal experience can constitute both a broad sampling of individual differences and probe the depths of a long-standing, profoundly intimate relationship. Because everyone knows only his or her own activities, and for the most part imagines what others are up to, myths abound.

Each generation and most people discover anew the exhilaration of a good sexual experience. In a perverse game played among the generations, a variety of contradictory rules for sexual relationships are dogmatically advocated. Accusations are formulated, anxieties created, and health disturbed.

Good feelings are what sex is all about. But the good feelings go beyond the pleasurable physical sensations of sexual arousal. Feeling good about yourself, your partner, intimacy — these are feelings you need for sex to be its most satisfying and pleasurable. A number of factors may undercut these good feelings, but only a few are related to sexual function itself. Anxiety or depression from any cause may result in problems with sex.

MYTHS AND ANXIETIES

Attitudes toward sex create problems, usually unnecessarily. We should expect anxiety about sex, especially in the learning stage, because it is a universal phenomenon. But this normal anxiety has been made worse by the two dominant approaches toward sex today.

The first approach considers sex as unspeakable. Some people thus develop moralistic fantasies that they feel they should suppress by will power, but can't. If you avoid feeling guilty about your natural fantasies, you promote your sexual health. The second approach occurs when a person views a sexual partner as an orgasm machine and becomes preoccupied with technique rather than feeling. The result is a depersonalized sexual relationship. Between them, these attitudes have given rise to many myths about sex without allowing sensible answers to be discussed.

Virility is one major area of myth. We frequently encounter patients who have fears that they have sex too often, or not often enough. Part of this problem stems from publicity about large-scale sex surveys and the average figures they report. People who find that their practices are far from the averages are often concerned. Relax. People can have healthy sex eight times a day or eight times a year. The only rule worth remembering is that in a stable relationship, the frequency of sexual activity should be a workable compromise between the partners.

Another area of anxiety concerns the sexual equipment. Men worry about the size of their penis. Women worry that their breasts are too big or too small, their legs too fat or too thin. Men worry about a pigeon chest, no hair on their chest, or too much hair on their chest. Women are concerned that their hair doesn't properly frame their face, that they have hairs around the nipples, or that their total image is too dowdy, too awkward, or too cheap. There is little worthwhile in such concerns.

Some individuals are more attractive than others. Some are more sensual than others.

However, the breadth of taste runs from thick to thin. Somebody likes you the way you are. Men may like large women or slender women who wear clothes well. Women may be excited by broad shoulders or by a thoughtful gesture. Whether this whole business is due to cultural indoctrination or to innate differences between individuals, the point is the same. Usually, the sexual equipment is the least important part of the problem! If you fear that you weren't created as the most attractive of creatures to the opposite sex, you will find that this obstacle can be reduced by warmth, affection, and humanity. In sex, how you feel about each other is more important than how you feel to each other.

The man frequently worries unnecessarily about penis size. In fact, there is little difference in size of the erect penis among different men, although there are significant differences in the resting state. Moreover, the vaginal canal, which accommodates birth, is potentially much larger than the thickest of penises. The size and rigidity of the penis will vary for the same man at different times. Some factors affecting erect penile size are physical — such as the length of time since previous intercourse — and some are psychological.

Impotence, or the inability of a man to have an erection, is seldom due to disease of genitalia, nerves, or blood vessels. No male is equally potent at all times, and all males are, on some occasions, impotent. Chronic impotence implies chronic anxiety, at least partially compounded by worry over the impotence.

Premature ejaculation refers to when a man ejaculates earlier in the sex act than is convenient or desired. While physically the opposite of impotence, it has the same cause: anxiety. Again, relaxation is usually a solution. There are some other potential aids.

A firm pinch on the tip of the penis will delay ejaculation. A condom usually decreases sensation so that ejaculation is delayed. Seldom are such measures necessary for more than a few occasions.

Female orgasm is the most written-about sexual phenomenon in recent years. This subject has been linked inseparably to aspects of the women's movement. It has been held that equality of orgasm is a principal requirement for sexual equality. It has been pointed out that some women may climax several times during a single intercourse, while men do so once. On the other hand, it has been observed that a large number of women don't have orgasms with regularity. The emerging sexual myth is that these women are in some way abnormal.

In fact, many women relating deep and satisfactory sexual experiences don't report frequent orgasms as a significant feature. If you let others tell you what you should be doing and then allow guilt to develop when you don't meet false "norms," you are promoting these myths. Of all human activities, sexual activity, more than any other, should be directed by the individual at his or her own pace and style.

SEXUAL PRACTICES

A variety of sexual practices have been recently reemphasized. These include sex with the aid of various appliances, oral sex, and sex in a virtual infinity of positions. Medically, there is no reason to either encourage or discourage sexual variety and experimentation. Such practices are recorded in all eras of human literature. Until recently advocates of sexual variety were discouraged by legal and ethical barriers. Now, in response to the fall of those barriers, people report the opposite problem: they feel guilty when their sex life doesn't have enough variety. Not everyone must conform to a hedonistic norm.

For example, the majority of heterosexual activity takes place in the "male-on-top" position. This position is often the most satisfactory for both partners because it allows the deepest penetration and the sensitivity value of being face to face. Recent ridicule of this technique as the "missionary position" illustrates ignorance of history and anatomy. The accusatory tone of the phrase suggests an attempt to make people feel guilt and anxiety about a normal practice.

Other individuals, for equally good reasons, prefer many different positions or find their greatest satisfaction with a particular alternative technique. There is no right way and no standard pattern for sexual expression. Averages are meaningless in a personal relationship between two individuals. Such relationships may be physically expressed in a wide variety of ways, none of which are any better than the others. You have personal freedom to be either ordinary or exotic — with pleasure, and without guilt.

There are sexual practices that do have risk, of course. Having multiple partners increases your risk of all sexually transmitted diseases, including AIDS. That risk is raised when you select these partners indiscriminately or when you have sex with those who are indiscriminate (such as prostitutes). Finally, anal sex increases the risk of AIDS transmission. The current public discussions of safer sex emphasize these points and the methods by which you may protect yourself (see pages 322–324).

Sex is not a competitive sport. Sexual health, for the great majority of individuals, comes down to common sense. If it feels good to both partners, do it. If it doesn't feel good, don't do it. Don't allow the fear of being "hung up" to become the major hang-up.

Individuals shouldn't allow other individuals, equally nonexpert, to define their satisfaction for them. There remain "different strokes for different folks."

PART III

Managing Your Professional Medical Care

CHAPTER 11

Working With Your Doctor and Your Health Care System

You should have one personal doctor in whom you trust and confide. This doctor should be your advocate and your guide through the complicated medical care system. You may require an additional consulting doctor from time to time, and your personal doctor should interpret and coordinate that consultant's recommendations. Good medical care usually doesn't result from having a different doctor for every organ of your body. Having too many doctors working in an uncoordinated manner often results in too many medications, too many medical procedures, too many side effects, and sometimes in opposing approaches to treatment. Your personal doctor doesn't need to be an expert in everything; he or she should readily seek advice from others when needed and guide you to other appropriate health professionals. But someone has to view the whole picture, to know everything that's going on. Someone needs to take responsibility for putting all the information together and making sure that nothing has been left out.

Finding the Right Doctor

What kind of doctor should your personal doctor be? He or she might appropriately be a:

- **Family practitioner** — specialist in family medicine
- **Internist** — specialist in internal medicine
- **Gynecologist** — specialist in female medicine or health
- **Geriatrician** — specialist in the medical care of older people

The family practitioner and the general internist are trained in dealing with the "whole patient" and in appropriate use of other consultants as required. Geriatrics is a relatively new specialty with practice limited to the senior population, and its practitioners take pride in recognizing the needs of the whole patient as well. Most internal medicine problems now occur after the age of 65, so the general internist has also become, in large part, a geriatrician.

If you have a particular major disease, such as heart disease or rheumatoid arthritis, it may be inefficient to have a general doctor who must frequently refer you to a specialist. See if it's possible for the specialist to serve as your primary doctor. As noted above, it's not a good idea to have two or more primary doctors at the same time.

The most important qualities that you want in a primary care doctor center around *communication* and *anticipation*. Communication is the human side of medicine. A good primary physician:

- **Takes time to listen.** You can help your doctor by explaining your problems clearly.
- **Takes time to talk with you.** The doctor will explain his or her suggested course of action clearly.
- **Plans ahead to prevent problems.** A substantial part of your conversation should be about how to prevent future illnesses. Problems will be anticipated and plans made before the problems become severe.
- **Reviews your total health program regularly.**
- **Has your trust and confidence.** If you can't communicate with your doctor, try another. Often two people just happen to operate on different frequencies. You want to keep the same doctor for a long time, so if a relationship with a particular doctor isn't working, find a new one early on. When you find the right doctor, stay with him or her unless there's a substantial change in your medical needs and you require a doctor with different skills.
- **Is available by telephone.** Simple questions can often be answered by phone. And you don't want to make a doctor visit just to get a prescription refilled.
- **Makes house calls.** This service is hard to find these days, but if available it's a plus.

There's a technical side of medicine too, and for some individuals this will represent the most important part of modern medicine. Perhaps you need an operation on your blood vessels or your brain. Perhaps you need surgery inside your middle ear. Perhaps you need replacement of your hip joint, kidney dialysis, or even an organ transplant. In these situations your standards for excellence in your consulting doctor are a little different.

You're still interested in anticipation and communication, but you also want to pay a great deal of attention to the *technical skill* of the individual.

You'd like to know if a particular surgeon, for example, gets better or worse results than average. This is often a little hard to judge, but there are two key tests you can apply.

- Does the specialist have the complete confidence and approval of your primary doctor? Talk with your primary doctor about possible alternative physicians, and ask about the advantages and disadvantages of each.

- Ask how frequently the specialist performs the particular procedure. Technical results are generally better at institutions and with doctors who perform a technical procedure frequently. As a general rule, results are substantially better where the procedure is done at least 50 times each year, and are not as good where the procedure is done only occasionally.

These considerations don't apply only to surgical specialists. Increasingly the line between surgery and medicine has blurred. There are now "invasive cardiologists" who perform marvelous but sometimes hazardous tasks using long tubes manipulated through your blood vessels under X-ray control. The gastrointestinal "endoscopist" can now use long, flexible, lighted tubes to look at (and sometimes treat) a surprising amount of your insides from the outside. An arthroscopist can perform surgery inside a joint, needing only a small cut in the skin to admit a lighted tube with which to see the joint's interior. Arteriographers, often radiologists, use dye injected through long catheters to visualize your blood vessels on X-ray film. New imaging techniques include computed axial tomography (CT or CAT scans) and magnetic resonance imagery (MR or MRI). These techniques require skill both for performing the procedure and for interpretation of the results. Again, apply your two tests. Does the specialist who will do the procedure have the full agreement and confidence of your primary doctor? Does the specialist perform the procedure frequently?

Communicating with Your Doctor

You and your doctor must be able to listen, explain, ask questions, understand each other, and choose options wisely. Put simply, you and your doctor must be able to talk and work together as partners.

THE MEDICAL HISTORY

When you visit your doctor, it's essential for you to give a concise, organized description of your illness. Tell it like it is. If you want to report a sexual problem, don't say that you're "tired and run down." If you're afraid that you have cancer, don't say that you came "for a checkup." Patients who ramble or don't mention their real concerns are their own worst enemies. The ability to give a good medical history helps to preserve your health and your dollars.

Most people don't realize that every doctor uses a similar process to learn a patient's medical history and to organize those facts so as to be able to remember and analyze them. Knowing that process can help you give accurate information. Your primary physician may not go through your entire medical history on a repeat visit, but doctors will do so during a first visit or a comprehensive evaluation. Be prepared to give your doctor information under these five headings.

- **Chief complaint.** After greeting you, the doctor usually asks about your chief complaint. This question may take several forms: "What bothers you the most?" "What brings you here today?" "What's the trouble?" Your answer establishes the priorities for the rest of the visit. Be sure you express your problem clearly. Know in advance how to state your chief complaint: "I have a sore throat." "I have a pain in my lower right side." "I seem to have three problems: sore throat, skin rash, and cloudy urine." Think of the chief complaint as the *title* for the story you're about to tell the doctor. Any of the problems listed in Part II may be your chief complaint, and there are hundreds of less common problems.

- **Present illness.** Next your doctor will want to hear the story behind your chief complaint: "When did this problem begin?" "When were you last entirely well?" "How long has this been going on?" Think about these questions in advance so you can give a clear answer: "Yesterday." "On June 4th." "About the middle of May." If you're uncertain about the date that the problem began, state the uncertainty and tell what you can. "I'm not sure when these problems began. I began to feel tired in the middle of February, but the pain in the joints didn't begin until April." After you define the starting point for the problem, the doctor will want to establish the sequence of events from that time until the present. Tell the story in the order it occurred. Try not to use "flashbacks" or irrelevant details; you'll only confuse yourself and your doctor. The doctor may interrupt to ask specific questions or at the end ask questions about problems that you haven't mentioned.

- **Past medical history.** Your doctor may want more background information about your general health. Information that didn't appear important earlier may be relevant. The doctor will ask specific questions about your general health, childhood illnesses, hospitalizations, operative procedures, allergies, and medications. Give direct, reasonably brief answers. If you report a drug "allergy," describe the specific reaction you experienced; many reactions to drugs (such as nausea, vomiting, or ringing in the ears) are not allergies but common side effects. Be thorough when reporting medications, including birth control pills, vitamins, pain relievers, and laxatives.

- **Review of systems.** In a complete medical exam, your doctor will usually review symptoms related to the different body systems, asking standard questions for each system.

- **Social history.** In a complete medical exam, your doctor may ask about your job, family, interpersonal stresses, smoking, drinking, use of drugs, sexual activity, even exposures to chemical or toxic substances. These questions are sometimes intensely personal. However, the answers can be of the utmost importance in determining your illness and how it can be best treated.

Supporting information can be extremely important. Know which medications you've taken before and during the course of your illness. Often it's helpful to bring the medication bottles to the doctor. Mention any allergic reactions that you have to drugs. If you're pregnant or could be pregnant, tell the doctor. If X-ray studies or laboratory tests have been performed during the course of the illness, try to make the results available to the doctor. If you've consulted other doctors, bring those medical records with you. Be a careful observer of your own illness. Your observations, carefully made and recounted, are more valuable than any other source of information.

Understanding Your Health Plan

The present variety of medical plans is somewhat bewildering. This section defines the major types of medical plans that have emerged, ranging from fee-for-service to prepayment.

"Managed care" techniques are an increasing part of all plans. In such an arrangement your care is "managed" by the health plan, which rules on whether it will pay for particular parts of your care. The health plan's representative may have to approve your surgery beforehand, or make sure that you don't stay in the hospital too long. The purpose of managed care is to save money for the health plan. It is sometimes argued that managed care improves the quality of care through its surveillance techniques and that it prevents unnecessary surgery.

- **Traditional Indemnity.** This is the traditional type of medical insurance. Your medical care charges are paid at a specified rate. Often there are deductibles (you must pay for a certain amount on your own before coverage begins) and co-payments (you must pay a certain percentage of charges up to a specified limit) as a part of these plans. Increasingly these plans include elements of managed care techniques.

- **Preferred Provider Organization (PPO).** The medical plan provides a list of "preferred doctors." If you choose one of these doctors, you'll pay less than if you choose a doctor or hospital not on the list because those on the list charge the medical plan less. Sometimes the plan may be an Exclusive Provider Organization (EPO). This is similar to a PPO except that you'll pay essentially *all* the medical costs if you don't use a doctor or hospital on the list given by the medical plan.

- **Health Maintenance Organization (HMO).** This is the original form of prepaid medical care. Virtually all HMOs today combine prepayment (sometimes called "capitation") with managed care techniques. Doctors who provide care for HMOs may be employed exclusively by the HMO or may contract to provide care for HMO patients while still providing care for patients in other medical plans. Usually HMOs won't pay for any care given by physicians or hospitals that aren't part of their HMO system except in emergencies or when you're traveling.

- **Point-of-Service Plans.** Recognizing that choice is important to many people, some plans will let you choose among plans when you go for care, i.e., at the point of service. In other words, you can wait until you need care to decide whether you'll use traditional indemnity, an EPO, or your favorite physician. However, if you choose a doctor or hospital that costs the health plan more, you will pay more. You get more freedom of choice, but at a cost.

- **Medical Savings Accounts (MSA).** These relatively new plans most often will be the least expensive for people who take care of themselves. Your insurance premium is broken into two parts. The first goes to buy an insurance policy against catastrophic illness with a high deductible, perhaps $3,000. The remainder, perhaps $2,000, goes into your medical savings account, and you use it to pay medical costs below the deductible. If you don't spend all the money in your medical savings account, you get to keep it. Be sure, however, that you don't delay care that you really need just to save money. Follow the guidelines of this book.

Getting the Most Out of Your Visit to the Doctor

ASKING QUESTIONS

To use your time with the doctor effectively, make a list of your questions before the visit. Write out your questions. Date the list. Leave space to jot down answers while you're talking with the doctor. If someone is accompanying you on the visit, perhaps he or she can write down the answers for you. Take the list to your doctor and ask each question. Go over the list and the answers again after you get home. Save the list as part of your own records. A written record can be very useful for you.

Table 11 suggests some questions that you may want to ask your doctor. As you make up your list for a particular visit, run through this list

TABLE 11   *A Question List*

General questions to ask:
- What is my problem?
- Is it a common problem?
- What does the diagnosis mean?
- What is likely to happen?
- Can you tell me what these words [any words you don't understand] mean?
- Could the problem be anything else?
- How likely is that?
- What are my options for the next step?
- What are the benefits, risks, and cost of each choice?

If the doctor suggests tests:
- What will we learn from these tests?
- Will they be uncomfortable?
- Do I need to make special arrangements (such as fasting before the test or planning transportation home)?

If the doctor suggests medication:
- How will the medication help?
- Does it have any side effects I should know about?
- Is it available in a generic form?
- Might it interact badly with other drugs or with foods?
- What can I expect in the next few weeks and also over the long term?

If the doctor suggests surgery or other medical procedures:
- What are the risks of the procedure?
- How frequently does this procedure relieve this kind of problem?
- Must the procedure be done right away? Why?
- Can this be done safely as an outpatient procedure?
- How frequently do you do this procedure?
- I would feel more comfortable with another opinion. Could you recommend someone for me to check with?

If the doctor suggests hospitalization:
- Can I have the tests or treatment done as an outpatient?
- What are the risks of being in the hospital?
- Which hospital do you suggest and why?
- Does the hospital staff perform this treatment frequently?
- Can I recover at home and shorten the hospital stay?
- What should I do at home?
- Is there anything I shouldn't do?
- When should I check back with you?
- Should I avoid aspirin for a week or more before the procedure?

and see which questions you want to include. After the table has helped you get started, think of other questions that you may also find useful; don't just limit yourself to these.

The figure below shows what your list might look like if you made a visit to Dr. Johanson because of a problem with dizziness when standing. Your questions on the left will probably be handwritten in full and the answers on the right jotted down, so this example will give you a general idea of the process.

It's not necessary to limit a valuable doctor visit to your most recent problem. You may have a lot of questions. The doctor visit is a good place to begin thinking about them, together with a knowledgeable expert. Table 12 lists a few of the subjects you may wish to discuss.

You must understand all instructions the doctor gives you. If you're confused, ask more questions: "Could you go over that again?" "I don't understand how to use this medication." "How long should I apply the ice pack?" "Are there any risks to this?" Ask your doctor to write out the instructions, or write them down yourself. Do *not* depend on your memory.

Problem List for Dr. Johanson, June 19, 1996

Questions	Answers
1. Dizziness when standing?	• Low blood pressure. Decrease Aldomet to 2/day. Will check blood counts.
2. Wonder about aspirin or fish oil capsules for heart attacks?	• Not yet. Diet first. Will check cholesterol.
3. Leg cramps?	• Warm baths and massage.
4. Gray splotches on skin?	• Just age spots — OK.
5. Move to Arizona for joint pains?	• Probably not. Try vacation to hot, dry area first; see if it feels better.
6. Cost of blood pressure pills?	• Reducing dose anyway because of dizziness. Try AARP pharmacy services.

TABLE 12

Some Subjects to Discuss

- Exercise
- Sexual problems
- Diet
- Weight
- Calcium
- Smoking
- Drug or alcohol use
- Estrogen for women after menopause
- Medication program
- Mammography for women
- Screening tests
- Any immunizations needed

Understand the importance of each drug. In some instances it doesn't matter if you take the medicine regularly because the drug gives only symptomatic relief and should be discontinued as soon as possible. Be sure that you understand whether or not it's necessary to continue the medication after you feel well.

Consider the entire prescribed program. You may already be taking medications your doctor doesn't know about. Perhaps you have trouble taking a medication at work, or you anticipate trouble with a diet the doctor prescribes. If the doctor prescribes more than one medication, you may want to take them all at once — is this okay? An upcoming trip could interfere with a treatment program, or you may worry about starting exercise in the winter. When such questions arise, ask the doctor in advance. Often if you raise these questions with your doctor, your treatment program can be modified so that you feel more comfortable. Be frank. Don't say that you'll do something that you know you won't. Express your worries. You don't have to be a "perfect" patient; it's all right to be persistent until your questions are answered.

CARRYING OUT YOUR TREATMENT PROGRAM

After you and your doctor have agreed on a program, follow it closely. If you notice possible side effects from the program, call the doctor and ask about them. If the side effects are serious, return for an examination.

Make a chart of the days of the week and the times when you are to take medications. Note on the chart when you take them; such charts are universally used in hospitals to ensure that medication schedules are maintained accurately. At home you and your family are the custodians of your health. Don't view the task of taking medication more lightly than it is viewed by professionals. More importantly, if you find that you can't carry out the program, you and your doctor must make changes.

When you have pills left over at the end of a course of therapy, flush them down the toilet. A medicine chest containing old prescription medicines presents multiple hazards. Every year children and adults die from taking leftover drugs. Children take birth control pills, adults brush their teeth with corticosteroid creams, and people take the wrong medication because they mistake one bottle for another. If, for example, you give your leftover tetracycline to your children with their next cold, you may cause mottling (gray spotting) of their teeth. Taking outdated tetracycline may cause liver damage. When a new illness occurs and you take leftover medications, your condition may then confuse your doctor; sometimes it will be impossible to make an accurate identification of a bacterium by culture, or the clinical picture of the disease may be changed by the medicine.

The doctor-patient encounter is your most reliable protection against serious illness. Value the opportunity for such attention, use it effectively, and follow the program that you and your doctor develop to the maximum extent possible.

Choosing the Right Medical Facility

HOSPITALS

The hospital is expensive. It's not a home or a hotel. Lives are saved and lost here. At some times you must use the hospital, and at other times you must avoid it. To manage these contradictions, you and your family must carefully consider the need for hospitalization in each instance.

Don't use the hospital if services can be performed elsewhere. The acute (short-term) general hospital provides acute general medicine; it doesn't perform other functions well.

Don't use the hospital for a rest; it's not a good place to go for rest. It's busy, noisy, and populated with unfamiliar roommates. Its nights are punctuated with interruptions, and it has an unusual time schedule. It has many employees, a few of whom will be less thoughtful than others.

Don't use the hospital for the "convenience" of having a number of tests done in just a few days. It doesn't provide tests in the most efficient manner; indeed, many hospital laboratories and special X-ray facilities aren't open on the weekend, and just to schedule special procedures may require several days.

In our present age, evidence suggests that for many conditions, treatment at home may work better than treatment in the hospital. Even home treatment for minor heart attacks in the elderly has been reported as possibly better than hospital treatment. It's apparent to most hospital visitors that the crisis atmosphere of the short-term acute hospital doesn't promote the calmest state of mind for the patient. Many therapeutic features of the home, such as familiar, comfortable surroundings, can't be duplicated in the hospital.

EMERGENCY ROOMS

The emergency room has become the "doctor" for many people. Those who can't find a doctor at night, or who don't know where else to go, increasingly go to emergency rooms. Thus, the typical emergency room is now filled with nonemergency cases. Various problems are all mixed together: trivial illnesses that could have been treated with the aid of this book, routine problems more easily and economically handled in a doctor's office, specialized problems that should have been dealt with at a time when the hospital facilities were fully available, and true emergencies. Although the emergency room isn't designed for the purpose it now serves, it does a surprisingly good job of delivering adequate care.

However, there are five major disadvantages to using an emergency room as your sole medical contact.

■ Emergency rooms make little or no provision for continued care. You'll usually be seen by a different doctor each time. The emergency room doctor will attend to the chief problem you report but seldom has enough time to complete a full examination or to deal with underlying problems.

■ Although simple X-ray facilities are available, procedures such as gallbladder studies and upper G.I. (gastrointestinal) series are difficult to arrange. Thus, emergency rooms aren't the right place for evaluating complicated problems.

■ When a true emergency occurs, patients with less urgent problems are shunted aside. You can't estimate with any certainty how long you'll have to wait for treatment in an emergency room.

■ Emergency room fees, because they support equipment required to handle true emergencies, are higher than those for standard office visits.

■ Emergency room services aren't always covered by medical insurance, even when the policy states that the costs of emergency care are included. With many policies, the *nature of the illness* determines whether or not it's covered. In other words, the medical plan will pay for emergency room care only in a true emergency. You may end up paying a large bill out of your own pocket if you go to the emergency room with a sore throat.

The smoothly functioning emergency room provides one of the finest and most dramatic examples of a service profession at work. Following the procedures outlined in this book, you can use this valuable resource appropriately.

OTHER MEDICAL FACILITIES

Short-term Surgery Centers

A number of facilities specially designed for short-term surgery (requiring only a short stay, overnight at the most) have recently appeared. Obviously the surgery performed is relatively minor, and the patient must basically be in good health. Because such centers can avoid some of the overhead of a hospital, they often charge less. But because they don't have the capability to handle difficult cases or complications, you should use them only for minor procedures. The growing experience with these centers has been positive.

Walk-in Clinics

Similarly, some medical problems can be managed at walk-in or "drop-in" clinics. If you have a new, uncomplicated problem (for example, a sore throat or a minor injury), such clinics can be excellent. The decision charts in Part II will help you to determine if you should visit the doctor. Appointments at walk-in clinics aren't usually necessary, and service is swift and efficient. Often these clinics are open for long hours, including evenings and weekends. When available, such clinics should be used for nonemergency care in preference to emergency rooms. The problem with these clinics is with follow-up and sometimes with cost. Costs are rising and now approach those of emergency rooms. If you've had your problem for more than six weeks, or if you expect that it will require multiple visits and more than six weeks to clear up, we think you should see your regular doctor.

Long-term Care Facilities

Nursing homes and various types of rehabilitation facilities provide for the patient who doesn't require hospital care but can't be adequately managed at home. The quality of these facilities ranges from superb to horrible. In the best circumstances, with dedicated nursing and regular doctor attendance, a comfortable and homelike situation for the patient can accelerate the healing process. In other cases, uninterested personnel, inadequate facilities, and minimal care are the rule. Before choosing a nursing home facility, visit the facility or have a friend or relative visit it for you. In the long-term care setting, your comfort with the arrangements is essential.

Hospice Care

For patients with terminal diagnoses (usually a life expectancy of less than six months), the hospice movement tries to provide humane, caring, medically sound treatment without all the technological trappings of the hospital. This can occur either at home with professional personnel or in a hospice facility. The care approach emphasizes improving the patient's comfort. Hospice and home-care programs are becoming more available and are worthwhile. Check out a hospice facility in the same way you would a nursing home; most are good, but some aren't.

Reducing the Cost of Medications

Legal drugs are a multibillion-dollar industry, but your contribution to this industry is largely voluntary. The size of your contribution is determined by your doctor, your pharmacy, and you.

Drugs are at the same time lifesaving and dangerous, curative and fraught with side effects, painful and pain-relieving, and easy to misuse. Most drugs act to block one or more of the natural body defense mechanisms, such as pain, cough, inflammation, or diarrhea. Drugs can interact with other drugs, causing hazardous chemical reactions. They can have direct toxic reactions on the stomach lining and elsewhere in the body. They can cause allergic rashes and shock. They can have severe toxic effects when taken in excess. Some drugs can decrease the ability of the body to fight infections.

You don't want to take any medications you don't truly need. If you don't receive a prescription or a sample package of medication from your physician, consider this good news rather than rejection or lack of interest on the part of the doctor. Take the fewest possible drugs for the shortest possible time. When drugs are prescribed, take them regularly and as directed, but expect that your medication program will be thoroughly reviewed every time you see your doctor.

Most of today's drugs are "symptomatic medications" — that is, they don't cure your problem but give partial relief for the symptoms. The symptoms that may be relieved include pain, cough, inflammation, insomnia, stress, diarrhea, or constipation. If you report a different symptom every time you see your doctor and urgently request relief from that symptom, you're likely to be given additional medications. You're unlikely to feel much better as a result, and you may function at a lower level. Unless you have a serious illness, you'll seldom need to take more than one or two medications at a time. Many perceptive observers have argued that our present practice of using drugs to control symptoms is only a temporary phase in the history of medicine.

YOUR DOCTOR CAN HELP

Your doctor plays a major role in the cost of drugs by choosing the drugs to be prescribed. For example, if you have an infection due to bacteria, you may be given tetracycline or erythromycin. Tetracycline may cost about 10¢ a capsule, whereas erythromycin costs about 80¢. At the doctor's option, a corticosteroid prescription for asthma may be prednisone at 8¢ per tablet or methylprednisolone at 50¢ per tablet. These drugs have similar effectiveness.

If your doctor prescribes a drug by its trade name, in some states the pharmacist must fill the prescription with that particular brand-name product. The brand-name product frequently costs many times more than its generic equivalent. Does your doctor know the relative cost of alternative drugs? Many doctors don't.

The drug-prescribing habits of different doctors can be divided into two types: the "additive" and the "substitutive." With each visit to an "additive" doctor you receive a medication in addition to those you already have. With a "substitutive" doctor, a medication you were previously taking is discontinued, and a new medicine is substituted. Usually the "substitutive" practice is better for your health as well as your pocketbook. Even better is a doctor who likes to *decrease* the number of medications you take.

Most of the time you can take medication by mouth. Sometimes a doctor gives medication by injection because of uncertainty that you'll take it as prescribed. However, as a thoughtful and reliable patient, you can assure your doctor that you will comply with an oral regimen. Taking medication by mouth is less painful, less likely to result in an allergic reaction, and usually far less expensive. There are exceptions, but whenever possible you should take medication by mouth rather than by injection.

If it's clear that you must take a medication for a prolonged period, ask the doctor to allow refills on the prescription. With many drugs it's not necessary to incur the expense of an additional doctor visit just to get a prescription written. However, under some circumstances the doctor may prefer to examine you before deciding whether the drug can be safely continued or is still required.

The careful doctor will ensure that you fully understand the nature of each drug you're taking, the reasons you're taking it, the side effects that may arise, and the length of time that you can expect to take it. You and your doctor should arrange a daily medication schedule that's convenient as well as medically effective. If the program is confusing, ask for written instructions. It's crucial that you understand the why and how of your drug therapy. Don't leave the doctor's office for the pharmacy without understanding your medications.

YOUR PHARMACIST CAN HELP

Studies indicate that the pharmacy you choose is a very important factor in drug costs. For the most part, the pharmacist no longer weighs and measures individual chemical formulations. Much of the activity in the pharmacy consists of relabeling and dispensing manufactured medication. Medication is thus usually identical at different pharmacies; you should choose the least expensive and the most convenient place that your medical plan allows.

Comparison shop beforehand. Discount stores often sell the same medication at significantly lower prices. If a considerable sum of money is involved, you should compare prices by telephone before purchasing the medication. Don't buy from a pharmacy that won't give you price information over the phone.

Unfortunately, even when your doctor writes a prescription by generic name rather than brand name, the pharmacist often isn't required to give you the cheapest alternative. The pharmacy often stocks only one manufacturer's formulation of each drug. Thus, even though your doctor has been careful to permit a less expensive preparation, the pharmacist may substitute the more expensive alternative that's in stock. There's no way to detect this problem except to get direct price quotes from different pharmacies. Once you have found a pharmacy with fair prices and helpful pharmacists, stay with it.

Your pharmacist can help you understand your medications. If you forget to ask your doctor some of the key questions above (see Table 11), the pharmacist can often help you with the answers. If you use the same pharmacy all of the time, the pharmacist can often spot problems in your overall treatment, such as taking two drugs that don't go well together.

YOU CAN HELP

Nowadays, visits to the doctor frequently are requests for medication. If your satisfaction with the doctor depends on whether or not you're given medication, you're working against your own best interest. If you go to a doctor because of a cold and request a "shot of penicillin," you're asking for poor medical practice. (Penicillin should only rarely be given by injection, and it shouldn't be given for uncomplicated colds.) Your doctor knows this but may give in to your request.

The most frequently prescribed medications in the United States, making up the bulk of drug costs, are tranquilizers, minor pain relievers, and sedatives. These drugs cause the greatest number of side effects, and they aren't really scientifically important medications. Our national prescription pattern arose, at least in part, because of ill-advised consumer demand. You can decrease the cost of medications by using some of the techniques discussed previously; you can eliminate them almost completely by decreasing your pressure to receive and take medications that you don't need.

Fortunately, our bodies heal most problems if we curb our impatience a little. The policy of "watchful waiting" without medication is usually the best one. Follow the guidelines of this book to identify the more serious situations. Doctors have a name for this most useful treatment of all; they call it "tincture of time."

Keeping Your Family's Medical Records

Use the forms on the following pages to keep track of your family's medical care. The Immunizations table reflects the most up-to-date recommendations of the medical profession. The Childhood Diseases entries will help you to keep track of every member of the family who has had particular contagious diseases. People who have had a confirmed case of these diseases or an up-to-date immunization are out of danger.

Note your family members' blood types and any allergies they have been diagnosed as having. This information may be very important in emergencies. Take this book to the doctor if that's the best way to make sure the information is available when you need it. Right after you come home from the doctor with a new immunization or a diagnosis, write it down in this book so your records remain up-to-date.

Immunizations: A Family Record

DPT = Diphtheria, pertussis (whooping cough), and tetanus (lockjaw)
DTap = Diphtheria, tetanus, acellular pertussis
HIB = *Hemophilus* influenza type B
Measles = Measles

Mumps = Mumps
OPV = Oral polio virus
Rubella = German measles (three-day measles)
T(d) = Tetanus and adult diphtheria
Hepatitis B = Hepatitis B

Name: _____ _____ _____ _____ _____ _____

Recommended Age	Date	Date	Date	Date	Date	Date
Newborn						
Hepatitis B	___	___	___	___	___	___
2 months						
DPT #1	___	___	___	___	___	___
OPV #1	___	___	___	___	___	___
HIB #1	___	___	___	___	___	___
4 months						
DPT #2	___	___	___	___	___	___
OPV #2	___	___	___	___	___	___
HIB #2	___	___	___	___	___	___
6 months						
DPT #3	___	___	___	___	___	___
OPV #3	___	___	___	___	___	___
HIB #3	___	___	___	___	___	___
15 months						
Measles #1	___	___	___	___	___	___
Mumps #1	___	___	___	___	___	___
Rubella #1	___	___	___	___	___	___
18 months						
DPT #4	___	___	___	___	___	___
OPV #4	___	___	___	___	___	___
HIB #4	___	___	___	___	___	___
4–6 years						
OPV #5	___	___	___	___	___	___
DTap	___	___	___	___	___	___
5–18 years						
Measles #2	___	___	___	___	___	___
Mumps #2	___	___	___	___	___	___
Rubella #2	___	___	___	___	___	___
Every 10 years*						
T(d)	___	___	___	___	___	___
	___	___	___	___	___	___
	___	___	___	___	___	___
	___	___	___	___	___	___

Have an additional tetanus booster for contaminated wounds more than 5 years after the last booster.

Childhood Diseases

Whooping Cough

Name	Date	Place	Remarks
_____	_____	_____	_____
_____	_____	_____	_____
_____	_____	_____	_____

Chicken Pox

Name	Date	Place	Remarks
_____	_____	_____	_____
_____	_____	_____	_____
_____	_____	_____	_____

Measles

Name	Date	Place	Remarks
_____	_____	_____	_____
_____	_____	_____	_____
_____	_____	_____	_____

Mumps

Name	Date	Place	Remarks
_____	_____	_____	_____
_____	_____	_____	_____
_____	_____	_____	_____

Childhood Diseases

Rubella

Name	Date	Place	Remarks

Hepatitis

Name	Date	Place	Remarks

Other Diseases: _____

Name	Date	Place	Remarks

Other Diseases: _____

Name	Date	Place	Remarks

Other Diseases: _____

Name	Date	Place	Remarks
_____	_____	_____	_____
_____	_____	_____	_____
_____	_____	_____	_____
_____	_____	_____	_____

Other Diseases: _____

Name	Date	Place	Remarks
_____	_____	_____	_____
_____	_____	_____	_____
_____	_____	_____	_____

Family Medical Information

Name	Blood Type	Rh Factor	Allergies (including drug allergies)
_____	_____	_____	_____
_____	_____	_____	_____
_____	_____	_____	_____
_____	_____	_____	_____
_____	_____	_____	_____
_____	_____	_____	_____
_____	_____	_____	_____
_____	_____	_____	_____
_____	_____	_____	_____
_____	_____	_____	_____

Hospitalizations

Name _____ Date _____ Hospital _____
Address _____ Reason _____

Name _____ Date _____ Hospital _____
Address _____ Reason _____

Name _____ Date _____ Hospital _____
Address _____ Reason _____

Name _____ Date _____ Hospital _____
Address _____ Reason _____

Name _____ Date _____ Hospital _____
Address _____ Reason _____

Name _____ Date _____ Hospital _____
Address _____ Reason _____

Name _____ Date _____ Hospital _____
Address _____ Reason _____

Name _____ Date _____ Hospital _____
Address _____ Reason _____

Name _____ Date _____ Hospital _____
Address _____ Reason _____

Name _____ Date _____ Hospital _____
Address _____ Reason _____

Name _____ Date _____ Hospital _____
Address _____ Reason _____

Name _____ Date _____ Hospital _____
Address _____ Reason _____

Additional Reading

Books

American College of Obstetrics and Gynecologists. *Planning for Pregnancy, Birth, and Beyond*. Washington, D.C., 1990.

Dubos, R. *Mirage of Health: Utopias, Progress, and Biological Change*. New York: Harper & Row, 1959.

Farquhar, J. W. *The American Way of Life Need Not Be Hazardous to Your Health*. Reading, Mass.: Addison-Wesley, 1987.

Ferguson, T. *Medical Self-Care: Access to Health Tools*. New York: Summit Books, 1980.

Frank, J. F. *Persuasion and Healing*. New York: Schocken Books, 1963.

Fries, J. F. *Living Well*. Reading, Mass.: Addison-Wesley, 1994.

Fries, J. F. *Arthritis: A Take Care of Yourself Health Guide*, 4th ed. Reading, Mass.: Addison-Wesley, 1994.

Fries, J. F., and L. Crapo. *Vitality and Aging*. San Francisco: W. H. Freeman, 1981.

Fries, J. F., and G. E. Ehrlich. *Prognosis: A Textbook of Medical Prognosis*. Bowie, Md.: The Charles Press Publishers, 1983.

Fuchs, V. R. *How We Live*. Cambridge, Mass.: Harvard University Press, 1983.

Knowles, J. H. *Doing Better and Feeling Worse: Health in the United States*. New York: W. W. Norton, 1977.

Lorig, K., and J. F. Fries. *The Arthritis Helpbook*, Rev. ed. Reading, Mass.: Addison-Wesley, 1990.

Lowell, S. L., A. H. Katz, and E. Holst. *Self-Care: Lay Initiatives in Health*. New York: Prodist, 1979.

McKeown, T. *The Role of Medicine: Dream, Mirage, or Nemesis?* Princeton, N.J.: Princeton University Press, 1979.

Pantell, R., J. F. Fries, and D. M. Vickery. *Taking Care of Your Child*, 4th ed. Reading, Mass.: Addison-Wesley, 1993.

Riley, M. W. *Aging from Birth to Death: Interdisciplinary Perspectives*. Boulder, Colo.: Westview Press, 1979.

Silverman, M., and P. R. Lee. *Pills, Profits and Politics*. Berkeley, Calif: University of California Press, 1974.

Sobel, D. S., and T. Ferguson. *The People's Book of Medical Tests*. New York: Summit Books, 1985.

Totman, R. *Social Causes of Illness*. New York: Pantheon Books, 1979.

Urquhart, J., and K. Heilmann. *Risk Watch. The Odds of Life*. New York: Facts on File Publications, 1984.

U. S. Department of Health and Human Services. Healthy People 2000: National Health Promotion and Disease Prevention Objectives. 1991. DHHS No. 91-50213. U. S. Government Printing Office, Wash., D.C. 20402.

Vickery, D. M. *Taking Part: A Consumer's Guide to the Hospital*. Reston, Va.: The Center for Corporate Health Promotion, Inc., 1986.

Vickery, D. M. *Lifeplan: Your Personal Guide to Maintaining Health and Preventing Illness*. Reston, Va.: Vicktor, 1990.

Articles

American Cancer Society. *The Cancer-Related Health Checkup.* 8 February, 1980.

Betz, B. J., and C. B. Thomas. "Individual Temperament as a Predictor of Health or Premature Disease." *Johns Hopkins Med. J.* 144(1979):81–89.

Breslow, L., and A. R. Somers. "The Lifetime Health-Monitoring Program." *N. Engl. J. Med.* 296(1977):601–08.

Brody, D. S. "The Patient's Role in Clinical Decision Making." *Ann. Intern. Med.* 93(1980):718–22.

Camargo, Jr., C. A., P. T. Williams, K. M. Vranizan, J. J. Albers, and P. D. Wood. "The Effect of Moderate Alcohol Intake on Serum Apolipoproteins A-I and A-II." *JAMA* 253(1985):2854–57.

Creagan, E. T., et al. "Failure of High-Dose Vitamin C (Ascorbic Acid) Therapy to Benefit Patients with Advanced Cancer." *N. Engl. J. Med.* 301(1979):687–90.

Danis, M., L. I. Southerland, J. M. Garrett, J. L. Smith, F. Hielema, C. G. Pickard, D. M. Egner, D. L. Patrick. "A Prospective Study of Advance Directives for Life-Sustaining Care." *N. Engl. J. Med.* 324(1991):882–88.

Delbanco, T. L., and W. C. Taylor. "The Periodic Health Examination: 1980." *Ann. Intern. Med.* 92(1980):251–52.

Dinman, B. D. "The Reality and Acceptance of Risk." *JAMA* 244(1980):1226–28.

Farquhar, J. W. "The Community-Based Model of Life Style Intervention Trials." *Am. J. Epidemiol.* 108(1978):103–11.

Farquhar, J. W., S. P. Fortmann, J. A. Flora, C. B. Taylor, W. L. Haskell, P. T. Williams, N. Maccoby, P. D. Wood. "Effects of Communitywide Education on Cardio-vascular Disease Risk Factors." *JAMA* 264(1990):359–65.

Fletcher, S. W., and W. O. Spitzer. "Approach of the Canadian Task Force to the Periodic Health Examination." *Ann. Intern. Med.* 92(1980):253.

Franklin, B. A., and M. Rubenfire. "Losing Weight Through Exercise." *JAMA* 244(1980):377–79.

Fries, J. F. "Aging, Natural Death, and the Compression of Morbidity." *N. Engl. J. Med.* 303(1980):130–35.

Fries, J. F. "Compression of Morbidity: Near or Far?" *Milbank Quarterly* 67(1990):208–232.

Fries, J. F., D. A. Bloch, H. Harrington, N. Richardson, R. Beck. "Two-Year Results of a Randomized Controlled Trial of a Health Promotion Program in a Retiree Population: The Bank of America Study." *Am. J. Med.* 94(1993):455–62.

Fries, J. F., S. T. Fries, C. L. Parcell, and H. Harrington. "Health Risk Changes with a Low-Cost Individualized Health Promotion Program: Effects at Up to 30 Months." *Am. J. Health Promotion* 6(1992):364–71.

Fries, J. F., L. W. Green, and S. Levine. "Health Promotion and the Compression of Morbidity." *Lancet* 1(1989):481-83.

Fries, J. F., H. Harrington, R. Edwards, L. A. Kent, N. Richardson. "Randomized Controlled Trial of Cost Reductions from a Health Education Program: The California Public Employees' Retirement System (PERS) Study." *Am. J. Health Promotion* 8(1994):216-23.

Fries, J. F., C. E. Koop, C. E. Beadle, P. P. Cooper, M. J. England, R. F. Greaves, J. J. Sokolov, D. Wright, and The Health Project Consortium. "Reducing Health Care Costs by Reducing the Need and

Demand for Medical Services." *N. Engl. J. Med.* 329(1993):321–25.

Fries, J. F., G. Singh, D. Morfeld, H. B. Hubert, N. E. Lane, and B. W. Brown. "Running and the Development of Disability with Age." *Ann. Intern. Med.* 121(1994)502–09.

Glasgow, R. E., and G. M. Rosen. "Behavioral Bibliotherapy: A Review of Self-Help Behavior Therapy Manuals." *Psych. Bull.* 85(1978):1–23.

Goldman, L., and E. F. Cook. "The Decline in Ischemic Heart Disease Mortality Rates." *Ann. Int. Med.* 101(1984):825–36.

Greco, P. J., K. A. Schulman, R. Lavizzo-Mourey, and J. Hansen-Fluscher. "The Patient Self-determination Act and the Future of Advance Directives." *Ann. Intern. Med.* 115(1991):639–43.

Hayward, R.S.A., E. P. Steinberg, D. E. Ford, M. F. Roizen, and K. W. Roach. "Preventive Care Guidelines, 1991." *Ann. Intern. Med.* 114(1991):758–83.

Herbert, P. N., D. N. Bernier, E. M. Cullinane, L. Edelstein, M. A. Kantor, and P. D. Thompson. "High-Density Lipoprotein Metabolism in Runners and Sedentary Men." *JAMA* 252(1984):1034–37.

Huddleston, A. L., D. Rockwell, et al. "Bone Mass in Lifetime Tennis Athletes." *JAMA* 244(1980):1107–09.

Hughes, B. D., G. E. Dallal, E. A. Krall, L. Sadowski, N. Sahyoun, S. Tannenbaum. "A Controlled Trial of the Effect of Calcium Supplementation on Bone Density in Postmenopausal Women." *N. Engl. J. Med.* 323(1990):878–83.

Huttenen, J. K., et al. "Effect of Moderate Physical Exercise on Serum Lipoproteins." *Circulation* 60:(1979):1220–29.

Kaplan, N. M. "Non-Drug Treatment of Hypertension." *Ann. Intern. Med.* 102(1985):359–73.

Kromhout, D., E. B. Bosschieter, and C. DeLezenne Coulander. "The Inverse Relation Between Fish Consumption and 20-Year Mortality from Coronary Heart Disease." *N. Engl. J. Med.* 312(1985):1205–09.

Lane, N. E., D. A. Bloch, H. B. Hubert, H. Jones, U. Simpson, and J. F. Fries. "Running, Osteoarthritis, and Bone Density." *Am. J. Med.* 88(1990):452–59.

Langford, H. G., et al. "Dietary Therapy Slows the Return of Hypertension After Stopping Prolonged Medication." *JAMA* 253(1985):657–64.

Leigh, J. P., and J. F. Fries. "Health Habits, Health Care Utilization, and Costs in a Sample of Retirees." *Inquiry* 29(1992):44–54.

Lipid Research Clinics Program. "The Lipid Research Clinics Coronary Primary Prevention Trial Results. I. Reduction in Incidence of Coronary Heart Disease." *JAMA* 251(1984):351–64.

Lipid Research Clinics Program. "The Lipid Research Clinics Coronary Primary Prevention Trial Results. II. The Relationship of Reduction in Incidence of Coronary Heart Disease to Cholesterol Lowering." *JAMA* 251(1984):365–74.

Lorig, K., R. G. Kraines, B. W. Brown, and N. Richardson. "A Workplace Health Education Program Which Reduces Outpatient Visits." *Medical Care* 23(1985):1044–54.

Moore, S. H., J. LoGerfo, and T. S. Inui. "Effect of a Self-Care Book on Physician Visits." *JAMA* 243(1980):2317–20.

Multiple Risk Factor Intervention Trial Research Group. "Multiple Risk Factor Intervention Trial. Risk Factor Changes and Mortality Results." *JAMA* 248(1982):1465–501.

Paffenbarger, R. S., et al. "A Natural History of Athleticism and Cardiovascular Health." *JAMA* 252(1984):491-95.

Phillipson, B. E., et al. "Reduction of Plasma Lipids, Lipoproteins, and Apoproteins by Dietary Fish Oils in Patients with Hypertriglyceridemia." *N. Engl. J. Med.* 312(1985):1210–16.

Relman, A. S. "The New Medical-Industrial Complex." *N. Engl. J. Med.* 303(1980):963–70.

Rimm, E. B., M. J. Stamper, A. Ascherio, E. Giovannucci, G. A. Colditz, W. C. Willett. "Vitamin E Consumption and the Risk of Coronary Heart Disease in Men." *N. Engl. J. Med.* 328(1993):1450–56.

Simonsick, E. M., M. E. Lafferty, C. L. Phillips, C. F. Mendes de Leon, S. V. Kasl, T. E. Seeman, G. Fillenbaum, P. Hebert, J. H. Lenke. "Risk Due to Inactivity in Physically Capable Older Adults." *Am. J. Public Health* 83(1993):1443–50.

Stallones, R. A. "The Rise and Fall of Ischemic Heart Disease." *Scientific Amer.* 243(1980):53–59.

Stamper, M. J., C. H. Hennekens, J. E. Manson, G. A. Colditz, B. Rosner, W. C. Willett. "Vitamin E Consumption and the Risk of Coronary Heart Disease in Women." *N. Engl. J. Med.* 328(1993):1444–49.

Taylor, W. C., and T. L. Delbanco. "Looking for Early Cancer." *Ann. Intern. Med.* 93(1980):773–75.

Vickery, D. M. " Medical Self-Care: A Review of the Concept and Program Models." *Am. J. Health Promotion* 1(1986):23–28.

Vickery, D. M. and T. Golaszewski. "A Preliminary Study on the Timeliness of Ambulatory Care Utilization Following Medical Self-Care Interventions." *Am. J. Health Promotion* (Winter 1989):Vol. 3, No. 3, 26–31.

Vickery, D. M., T. Golaszewski, et al. "The Effect of Self-Care Interventions on the Use of Medical Service Within a Medicare Population." *Medical Care* (June 1988):580–88.

Vickery, D. M., T. Golaszewski, et al. "Life-Style and Organizational Health Insurance Costs." *Journal of Occupational Medicine* 28(Nov. 1986):1165–68.

Vickery, D. M., H. Kalmer, D. Lowry, M. Constantine, E. Wright, and W. Loren. "Effect of a Self-Care Education Program on Medical Visits." *JAMA* 250(1983):2952–56.

Weinstein, M. C. "Estrogen Use in Post-menopausal Women—Costs, Risks, and Benefits." *N. Engl. J. Med.* 303(1980):308–16.

Zook, C. J., and F. D. Moore. "High-Cost Users of Medical Care." *N. Engl. J. Med.* 302(1980):996–1002.

Index

For advice on a common medical problem, look up the primary symptom in this index. Numbers in **boldface** indicate the pages where you can find the most information on each subject. These are usually the pages with decision charts and advice on home treatment and when to see a doctor.

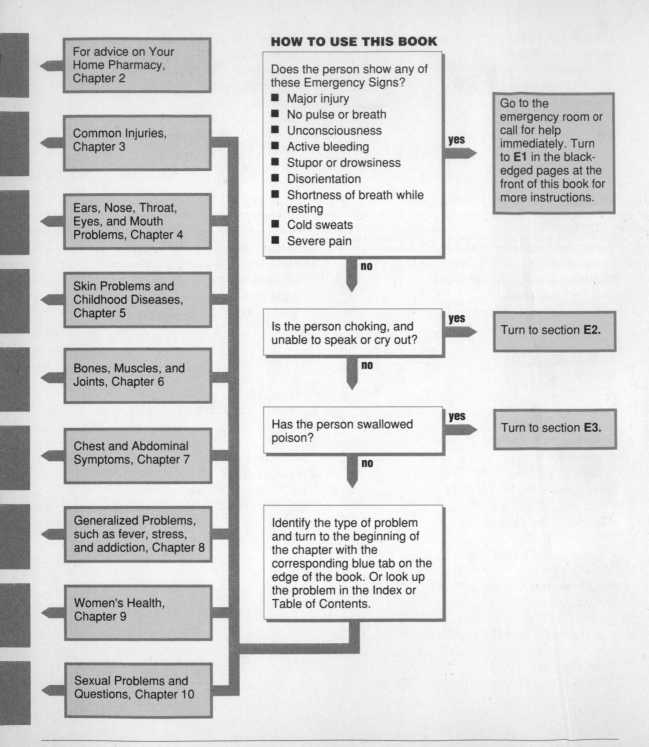

For advice on Your Home Pharmacy, Chapter 2

Common Injuries, Chapter 3

Ears, Nose, Throat, Eyes, and Mouth Problems, Chapter 4

Skin Problems and Childhood Diseases, Chapter 5

Bones, Muscles, and Joints, Chapter 6

Chest and Abdominal Symptoms, Chapter 7

Generalized Problems, such as fever, stress, and addiction, Chapter 8

Women's Health, Chapter 9

Sexual Problems and Questions, Chapter 10

HOW TO USE THIS BOOK

Does the person show any of these Emergency Signs?
- Major injury
- No pulse or breath
- Unconsciousness
- Active bleeding
- Stupor or drowsiness
- Disorientation
- Shortness of breath while resting
- Cold sweats
- Severe pain

yes → Go to the emergency room or call for help immediately. Turn to **E1** in the black-edged pages at the front of this book for more instructions.

no

Is the person choking, and unable to speak or cry out?

yes → Turn to section **E2**.

no

Has the person swallowed poison?

yes → Turn to section **E3**.

no

Identify the type of problem and turn to the beginning of the chapter with the corresponding blue tab on the edge of the book. Or look up the problem in the Index or Table of Contents.